Clinical PET and PET/CT

Clinical PET and PET/CT

With 145 Figures

H. JADVAR, MD, PhD, FACNM
Assistant Professor of Radiology and Biomedical Engineering,
Keck School of Medicine, University of Southern California,
Loa Angeles, CA, USA,
and
Visiting Associate in Bioengineering,
California Institute of Technology,
Pasadena, CA, USA

J.A. PARKER
Associate Professor of Radiology,
Department of Radiology, Harvard Medical School,
Boston, Massachusetts, USA

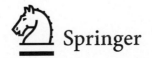 Springer

H. Jadvar, MD, PhD
Assistant Professor of Radiology and Biomedical Engineering, Keck
School of Medicine, University of Southern California, Los Angeles,
CA, USA, *and* Visiting Associate in Bioengineering, California Institute
of Technology, Pasadena, CA, USA

J.A. Parker, MD, PhD
Associate Professor of Radiology, Department of Radiology,
Beth Israel Deaconess Medical Center, Harvard Medical School,
Boston, MA, USA

British Library Cataloguing in Publication Data
A catalogue record for this book is available from the British Library

Library of Congress Cataloging-in-Publication Data
Jadvar, H.
    Clinical PET and PET/CT / H. Jadvar and J.A. Parker.
      p. ; cm.
    Includes bibliographical references and index.
    ISBN 1-85233-838-5 (alk. paper)
      1. Tomography. 2. Tomography, Emission. I. Parker, J. Anthony. II. Title.
    [DNLM: 1. Tomography, Emission-Computed–methods. 2. Tomography,
    X-Ray Computed–methods. WN 206 J21c 2005]
    RC78.7.T6.J346 2005
    616.07′57–dc22
                                                      2004058913

ISBN 1-85233-838-5 Springer London Berlin Heidelberg
Springer Science+Business Media
springeronline.com

Typeset by EXPO Holdings Sdn Bhd
Printed and bound in the United States of America
28/3830-543210   Printed on acid-free paper   SPIN 10950500

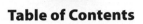

Table of Contents

Foreword: Imaging Marches Forward

The field of molecular imaging/nuclear medicine continues to build excitement for the medical community as a whole. To be able to visualize fundamental molecular and biochemical processes in patients in a meaningful way has truly become reality. Of all the available molecular probes and tools it is clear that FDG with PET-CT is one of the true clinical success stories. Very few would have been able to predict the eventual impact of a simple glucose analog as a marker for imaging cancer, hibernating myocardium, Alzheimer's disease, epilepsy and many other important disease processes. Although relatively well entrenched in the imaging research community there is a growing need to better explain the use of FDG in everyday clinical applications. As more radiologists become involved in the daily interpretation of FDG PET-CT scans, it is important that they understand this technology. With the continued expansion of reimbursement for FDG PET it is important to point out both the advantages and limitations of this technology in the routine management of patients.

This book is a concise summary of the use of FDG PET/PET-CT for the practicing Radiologist/Nuclear Medicine Physician. In this regard it fills an important void of being relevant to the clinical imaging community with an emphasis on the *practical* utility of FDG across many areas including oncology. The consistency between chapters and the highly relevant clinical examples make this book a true pleasure to read. The use of figures with both anatomical and functional information truly helps to make case presentations very clear. The specific attention to pediatric FDG PET-CT is also particularly a refreshing welcome.

Drs. Jadvar and Parker have done a wonderful job in putting together a textbook that is clear, concise and timely. I hope the readers will find it a useful resource for becoming state-of-art practitioners in the rapidly growing and exciting field of FDG PET-CT.

Sanjiv Sam Gambhir M.D., Ph.D.
Director, Molecular Imaging Program at Stanford
Head, Nuclear Medicine
Professor of Radiology & Bio-X
Stanford University
Stanford, California, USA

Preface

Medical imaging has undergone remarkable evolution over the past century. Since the discovery of the x-rays by Wilhelm Röntgen, for which he received the Nobel Prize in 1901, there have been many other important discoveries and technical developments that have culminated in our current sophisticated multi-modality imaging systems. Nobel Prizes have been given for the discoveries of radioactivity (Marie Curie, Pierre Curie, and Henri Becquerel in 1903) and the positron (Carl Anderson in 1936) and for technical developments such as the radiotracer concept (George De Hevesy in 1943), computed tomography (Godfrey Hounsfield and Alan Cormack in 1979), and magnetic resonance imaging (Paul Lauterbur and Peter Mansfield in 2003).

In keeping pace with these milestones in the evolution of medical imaging, positron emission tomography (PET), and more recently integrated positron emission tomography-computed tomography (PET-CT), have now emerged not only as important research tools but also as significant diagnostic imaging systems in clinical medicine. There is little doubt that in the near future PET and PET-CT will become even more important as clinical imaging tools for the evaluation of many disease processes. PET and PET-CT will also aid in the evolution from the current nonspecific imaging methods toward patient-specific imaging evaluation based on morphologic, physiologic, molecular, and genetic markers of disease. Ultimately, the use of multi-modality imaging systems and "smart" specific imaging agents will achieve the key tasks of accurate diagnosis, treatment evaluation, surveillance, and prognosis in individual patients.

Toward this goal, we have attempted to compile a relatively short book that reviews the current state of affairs for PET and PET-CT. Each chapter of the book is intended to be independent, so that a reader may refer to any particular chapter of interest without loss of continuity. Therefore, some repetitions of concepts may be noted. Another difference from other books is that instead of referring to various sources by a reference number in the text, we list all the references alphabetically in the bibliography of each chapter and no specific referrals are made in the text. We preferred this format as we intended to consolidate and summarize the information from various sources for the reader. The book is nearly entirely based on the use of [F-18]fluorodeoxyglucose (FDG) as the radiotracer, but in some cases the uses of other relevant PET radiotracers in specific clinical situations are also included.

The book is organized into 18 chapters. Chapters 1 and 2 review PET physics, instrumentation, and radiotracers. The clinical chapters, 3–17, emphasize the oncology applications of FDG for various organ systems or disease processes (5 through 15) but also review cardiac applications (chapter 3), neurology and psychiatry applications (chapter 4), and the emerging role of PET in infection and inflammation imaging (chapter 16) and in pediatrics (chapter 17). The book concludes with a brief discussion of variants and pitfalls.

It is important to note that although many third-party payers continue to cover PET for various conditions in individual cases but the current list of indications approved by the Centers for Medicare and Medicaid Services include myocardial perfusion studies, myocardial viability assessment, pre-surgical evaluation of seizure disorders, evaluation of some patients suspected of having Alzheimer's disease or fronto-temporal dementia, characterization of solitary pulmonary nodule, and evaluations of breast cancer, colorectal cancer, esophageal cancer, head and neck cancer, non-small cell lung cancer, lymphoma, and melanoma.

We hope that the book will appeal to all those who would like to learn about PET and PET-CT quickly and concisely. We regret any potential errors and omissions, and we will make certain to remedy the shortcomings in any future editions.

Both authors would like to thank the Springer-Verlag staff, including Melissa Morton, Eva Senior, and Lesley Poliner, for their expert work in the design, editing, and production of this book. H. Jadvar dedicates this book to his very understanding and patient wife, Mojgan, and his lovely infant daughter, Donya. J.A. Parker dedicates this book to the great joy of his life, his children, Scott, Meg, and Bidget.

October 2004

H. Jadvar
Keck School of Medicine
University of Southern California

J.A. Parker
Beth Israel Deaconess Medical Center
Harvard Medical School

PET Physics and Instrumentation

POSITRON DECAY

Radioisotopes that have an excess of protons may decay by electron capture or positron decay. During **electron capture**, one of the orbital electrons—usually a k-shell electron—is captured by the nucleus and a proton is converted into a neutron. Electron capture can be written with the equation:

$$P^+ + e^- \rightarrow N + \nu + E$$

where P^+ is a proton, e^- is an electron, N is a neutron, ν is a neutrino, and E represents the excess energy released during decay. Isotopes undergoing electron capture cannot be imaged with a PET scanner.

In order to decay by positron decay, an isotope must have at least 1.02 million electron volts (MeV) more energy than the isotope to which it decays. Isotopes that transition with less than this energy cannot undergo positron decay and will decay only by electron capture. Isotopes with enough energy to undergo positron decay can decay by either positron decay or electron capture. For most commonly used positron emitters the probability of undergoing electron capture is small enough that it can be ignored. In a few cases, however, an important fraction of the isotope decays by electron capture.

Positron decay can be written with the equation:

$$P^+ \rightarrow N + \beta^+ + \nu + E$$

where P^+ is a proton, N is a neutron, β^+ is a positron, ν is a neutrino, and E represents excess energy. A **positron** is the antiparticle that corresponds to the electron. A **neutrino** has very little interaction with matter, and it can be ignored for positron emission tomography (PET). The excess energy is shared between the positron and the neutrino with different amounts of energy going to each particle during decay.

An easy way to check a decay equation is to use **conservation laws**. As one might expect, the charge needs to be conserved. There is one positive charge on the left side of the positron decay equation, P^+, and one positive charge on the right side of the equation β^+. Nucleons such as the proton and neutron belong to a group called baryons. Less well known is that the baryons must be conserved. There is one baryon, P^+, on the left side and one baryon, N, on the right side. Electrons, positrons, and neutrinos belong to a group called leptons. They must also be conserved. There are zero leptons on the left side of the equation. On the right side, the antiparticle β^+ cancels out the other lepton, ν, giving a net of zero leptons on the right side. It is often difficult to remember which particle goes with which in these equations. The conservation laws provide an easy way to get the decay equations right without having to memorize each individual decay equation.

The excess energy that the positron receives during decay is expressed as kinetic energy, the energy of motion. The positron follows a jagged path

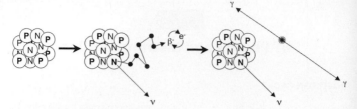

Figure 1: Positron Decay. During positron decay a proton, P, is converted to a neutron, N, a positron, β^+, and a neutrino, ν. After losing energy in the tissue, the positron combines with a tissue electron, e^-, to form positronium. The positron, which is the antimatter analog to the electron, and the electron annihilate each other, giving rise to two nearly back-to-back gamma ray photons, γ, of 511 keV.

through tissue, losing its energy by ionizing surrounding molecules, just like any high-energy charged particle. When it has slowed down so that it is moving at the same speed as the surroundings, the positron will form positronium with a tissue electron. **Positronium** is analogous to a hydrogen atom, but in positronium the electron and positron, which are equal in weight, circle each other. The positronium is very short lived, and the antimatter positron and the electron annihilate each other, giving rise to two gamma rays that travel in nearly opposite directions. The **resting mass** of an electron and a positron are both equal 511 thousand electron volts (keV). (Masses for atomic particles are usually given in terms of the equivalent energy using Einstein's famous formula, $E = mc^2$.).

Figure 1 shows positron decay schematically. One of the protons in the nucleus changes to a neutron, and a positron and a neutrino are emitted from the nucleus. The positron losses energy in the tissue and then forms the short-lived positronium with a tissue electron. The positron and electron annihilate each other, producing two nearly back-to-back photons of 511 keV.

Radioactive Decay Equation.   Radioactive decay is described by an exponential equation:

$$A(t) = A_0 \cdot e^{-\lambda \cdot t}$$

where $A(t)$ is the activity present at time equal to t, A_0 is the amount of activity present at time equal to zero, and λ is the **decay constant**. The decay equation can be derived from the fact that the rate of decay is a constant fraction of the amount of activity present. (Like radioactive decay, it is common for simple physical systems to depend only on the current state and not to have any memory of prior states. It is possible to show mathematically that all memoryless systems are exponential or sinusoidal. Since these simple memoryless systems are very common, exponential and sinusoidal systems are common in nature.)

The **decay constant** is proportional to the reciprocal of the half-life:

$$\lambda = \ln(2)/T_{1/2}$$

where $\ln(2)$ is the natural logarithm of two (approximately 0.693), and $T_{1/2}$ is the half-life. Larger decay constants are associated with shorter half-lives. The

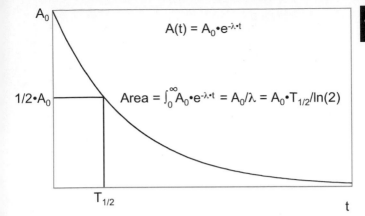

$$A(t) = A_0 \cdot e^{-\lambda \cdot t}$$

$$\text{Area} = \int_0^\infty A_0 \cdot e^{-\lambda \cdot t} = A_0/\lambda = A_0 \cdot T_{1/2}/\ln(2)$$

Figure 2: Exponential Decay. The activity, $A(t)$, during radioactive decay is an exponential function of time, t. At time equal to zero, the activity is equal to A_0. The half-life, $T_{1/2}$, is the time when the activity has decayed to one-half of the initial activity. The decay constant, λ, is equal to the natural logarithm of two, $\ln(2)$, divided by the half-life, $T_{1/2}$. The area of the decay cure is A_0/λ.

half-life is the amount of time it takes for the activity to decrease to one-half of the original activity. Figure 2 shows the exponential decay curve. The area under the decay curve is equal to $A_0 \cdot T_{1/2}/\ln(2)$.

COINCIDENCE DETECTION

The two nearly back-to-back gamma rays are key to positron emission tomography. If two detectors on opposite sides of the patient record an event at nearly the same time, then the annihilation event must have happened somewhere on a straight line between the two detectors. Two detectors are said to be "in coincidence" when the camera detects events in both detectors at nearly the same time. Key to a PET camera is this ability to identify these coincident events.

Single photon imaging depends on a collimator to make an image of the object. The collimator only allows rays that are traveling perpendicular to the detector to pass. Coincidence detection is different from single photon imaging; it does not need a collimator to make an image. Two points, the locations of the detectors, define the line-of-response along which the annihilation must have occurred.

Many current positron cameras are constructed as annular arrays of small crystals. Crystals on either side of the patient stop the gamma rays from the annihilation reaction. The left side of Figure 3 shows two back-to-back gamma rays produced by the electron/positron annihilation. If a detector on each side records an event at nearly the same time, then the annihilation must have occurred on a straight line between the detectors. This straight line between the detectors is called the **line-of-response**. The right side of the figure shows that there is actually a tubular region between the two detectors. A detected annihilation could have come from anywhere in this tubular region.

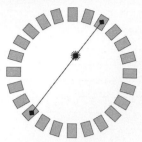 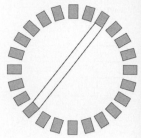

Figure 3: Coincidence Detection. The diagram on the left shows a positron annihilation resulting in two back-to-back photons, which strike crystals on opposite sides of the ring of detectors. The diagram on the right shows the area defined by two crystals. An annihilation from anywhere in this area could result in the two crystals' recording an event at nearly the same time. Outside of this area, it is not geometrically possible for the back-to-back photons to strike both crystals.

Since the lines-of-response are determined geometrically, the lines-of-response are not dependent on the separation between the detectors. To the extent that the gamma rays are back-to-back, the distance of the detectors from the patient does not affect the resolution. This lack of dependence on being close to the patient is another difference between single photon and PET cameras.

In single photon scanning, **patient–detector distance** is an essential factor in good scan quality. Placing the collimator as close as possible to the patient is a key principle that cannot be over emphasized. However, in coincidence scanning, the patient–detector distance is relatively unimportant.

PHYSICS LIMITS OF RESOLUTION

Positron Range. A positron does not undergo annihilation with tissue electron immediately after emission. First the positron follows a jagged path through the tissue as it interacts by producing ionization. The position of the positron-electron annihilation will be at some distance from the position of the decay. The average distance will depend on the initial energy of the positron and the composition of the tissue, particularly the tissue density. For example, the distance in lung tissue will be about three times the distance in soft tissue, since the density of lung tissue is about one-third of soft tissue.

The initial energy of the positron will vary depending on the distribution of energy between the positron and the neutrino. The path of the positron through the tissue will be governed by the statistical interaction probabilities. Thus, there will be a range of distances from the initial site. For low-energy positron emitters, such as fluorine-18, this distance in soft tissue is small (see Table 1). For high-energy positron emitters, such as rubidium-82, this distance will cause a noticeable loss of resolution.

Non-Colinearity of the Gamma Rays. Before the positron can combine with a tissue electron to form positronium, it must lose almost all of its energy. At that point it is said to be thermal, i.e., have about the same kinetic energy as

Clinical PET and PET/CT

Table 1: Positron Range

	Max β⁺ Energy (MeV)	Average Range (mm)	Extrapolated Range (mm)
F-18	0.64	0.64	2.3
C-11	0.96	1.03	3.9
N-13	1.19	1.32	5.1
O-15	1.72	2.01	8.0
Rb-82	3.35	4.29	16.5

After Sherry SR, Sorenson JA, Phelps ME: Physics in Nuclear Medicine.

that due to the temperature of the tissue. Although the positronium is moving at thermal energies, the momentum of the positronium is not negligible. When it decays, the sum of the momentum of two photons must be the same as the positronium, and since photons have relatively little momentum compared to energy, this small momentum has an effect.

If the positronium was moving in the direction of one of the emitted photons, then that photon will have slightly higher energy than the other photon. The spread in the energy of the 511-keV photons can be detected with high-resolution physics instruments but does not affect PET scanners (see Figure 4).

Mathematically, annihilation photons that are exactly back-to-back are called colinear. If the positronium was moving perpendicular to the annihilation photons, then the two photons would not be exactly 180 degrees apart. Due to conservation of momentum, the photons are slightly non-colinear. The non-colinearity is exaggerated in Figure 4. The average non-colinearity is typically on the order of less than one degree.

For a ring the size of a normal whole body PET scanner, this results in a loss of resolution of 1–2 mm. In small animal, micro-PET scanners, a smaller ring diameter is important for achieving the highest resolution, but for clinical scanning, ring diameter is relatively unimportant in terms of resolution. The major effect of ring diameter in clinical PET is its effect on cost; a larger ring requires more components.

Compton Scatter. Compton scatter, which often has the largest effect on resolution, is described below. Although Compton scatter is a basic physics

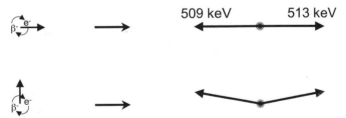

Figure 4: Conservation of Momentum. Before annihilation, if the positronium is moving in the direction of one of the annihilation photons, then that photon will have slightly higher energy than the other photon. Before annihilation, if the positronium is moving perpendicular to the direction of the annihilation photons, then the photons will not be exactly back-to-back. This effect is exaggerated in the diagram.

process, its effect on resolution of the final scan is dependent on many instrumental design considerations.

TYPES OF SCANNERS

Single Photon Detection. Positron-emitting radiopharmaceuticals can be imaged with a single photon system. One of the photons from the positron annihilation can be detected using a standard Anger gamma camera equipped with a collimator. Either planar or single photon emission computed tomography (SPECT) may be used.

Single photon detection has the advantage that it is possible simultaneously to collect data from more than one radioisotope, by using multiple pulse height analyzers. For example, fluorine-18 labeled FDG data, and Tc-99m-labeled sestamibi could be used simultaneously to collect myocardial metabolism and perfusion. Simultaneous data acquisition means that the distribution of the two pharmaceuticals is sampled at exactly the same time with the organ of interest in exactly the same position.

Although simultaneous measurement of two radiopharmaceuticals is a major advantage, both planar and SPECT imaging at 511 keV have considerably poorer resolution than PET imaging. Single photon imaging is not included in this book.

Dual-Use Cameras. Anger cameras with dual heads can be used to collect PET data if they are equipped with coincidence circuitry so that they can identify the two simultaneous annihilation photons. The major difference in configuration between this type of data collection and single photon data collection is that there is no need for a standard collimator.

These types of scanners can be used for both SPECT and PET data collection, so they have often been called dual-use cameras. Since coincidence circuits must be added to the SPECT system, this method has also been referred to as **coincidence detection**; however, this property does not distinguish them from the other PET systems. Many other names have also been used to describe this type of PET camera, e.g., **dual-head coincidence detection**.

One of the major advantages of the dual-use cameras is that the addition of coincidence circuitry to a SPECT camera is relatively inexpensive. Thus, it is possible to add a PET capability to a nuclear medicine department at a much lower cost than is necessary when purchasing a dedicated PET scanner. When starting up PET service, the volume may not be sufficient to purchase a dedicated camera, and a dual-use camera provides a method for introducing the PET technology.

The disadvantage of dual-use systems is that the resolution is lower; and even more importantly, the count rate is much lower. As a rule of thumb, dedicated PET scanners can detect many lesions of about 7 mm with good sensitivity; dual-use cameras require lesions to be about 15 mm for the same detection sensitivity. In many instances, that difference is very important clinically.

Although start-up of PET service was a very important niche for dual-use cameras as PET was becoming more wide spread, currently PET volume is such that reasonably sized nuclear medicine practices can move directly to dedicated PET systems. Therefore, this book will not cover dual-use systems.

Ring Geometry. Many PET scanners have been constructed using a ring or several rings of detectors. Each detector is compared with an arc of detectors on the far side of the ring in order to detect simultaneous or coincident events. The scanner may check for coincidence between a few or all of the adjacent rings (see "Axial Collimation" below). The detectors are generally made up of a very large number of column-shaped crystals. The crystals are narrow in the axial and transaxial directions, and relatively deep in the radial direction. Several crystals, say, eight by eight crystals, are viewed by a small number of photomultiplier tubes, often in a two-by-two array. The position of the crystal that scintillates is determined by Anger logic.

Figure 5 shows the ring geometry schematically. On the left, the in-plane view of the scanner shows the ring of crystals which define one plane. In a real camera there are more than 500 crystals per ring. On the right, the cross-plane view at right angles to the in-plane view shows the stack of rings. The black lines represent the annular septa that separate the planes. The out-of-plane septa are shown on the right using a crosshatched pattern. PET scanners of this type often have about 30 rings of detectors.

Septa: A major advantage of the ring design is that it allows for axial collimation. Axial collimation is provided by septa that are placed between the rings of detectors. The septa are made of a high-Z material such as tungsten that absorbs gamma rays that are not traveling in the plane of the detectors. The septa are annular plates, which only allow photons traveling approximately in a plane, to reach the ring of detectors. With septa in place, coincidences can only be recorded within a single ring or between adjacent rings. Higher-angle coincidences are stopped by the septa.

Block Detectors: Many scintillation crystals and a small number of photomultiplier tubes are often constructed as a block. A set of rings is then made up of many of these blocks arranged in a ring. The total number of possible coincidences between the crystals is proportional to the square of the number of crystals. In a camera with tens of thousands of crystals, this is a very large number, even for today's electronics. Therefore, the coincidence circuitry may identify coincidences between blocks of detectors rather than between each crystal

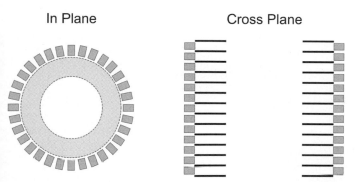

In Plane   Cross Plane

Figure 5: Multiple Ring PET Scanner. On the left is a view of a PET scanner from the plane of the crystal ring. On the right is a view along the axis of the scanner. The crystal rings are separated by septa, shown as heavy black lines on the right and as a cross-hatched annulus on the left.

individually. After a coincidence is determined, the individual crystals are then defined by Anger logic, and the specific line-of-response is determined by computer. If no coincidence is detected, then the other steps in detection do not need to be performed.

The use of a block design can also help with servicing. Hardware problems can be corrected relatively simply by replacing a single block. This was particularly important early in the development of commercial systems. The disadvantage of a block design is that there may be differences in the detector properties at the center and the edges of the block. Some current designs do not use a physical block design, but they still use the idea of a block of detectors for coincidence detection.

Partial Rings: Instead of a complete ring of detectors, a partial ring can be used. The advantage of a partial ring is a reduction in cost. In order to sample all of the lines-of-response, the partial ring needs to rotate about the patient. With a partial ring, a CT scanner can be positioned in the unused portion of the annulus.

Panel Geometry. Instead of constructing the PET scanner as a series of rings, the PET scanner can be constructed of opposing detector panels. Dual-use PET scanners are an example of this geometry. However, dedicated PET scanners may also be constructed this way. Because of edge effects, it is common for these systems to rotate. The advantage of a panel-type arrangement is that it may allow relatively long axial extent at lower cost. Like the partial ring systems, a CT scanner can be placed on the annulus if the panels do not make a complete ring.

PET/CT

A PET scanner can be combined with a CT scanner into a single machine. Metabolic information is obtained from the PET scanner and anatomic information is obtained from the CT scan. In addition, the CT scan can be used to provide information needed for attenuation correction. The current generation of PET/CT scanners all have a common bed, which travels from the PET gantry to the CT gantry. It may also be possible to design a scanner with both PET and CT on a single gantry.

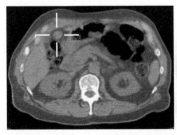 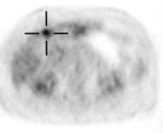

Figure 6: Colonic versus Nodal Uptake. The PET scan on the right shows a focus of FDG uptake in the anterior abdomen. From the PET scan, it would be reasonable to assume that this uptake was located in the transverse colon. The linked cursor on the corresponding CT slice on the left shows that instead the uptake was located in a lymph node.

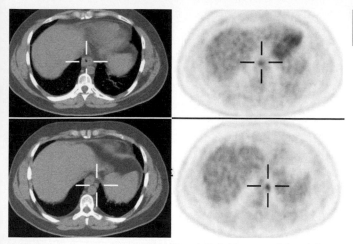

Figure 7: Gastroesophageal Junction Versus Lymph Node. The top panel shows a focus of activity in the center of the PET scan. The linked cursor shows that this location corresponds to the gastroesophageal junction. The bottom panel shows a similar focus of activity at a different level on the PET scan. The linked cursor shows that this location corresponds to a paraesophageal lymph node.

Nearly simultaneous anatomic data of the same part of the body is very useful for interpretation of PET images. For example, Figure 6 shows a focus of FDG activity below the liver in the anterior abdomen. This location would be typical of colonic uptake, which depending upon its pattern, is often incidental. However, the corresponding anatomic image shows that this uptake corresponds to a node that is not part of the colon.

The top panel of Figure 7 shows focal uptake of FDG that corresponds to the gastroesophageal junction. This location typically shows non-pathologic uptake. The bottom panel at a slightly different level in the same patient shows FDG uptake, which looks similar on the PET scan. However, the anatomic information from the CT shows that this uptake corresponds to a paraesophageal node. Distinguishing these adjacent locations is essential to proper interpretation of the PET images.

INTERACTION OF THE ANNIHILATION PHOTONS WITH TISSUE

In a PET scanner, the goal is to detect the two nearly back-to-back photons from the annihilation of the positron with a tissue electron. However, before the photons get to the detector they must pass through the patient, and some of the photons will interact with the tissue. This attenuation of photons by the tissue is what is measured in CT scanning. In PET scanning, attenuation is a problem that must be corrected. There are three interactions between the 511-keV annihilation photons and tissue—Rayleigh scattering, the photoelectric effect, and Compton scatter (see Figure 8).

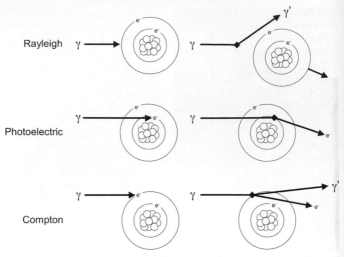

Figure 8: Interaction of Radiation with Matter. There are three processes by which 511-keV photons can interact with matter. During Rayleigh, or coherent, scattering, the photon, γ, bounces off atoms in the matrix, changing direction with a tiny change in energy. During the photoelectric interaction, the photon is completely absorbed. An inner shell electron, e⁻, is ejected from an atom. During Compton, or incoherent, scattering, the energy of the incoming photon is partially absorbed. A scattered photon leaves with lower energy. An outer shell electron, e⁻, is ejected from the atom.

Rayleigh, or Coherent, Scattering in the Patient. Rayleigh, or **coherent, scattering** is when a photon bounces off the atoms in the matrix without causing any ionization. Because the photon changes direction, there is a change in momentum, which must be transferred to the atoms in the matrix. But since the momentum of a photon is small, this change in momentum is associated with a small transfer of energy to the matrix. Thus, the outgoing photon has nearly the same energy as the incoming photon. Rayleigh scattering is quite infrequent at 511 keV in tissue and can be safely ignored.

Photoelectric Effect in the Patient. In the photoelectric effect, the annihilation photon usually interacts with an inner shell electron (generally a k-shell electron). The annihilation photon is completely absorbed. A small portion of the energy of the photon is used to overcome the binding energy of the electron. Most of the energy becomes kinetic energy of the photoelectron. The high-energy photoelectron loses its energy as it moves through the tissue by ionizing molecules in the tissue. The original atom returns to the ground state by giving off characteristic x-rays. In tissue most of these x-rays are very low energy and are absorbed locally. The photoelectric effect causes attenuation of photons and tissue dose, but it does not result in secondary high-energy photons.

Compton Scattering in the Patient. In Compton, or **incoherent, scattering**, the annihilation photon usually interacts with an outer shell electron. The annihilation photon looses a portion of its energy and scatters to a new direc-

---

tion. The angle between the annihilation photon and the scattered photon is a function of the energy lost during the interaction. Often in tissue, the angle of scatter is relatively small and the amount of energy lost is a relatively small fraction of the total energy. A small portion of the difference between the incoming and outgoing photon energies is used to overcome the binding energy of the outer shell electron. Most of the energy goes to the kinetic energy of the electron. As in the photoelectric effect, the high-energy electron looses energy by ionization in the surrounding tissue.

Compton scatter causes tissue dose like the photoelectric effect. The affect on attenuation is slightly more complicated than with the photoelectric effect. It is fairly common to have low-angle Compton scatter. Low-angle Compton scatter deposits a small fraction of the photon energy in the tissue and the scattered photon is only a little bit lower energy than the incoming photon. The Compton-scattered photon travels in approximately the same direction as the incoming photon and it has about the same energy as the incoming photon. Thus, it may fall within the photopeak in the detector and be counted as a photopeak event. The importance of these Compton-scattered events for resolution and quantization will be described below.

Because of these low-angle scattered photons, the apparent attenuation can be less than the real attenuation. The attenuation coefficient for 511-keV photons in tissue is approximately equal to 0.096 cm^{-1}. In the lung, the attenuation coefficient is approximately one-third of this value. The apparent attenuation coefficient depends on the geometry and the energy resolution of the system, and on the setting of the lower-level discriminator, but it may be more in the range of 0.09 or 0.085 cm^{-1}.

The real attenuation coefficient can be measured with an experimental setup that excludes almost all of the scattered photons. A narrowly collimated source and detector only allow the unscattered photons to reach the detector. This measured value is sometimes called the **narrow-beam attenuation coefficient**. A measured value in a setup that matches the PET scanner is sometimes called the **broad-beam attenuation coefficient**.

In some instances, the attenuation coefficient can be entered as a parameter used during reconstruction. A value lower than the real (narrow-beam) attenuation coefficient may be used to take into account the low-angle scatter. It may also take into account different composition of the tissue, especially the lung tissue.

ATTENUATION CORRECTION

Attenuation Equation.   The number of photons attenuated in a length of tissue is proportional to the number of photons impinging on the tissue. This relation is analogous to radioactive decay, and the attenuation equation is analogous to the radioactive decay equation:

$$I(x) = I_0 \cdot e^{-\mu \cdot x}$$

where $I(x)$ is the intensity of photons as a function of the distance, x, into the tissue; I_0 is the intensity at position x equal to zero; and μ is the **linear attenuation coefficient**. The linear attenuation coefficient is given by

$$\mu = \ln(2)/hvl$$

where ln(2) is the natural logarithm of 2 (approximately 0.693), and hvl is the half-value-layer. The **half-value-layer** is the length of tissue over which the intensity of the photons drops to one-half.

Attenuation of Two Photons: A PET scanner needs to detect both of the photons produced during an annihilation reaction. The probability that one photon will make it through a distance, x, in tissue is given by $e^{-\mu \cdot x}$; the probability that a second photon will make it through a distance, y, in tissue is given by $e^{-\mu \cdot y}$. The probability that both photons will simultaneously make it through is the product of these two attenuations. Mathematically, the product is equal to $e^{-\mu \cdot (x+y)}$. This mathematical result makes sense since it is the same probability as one photon traveling the whole distance x + y.

Importance of Attenuation.

Attenuation of photons decreases with an increase in the energy of the photon. The linear attenuation coefficient for the 140-keV photon of Tc-99m is about 0.15 cm^{-1}, and the coefficient for 511-keV annihilation photons is 0.096 cm^{-1}. The first impression is that the effect of attenuation is less for PET imaging than for single photon imaging with Tc-99m.

However, a PET scanner must detect both of the back-to-back photons, whereas with single photon imaging one needs only to detect one photon. Furthermore, when imaging an anterior organ using single photon imaging, an anterior image is used, and when imaging a posterior organ, a posterior image is used. In many instances the depth of the organ is only a few centimeters. However, in PET imaging most of the photons need to traverse the entire thickness of the patient. The attenuation factor for Tc-99m's 140-keV photon when imaging an organ that is 4 cm deep is about 0.5. The attenuation factor for a 511-keV photon across a body that is 30 cm thick is about 0.06.

Skin Effect.

There is an interesting geometric effect near the surface of any object. Figure 9 shows a sphere. At a point near the surface of a sphere, the tangential lines-of-response pass through little or no tissue. There are a moderate range of angles for which the lines-of-response have little attenuation. As the point moves into the sphere the tangential lines-of-response rapidly increase

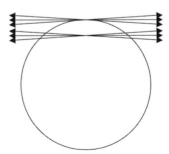

Figure 9: Skin Effect. Several nearly tangential lines-of-response are represented in this figure. Near the surface, they pass through very little tissue. A short distance below the surface, the amount of tissue through which these tangential lines-of-response pass is very much larger. Thus, there is a rapid increase in attenuation, moving from the surface to a short distance below the surface.

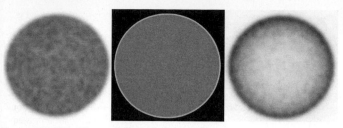

Figure 10: Uniform Phantom. The image on the left is an attenuation-corrected image of a uniform phantom. The image in the center is a CT scan of the phantom. The bright edge is the wall of the phantom. The image on the right is a non-attenuation-corrected image of the same phantom.

the amount of tissue through which they must pass. The tangential thickness of the sphere increases most rapidly at the edge. Toward the center the thickness changes only slowly as a function of depth.

The lines-of-response that are perpendicular to the surface pass through the whole sphere. And the amount of tissue does not change as the point moves into the sphere. Thus, as the point of interest moves into the surface of the object, there is a rapid increase in the total amount of attenuation, and the change in attenuation varies with the orientation of the lines-of-response.

Uncorrected Image: On a non-attenuation corrected image, the effect of the very low attenuation near the surface is to make this region appear much more intense than the interior of an object. Progressing toward the center of an object, there is further decrease in intensity, but the falloff is most rapid near the surface. The effect is to make the surface or the skin of the object appear very bright. Figure 10 shows a cylinder with uniform activity, which has been reconstructed with and without attenuation correction. The surface of the uncorrected image is very intense and the interior is much less intense.

Completely uncorrected images are difficult to view. Thus, it is useful to increase the intensity of the center with respect to the periphery. This can be done with a calculated attenuation correction (see below). If the exact contour of the body is not known, a contour that is larger than any part of the body can be used. (The attenuation coefficient can be set to a value that is lower than the real attenuation coefficient to compensate for the larger contour.) If the exact contour of the body is not known, this type of manipulation may correct for the overall attenuation, but cannot address the rapid changes near the surface. There is still a bright skin in images of this type, but the center of the body can be more easily visualized.

Clinical Implication: With accurate attenuation correction, there will be no skin effect in the final image. However, there are several reasons why attenuation correction may be inaccurate. If a calculated attenuation map is used, then the body contour may not be correctly outlined. If a measured map is used, there may be patient motion between the time of collection of the emission and transmission data. Or, there may just be inaccuracies in the transmission measurement.

Because of the relatively rapid change in attenuation at the surface of an object, inaccuracies in the attenuation measurement will often be most

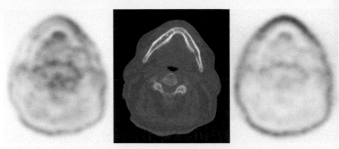

Figure 11: Artifact from Head Motion. The image on the left is an attenuation-corrected PET image; the image in the center is the CT scan used for attenuation correction; and the image on the right is a non-corrected PET image. There is a relatively small amount of motion between the time of the CT data collection and the PET data collection; however, on the corrected image, there is asymmetry in between right and left that is not seen in the non-corrected image. The effect is most marked at the surface.

dramatic toward the surface of the body. For example, Figure 11 shows a patient that moved his head between emission and transmission scans. The surface structures on one the left side of the face are overly intense and the surface structures on the right side are decreased in intensity.

In some diseases, such as melanoma, where there may be skin or subcutaneous lesions, these skin effects can emphasize or more importantly obscure a finding. One way to avoid this problem is to have both corrected and uncorrected images available during interpretation.

"Hot" Lungs. In the chest, the lung has about one-third the attenuation than the surrounding tissue. Non-corrected images will show "hot" lungs, whereas corrected images will show "cold" lungs (see Figure 12 opposite). When calculated attenuation correction is used, the same attenuation value is used for lung and soft tissue. In the lungs, there will be an overcorrection for attenuation, and the lungs will appear to have increased activity. Images with calculated attenuation correction may have particularly "hot" lungs.

Furthermore, there is a difference in attenuation near the edge of the lung. Adjacent to the mediastinum, there are few lines-of-response that pass entirely through lung tissue. As the point of interest moves toward the center of the lung, there is an increasing angle over which lines-of-response pass predominantly through lung tissue. Thus, the edge of the lung is not as "hot" as the center. This effect is analogous to a reverse skin effect. It tends to make the "hot" lungs appear smaller than they should, and the mediastinum to appear wider than it should be.

Distortion from Attenuation. At the surface of a sphere there is a rapid change in attenuation for the tangential lines-of-response, but no change in the radial lines-of-response. Inaccuracies in attenuation correction can easily result in more inaccuracy in one direction than in the other direction. If the lines-of-response in one direction are increased in intensity, a round hot spot can be distorted to appear to be an oval. If the lines-of-response are decreased in intensity, then a hot spot can be made to appear to be an oval in the other direction.

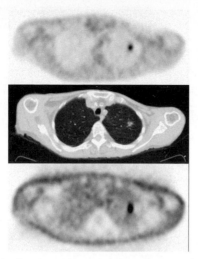

Figure 12: Distortion from Non-Uniform Attenuation. The top panel shows an attenuation-corrected PET axial slice of the chest. The middle slice shows the corresponding CT slice. The bottom panel shows the uncorrected PET slice. The round nodule on the corrected slice appears to be elongated in the anterior-posterior direction due to the variation in attenuation with direction. Also note the "cold" lungs on the corrected image and the "hot" lungs on the uncorrected image.

Furthermore, there can be distortion of structures from variations in the accuracy of attenuation correction in different directions. In the chest, the lines-of-response which are in the anterior-posterior direction often have very little attenuation compared with lines of response which go through the mediastinum or the chest wall at more oblique angles. In uncorrected images, the non-uniform attenuation in different directions can distort hot structures. Figure 12 shows a pulmonary nodule. In the top panel, the nodule appears circular in the attenuation corrected image. In the bottom panel, the nodule is elongated in the anterior-posterior direction due to the non-uniform attenuation.

Diaphragmatic Artifacts. There can be important artifacts around the diaphragm due to attenuation. Problems near the diaphragm tend to be more common with rapid attenuation measurements, especially using CT for attenuation measurement. If the attenuation is measured with a deep breath and the PET data is obtained during tidal breathing, then the measured attenuation for the upper portion of the liver will be much lower than it should be. The attenuation correction for the upper portion of the liver will be too small.

This situation can be very confusing because the artifact may have the appearance of normal anatomy. The upper portion of the liver, which is not adequately corrected, may appear to be the same intensity as the lung. The position of the diaphragm during the attenuation measurement will form an apparent upper border for the liver. This artifactual liver border will simulate the normal appearance of a liver border. The only clue that there is an artifact

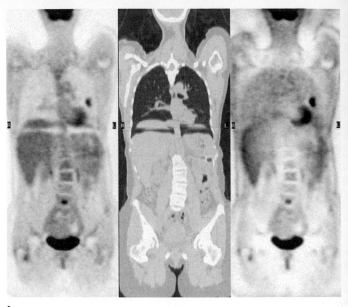

A

may be that the liver appears to be smaller on the PET scan than on a simultaneously acquired CT.

Although the dome of the liver is decreased in intensity, an intense liver lesion may still be seen. However, the lesion will appear to be located within the base of the lung. Similarly, if the attenuation data is collected on a deep expiration, a lung lesion may appear to be below the diaphragm.

These dramatic artifacts are relatively unusual. However, it is common to see some over- or undercorrection near the diaphragm. These artifacts may reduce detection of lesions near the diaphragm. In addition, movement during emission scanning may blur out small lesions. Thus, there are several reasons why the base of the lung is a difficult region for PET scanning. Figure 13 shows several artifacts due to diaphragmatic motion. The spiral CT in the center panel shows a fragmented dome of the diaphragm. The top portion of the diaphragm was collected during expiration. As the CT moved down, the patient took a large breath so that a portion of the lung appears in the midst of the liver. The attenuation-corrected PET image in the left panel has the same appearance as the CT. The low attenuation values of the lung decrease the liver activity so that it appears to be the lung. The uncorrected PET image in the panel on the right shows the true liver contour.

Physiologic Motion.   Figure 13 also shows another artifact from breathing. In Figure 13A there is an intense focus of FDG uptake in the left mid-lung field. There is no corresponding nodule seen on the corresponding CT slice. Figure 13B, several slices anterior to Figure 13A, shows the pulmonary nodule, but only faint FDG activity. A deep breath during the CT acquisition resulted in

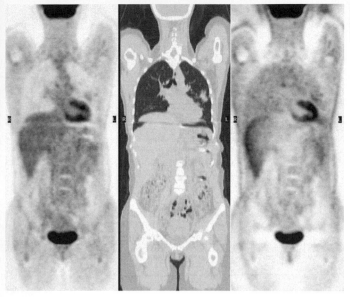

B

Figure 13: Diaphragmatic Motion. A. The coronal spiral CT scan in the middle panel shows marked diaphragmatic motion due to breathing. A few slices were obtained while the dome of the diaphragm was relatively high in the chest. Then the patient took a deep breath, and the next few slices include only lung. Finally the scan reenters the diaphragm. The attenuation-corrected PET scan on the left is obtained during tidal breathing when the diaphragm is mostly in the higher position. However, the activity in the liver appears to match the fragmented appearance of the CT scan. The uncorrected PET scan the right has a normal appearing, unfragmented liver. The pulmonary nodule which is seen best on this slice of the PET scan is not seen at all on the CT. It has moved anteriorly out of the plane of imaging due to respiration during the CT scan. (Incidentally, note a metastasis in the L5 vertebral body.) B. A more anterior slice of the same study. In this slice the pulmonary nodule is clearly shown on the CT scan.

anterior motion of the nodule with respect to its average position during the PET collection. Other physiologic motions—cardiac, gastrointestinal, etc.—can also cause miss-registrations between the attenuation collection data and the emission data.

Independence of Attenuation and Depth. Although the attenuation in PET imaging is high, there is a very important property of the attenuation—it is independent of the depth! Since both annihilation photons need to be recorded in order to detect an event, both photons need to escape the body without being attenuated. As described above, the probability that both photons will escape the body is equal to the probability that a single photon will traverse the whole body.

If an annihilation event occurs close to one side of the body, the photon on that side has little attenuation. The photon going the other way is highly

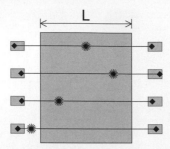

Figure 14: Independence of Attenuation with Depth. The gray box represents a patient with a thickness of L. Irrespective of the depth of the positron annihilation, the sum of the paths of the two photons is equal to L. Even if a positron source is placed outside the body, as shown on the last row, the path is L.

attenuated. For an annihilation event on the same line-of-response close to the other side of the body, the attenuation of the photons will be reversed. No matter what, the total attenuation will be equal to one photon traversing the whole path. This relation is shown in Figure 14.

If an annihilation event occurs outside the body, then the single photon that goes through the body will also have the same attenuation as an annihilation event anywhere along the same line-of-response. Thus, a positron source placed outside the body can be used to measure the attenuation. The difference in measurements made before and after the patient is placed in the scanner is due to the attenuation of the patient.

The ability to measure attenuation exactly in PET can be contrasted with SPECT. The attenuation in SPECT is directly related to the thickness of tissue along a ray from the source to the camera. There is no way directly to measure the attenuation from inside the patient. Instead it must be calculated. Furthermore, the primary SPECT data are the sum of sources at all different depths. Thus, the activity and the attenuation are mixed together. Correcting for attenuation is much more complicated in SPECT than in PET. The ability directly measure and correct for the attenuation for each line-of-response is the reason PET data has been known for its ability to produce quantitative measurements.

Types of Attenuation Correction. Calculated Attenuation Correction: The attenuation can be calculated given the contour of the body. The length of the path through the body can be determined from the contour and the attenuation calculated. The contour can be obtained from a preliminary uncorrected reconstruction of the PET data. The outer limits can be drawn or determined from a threshold, and then the data can be reconstructed again using this contour. If the tissues within the body are relatively constant in attenuation, this method can work well. It is particularly applicable to the brain. It works least well in the chest where there are major differences in density between the lungs and the other tissues.

Calculated attenuation correction can cause important artifacts such as the "hot" lungs described above. Given an awareness of these artifacts, calculated attenuation correction images can be used successfully in many situations. The major advantage of using calculated attenuation is that the time and expense of measuring attenuation correction can be avoided.

Pairs Transmission Scan: As described above, a point source of positrons outside the body can be used to measure the attenuation along each line-of-response. This type of measurement is often called a **transmission scan**. By comparison, scanning of the radiopharmaceutical from within the patient is called an **emission scan**.

For each line-of-response, a source outside the body has exactly the same total attenuation as the activity from any point in the body along that line-of-response. The sources for pairs attenuation correction are made of germanium-68. Germanium-68 has a 280-day half-life and decays by electron capture to gallium-68 without emitting a gamma ray. Gallium-68 has a 9.5-hour half-life and decays by positron emission. The annihilation radiation from the gallium-68 is used to measure the attenuation.

The germanium-68 is called a **rod source**. It is arranged as a rod in the axial direction; within each imaging plane the germanium-68 is a point source. Figure 15 shows three line sources as dots within the ring of the crystals. The lines-of-response for the line source at the top are shown.

One difficulty with pairs attenuation correction is that the small number of crystals nearest to the source receive a large number of unattenuated photons. (In Figure 15 all of the lines-of-response hit a single crystal.) The rate at which the data can be collected is limited by the rate at which these small number of crystals can collect data. This problem can be ameliorated by using three rods spaced 120 degrees apart. In this configuration, the rods do not interfere with each other and the data can be collected three times as fast.

A second problem with using coincidence pairs to collect the data is that the activity within the patient cannot be distinguished from the activity in the sources. Some early PET scanning protocols collected the attenuation data before the patient was injected with the radiopharmaceutical. Because of the problems with patient motion, these protocols have given way to collecting attenuation data at the same time as emission data, correcting the transmission data for the emission data.

The germanium-68 rod sources are moderately expensive (tens of thousands of dollars); and with a 280-day half-life, they need to be replaced every

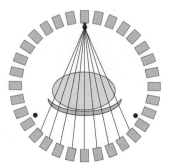

Figure 15: Rod Sources. Three rod sources of germanium-68 are shown as black dots. (The rods are points in the plane of the crystal rings.) The lines of response that are measured by the top source are shown diagrammatically.

year or so. It is often wise to include these sources as a part of the maintenance contract for the system.

Singles Transmission Scan: Instead of using coincidence imaging, it is possible to measure attenuation with a single photon method. A single photon traversing the whole patient will traverse the same tissue as the two photons detected during coincidence imaging. Using a single photon allows faster data collection. The collection rate is limited by the large number of detectors on the far side of the patient rather than the small number of detectors close to the source. Furthermore, the beam of photons is reduced by the attenuation before it gets to the detectors. And, single photon collection allows greater flexibility in the geometry of the source.

A positron emitter could be used as the source, collecting only the photon that pass through the body. However, it is also possible to use other isotopes. Cesium-137, with a 30-year half-life and a 662-keV photon, is often used for a single photon source. The energy resolution of most positron cameras is not good enough to separate completely the 662-keV photons of cesium-137 from the 511-keV annihilation photons; however, there is less contamination of the transmission data from the emission data when using cesium-137.

The attenuation of the 662-keV photons is generally proportional to the attenuation of the 511-keV photons. Therefore, translation of the attenuation measurement from 662- to 511 keV is more straightforward than the translation from low-energy photons such as those used in CT.

Segmentation: Both pairs and single transmission scans are photon limited. The attenuation data suffers from statistical noise. This noise can affect the attenuation-corrected imaging. Thus, it is common to process the transmission scan to improve statistical accuracy. One method that is used is segmentation. The reconstructed transmission scan is processed to identify different tissues.

Image-processing methods are used to join pixels together into larger, anatomically reasonable areas. Once identified, these different tissue regions are then regions are assigned an attenuation value. The methods used can be fairly complicated, but the basic idea is that the tissues are identified by the transmission scan, then a priori knowledge of the tissue attenuation is used during reconstruction.

Using segmentation to help calculate attenuation reduces the noise in the attenuation measurement and consequently reduces the noise in the final image. With segmentation, the transmission scan time can be reduced, and the increased noise is ameliorated by the noise reduction of the segmentation processing.

CT: A PET/CT scanner combines a CT scanner with a PET scanner. The CT can provide anatomical information near the time of the PET imaging. In addition the CT scanner can be used to measure the attenuation information. Some of the cost of the CT scanner can be offset if the attenuation subsystem is not included in the PET scanner.

The CT scan time is shorter than the singles transmission scan and much shorter than a pairs transmission scan. Thus throughput can be increased. A much higher photon flux is used during CT scanning than during single or pairs transmission scanning. Thus, very little statistical noise is added by attenuation correction with CT, especially when compared to the statistical noise added by singles or pairs attenuation correction.

A disadvantage of CT-measured attenuation correction is that it is more difficult to translate the attenuation of polychromatic x-rays used in CT to the attenuation of 511-keV photons as described in the next section. Many PET/CT protocols collect a whole CT scan followed by a whole PET scan. The last images of the PET scan may be collected considerably later than the attenuation data. This delay can result in patient or physiologic motion between the two scans, which can also lead to errors in attenuation correction.

Attenuation Versus Energy.   Attenuation of photons depends on the energy of the photons and the matter through which it passes. The relation between the energy of the photons and attenuation is complex. There is a jump in attenuation as the photon energy becomes greater than the electron binding energies. Below the binding energy, electrons in a particular shell cannot contribute to the photoelectric effect. Just above the binding energy, a photoelectric event is very likely. Thus, with a very small increase in energy, the attenuation may increase sharply. If this jump occurs at the k-shell binding energy, it is called a **k-edge**. The k-edge, which is the highest energy jump, is the most important for isotope imaging, but the other transitions can affect lower-energy x-rays that are included in the CT spectrum.

Except for these sharp increases in attenuation at the electron binding energies, the attenuation decreases with increasing photon energy. However, the rate of decrease in attenuation with energy is different for photoelectric and Compton interactions. The photoelectric event is most important at lower energies and Compton scatter is most important at higher energies. In tissue, Compton scatter predominates at both 140 keV (Tc-99m's principal photopeak) and 511 keV. The photoelectric interaction predominates at 140 keV in scintillation crystals. At 511 keV Compton scatter predominates in both the patient and the detector, although the fraction of Compton versus photoelectric interactions varies with the detector composition.

The electron binding energies vary with the composition of the matter. In addition, the photoelectric and Compton interactions and the relative importance of these two interactions vary with the composition of the matter. Thus, not only is the curve relating attenuation to energy complex, but also the curve varies depending on the composition of the matter.

Attenuation also varies within different body tissues. At 511 keV the major difference between body tissues is density. Thus, lung has about one-third the density of soft tissue. Bone has variable density, with compact bone having the highest density. At lower energies, such as those used in CT, the elemental composition of the tissue is more important. Thus, there is much higher contrast between the bone, which contains calcium, and other tissues.

In order to use attenuation measurements obtained at one energy to correct attenuation at another energy, it is necessary to characterize the material. This translation can be particularly complicated for polychromatic energies used in CT. In PET/CT scanners, the set of allowable peak CT voltages is often limited to a set where the translation has been characterized. Generally, the first step is to segment the CT data into different tissue regions, e.g., bone, soft tissue, lung. Then, the translation from the spectrum of energies in the CT beam to 511 keV is performed for each region.

Attenuation correction can be incorrect in the region of implanted metallic devices that may not have the same translation from the CT value to 511 keV.

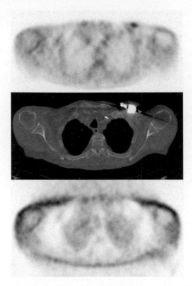

Figure 16: Pacemaker Artifact. The top panel shows a CT-corrected PET scan. The middle panel shows the CT scan. The bottom panel shows an uncorrected PET scan. The metal in the pacemaker causes the "hot spot" on the corrected scan.

Dense barium and dental amalgams may also result in incorrect attenuation correction. A barium-filled colon may incorrectly appear to have increased activity. The dilute barium typically used for CT scanning can, however, be used for PET/CT with relatively little problem.

Figure 16 shows the effect of a pacemaker when using a CT to correct for attenuation. The middle panel shows a CT scan with a pacemaker on the left. The top panel shows an FDG image that has been attenuation corrected using the CT data. Notice that there is an area of increased activity corresponding to the pacemaker. On the bottom is an uncorrected PET image, which shows decreased activity corresponding to the lesion. At the CT energies, the attenuation of the metal compared with tissue is much higher than the attenuation at 511 keV of the metal compared with tissue. Thus, the attenuation correction over corrects and makes the region of the metal appear hot.

When using CT data to correct for attenuation, there can be artifacts whenever there is unusual material present. An uncorrected image can be used to evaluate these regions, so that these artifacts can be properly identified.

IMAGE REGISTRATION

Interpretation of the metabolic information provided by PET is greatly aided by close correlation with anatomic information provided by CT or MRI imaging. Furthermore, display of PET scan data electronically linked to anatomic images improves interpretation compared with separate display of metabolic and anatomic images. The major advantage of PET/CT is that both metabolic and anatomic information for the same body region are obtained at nearly the same time. The PET and CT scans are physically aligned and the PET/CT viewing software allows close correlation of the images.

However, there may be patient motion between the PET and CT data collections, so the registration may not be perfect. In addition, it is useful to also compare data with prior studies, which are aligned with current images. In some instances another imaging method will provide better anatomical detail than CT. In all these cases, a workstation that provides image registration and linked display is valuable.

The images can be registered manually. In that case the workstation allows the user to move and rotate one image with respect to the other. If the software is cumbersome, this process can take a very long time. Even if the software very easy to use, this process can be a bit slow. Thus, there is appeal to automatic registration.

Automatic image registration was investigated in the 1970s for satellite imaging, especially the Landsat program, and for cruse missile development. Cruse missile development is in the classified literature, but the Landsat work is available in the open literature. Registration of images from different times of the year when the land cover is different and through the distortions of the atmosphere has much in common with radiological imaging. Recently, there has been a great deal of work on image registration for radiological images.

Types of Transformation.   During registration, one image is transformed so that it lines up with a second image. One decision that must be made is what type of transformations are allowed. **Rigid body transformation** allows the image to be translated and rotated, but does not allow stretching operations. Rigid body transformation works well if the voxels in both images have exactly the same size in all three dimensions. (A **voxel** is a volume element. It is a three-dimensional analog of a **pixel**, or picture element.) A rigid body transformation is defined by three translation distances and three rotation angles. The transformation can be limited to fewer degrees of freedom if it is known that one or more of these translations or rotations is not needed.

An **affine transformation** includes stretching and sheering in addition to the rigid body transformations. The translation is defined by three values. Rotation, stretching, and shearing transformations can be defined by a matrix of nine coefficients. In addition to the rigid body motion, the stretching of an affine transformation can correct for differences in voxel size. Shearing is a somewhat less common problem.

Motion of one part of the body with respect to another, such as during breathing, is a more complicated transformation. Rather than stretching the whole axis, a portion of the image needs to be stretched with respect to another portion. This type of operation is called a **warping transformation**. Since warping operations can be very complex, it is typical to limit the type of warping which is allowed. The types of warping that are allowed is often determined more by what is simple to implement mathematically than by what the expected motions are.

Image registration can be difficult and time-consuming. Using a transformation that uses the fewest parameters can make the process tractable. Thus, if it is known *a priori* that the only motion is a translation in one direction, it is best to limit the transformation process to that single parameter. The best results will be obtained if the model of the transformation is the simplest model that captures most of the difference between the images.

Similarity Measure. In order to register images automatically, it is necessary to know how well two images are lined up. That metric is often called a **similarity measure**. The idea is that when the two images are registered, they will be the most similar. As they move apart they will be less similar. A very simple similarity measure is to subtract the corresponding voxel values from images and then make a **sum of absolute differences**. This similarity measure works well when the two images have nearly the same values, for example, when registering two CT scans. When the images are perfectly aligned, this value would be zero, or nearly zero depending on the noise in the image.

A somewhat more robust similarity measure is **cross correlation**. For cross correlation, the voxel values are multiplied together and then summed. Both of these similarity measures depend on the voxel values having the same relation in the two images. A voxel that is white in one image should be white or nearly white in the other image; and similarly, dark voxels in one image should be dark in the other image. If the voxel values in the two pictures don't have any relation to each other, then these similarity measures will not work.

A similarity measure called **mutual information** has found considerable success in medical imaging. Mutual information requires that voxels with a particular value in one image correspond to voxels with a narrow range of values in the other image. The actual values in the two images do not need to be the same, rather there just needs to be a mapping of values from one image to the other. For example, if voxels corresponding to muscles are all white in one image, then they could be white, or gray or black in the other image; but they shouldn't be heterogeneous in intensity.

Someone who looks at two images that have high mutual information should identify similar region boundaries. The intensities within the boundaries need not be similar; only the boundaries of the regions should be similar. PET, CT, and MRI images often have very different values for different tissues; however, analogous tissue regions are often identifiable. Thus, different radiological modalities seem well suited for the use of mutual information as a similarity measure.

TYPES OF COINCIDENCE EVENTS

True Coincidence. Most of the description so far has dealt with true coincidence events. When the photons from an annihilation event reach crystals on either side of the ring and are detected as photopeak events, that event is called a true coincidence. However, there are other processes that will be recorded by the scanner as coincidence events that are not true coincidences.

Scattered Coincidence. One or both of the 511-keV annihilation photons can undergo Compton scattering in the patient's body. As described above, the scattered photon has decreased energy and leaves in a direction that is different from the incoming photon. The energy of the scattered photon may be below the lower-level discriminator of the detector. In that case, Compton scatter affects attenuation. However, frequently the scattered photon has enough energy that the detector will record it as a photopeak event. If the other photon is

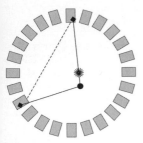 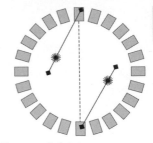

Figure 17: Scatter and Random Coincidence. The diagram on the left shows an annihilation event where one of the photons is scattered in the patient. The recorded line-of-response (dashed line) is far from the location of the annihilation in this scenario. On the right, two annihilation events occur at approximately the same time. One of the photons from each annihilation event is absorbed in the patient. The other photons produce a random coincidence. The line-of-response (dashed line) for this even does not pass near either of the true annihilations.

also detected, then a coincidence event will be recorded; however, the line-of response will be miss-positioned. Compton scatter events will result in a loss of resolution (see Figure 17).

Random Coincidence.   Because of geometry, attenuation, detector efficiency, limitations of the field-of-view, etc., the vast majority of the time only one photon reaches a detector. Thus, it is much more common to have a single event than a coincidence event. If two of these single events occur within the coincidence time of the camera, they will be recorded as a coincidence event even though these two photons have nothing to do with each other. Such an event is called a random coincidence. The diagram on the left of Figure 17 shows a random coincidence.

AXIAL COLLIMATION

Effect of Collimation.   The ratio of Compton scatter events to true coincidence events is called the **scatter fraction**. Collimation affects this ratio. Figure 18 shows two small detectors, which are set up to detect coincidence events. The only true coincidences that will be detected are those coming from annihilation events in a tube that connects the two detectors. For annihilation events outside of that tube, it is not geometrically possible for both of the back-to-back photons to strike the detectors. The top-left diagram of Figure 18 shows three annihilation events. Only the center annihilation event, which lies in the area-of-response between the two crystals, can result in a true coincidence.

There is no such geometrical limitation on the origin of Compton scattered events. For an event outside the area-of-response, one photon may go straight to one of the detectors; the second photon can be scattered by the angle necessary for it to strike the second detector. The bottom-left diagram of Figure 18 shows two annihilation events where one of the photons is scattered, and one annihilation event where both photons are scattered. It is possible for annihilation events in the whole area of the scanner to result in a scattered coincidence.

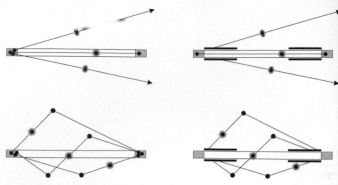

Figure 18: Area-of-Response. The diagram in the upper left shows two detectors. Lines connecting the edges of the detectors show the area-of-response of the detector. Geometrically, true coincidence events can only be detected from annihilations in this area. One annihilation event from this area is shown with both back-to-back photons detected in coincidence. Two annihilation events from outside this region result in detection of a single photon. The other photon is not detected. The diagram in the lower left shows three annihilations events with Compton scatter photons which reach the detector even though two of them are out of the area-of-response of the detector pair. The diagrams on the right show the effect of collimation. The true coincidence event is not affected by collimation, but the other events are affected by collimation.

A collimator placed outside the area-of-response will not affect any of the true coincidence events. Any pair of back-to-back photon that can be detected geometrically will not be affected by the collimation. The top-right diagram of Figure 18 shows that the true coincidence event is not affected by the collimation represented by the heavy lines. Many of the single photons from annihilations outside the tubular area-of-response will be stopped by the collimation.

By comparison, almost all of the Compton-scattered coincidence events will be eliminated by the collimator. Both of the photons need to be traveling in the directions defined by the collimators. Some very low angle events from within the tube between the detectors will make it through the collimators. Some double Compton events from outside that region will make it through the collimators. But the vast majority of Compton events will be stopped by the collimation. The bottom-right diagram of Figure 18 shows that the collimators stop many of the scattered photons, which would have struck the detectors.

The effect of collimation will be dependent on the distribution of activity between the two detectors in a complicated fashion; however, the number of Compton events that reach the detectors will be a function of the acceptance angle of the collimator. The Compton-scattered photons will decrease on the order of the acceptance angle of the collimation for each of the detectors separately. Thus, the Compton coincidence events will decrease on the order of the square of the acceptance angle of the collimators.

In this simple two-detector situation, collimation has a dramatic effect on the scatter fraction. The scattered events decrease as the square of the acceptance angle of the collimators, while the true events are not affected by the collimation! In more complicated situations, collimation also improves the scatter fraction.

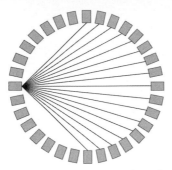

Figure 19: In-Plane Coincidence. This diagram shows a lines-of-response for a single crystal. An arc of crystals on the other side of the ring is put "in coincidence" with the single crystal. Each crystal in turn around the ring has a similar arc of crystals that are "in coincidence".

Only the annihilations, which occur within the axial field-of-view of the camera, can give rise to true coincidences. Out-of-field activity can result in scattered coincidence events as well as random coincident events. Thus, collimation of activity, which is totally out of field-of-view, is important. PET scanners have shields at either end of the machine to keep this out-of-field activity from striking the detectors.

"2D" and "3D" Imaging. A single pair of small detectors detects annihilation reactions from an area defined by a small tube connecting the detectors. It only detects the coincidence pairs that are traveling nearly parallel to the axis of tube. In order to increase sensitivity, a large number of detectors from one side of the patient need to be put in coincidence with a large number of detectors on the opposite side. The detectors are often arranged in a series of rings. Each crystal in the ring is put in coincidence with an arc of crystals on the other side of the patient. The size of the arc determines the active area of the camera. Figure 19 shows the lines-of-response within a plane of crystals.

Often PET scanners are made from a stack of crystal rings. In that case, a crystal in one plane may be placed in coincidence with crystals from a few or many planes of rings.

When a crystal is in coincidence with only crystals on the same or adjacent rings, the term "2D" imaging is used. When a crystal is in coincidence with crystals from all of the rings, the term "3D" imaging is used. Figure 20 shows the cross plane coincidences for a crystal in "2D" or "3D" mode. The terms "2D" and "3D" are misleading since modern multi-slice PET cameras always produce three-dimensional images of three-dimensional objects. Unfortunately, the terminology has become imbedded in common usage.

With "2D" imaging, it is possible to use axial collimation between the slices. Annular tungsten plates centered between the detector rings extend toward the center of the scanner (see Figure 5). These plates stop photons that are not traveling in the plane of the detector ring. With "3D" imaging, these septa need to be removed. "3D" imaging is more sensitive than "2D" imaging, since many more lines-of-response are sampled.

"2D"   "3D"

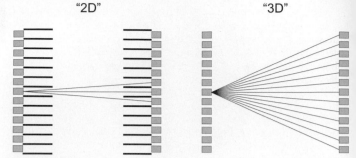

Figure 20: Cross-Plane Coincidence. This diagram shows the cross-plane coincidence for "2D" and "3D" imaging modes. In "2D" mode, axial collimation is provided by septa shown as heavy dark lines. The septa limit the coincidence to a single plane or the next adjacent plane. In "3D" mode, with no axial collimation, a crystal can be placed "in coincidence" with all of the planes.

Sensitivity Profile: The sensitivity profile for "3D" imaging changes markedly along the axis of the scanner. Radioactivity in the top or bottom plane can only be detected by the ring of detectors in that plane. For lines-of-response that are angled with respect to the plane, at least one of the photons will land outside the sensitive region. Radioactivity in the central ring of the scanner can be seen by the widest angle of detectors. On the left side of Figure 21 the many lines-of-response going through the center of the central plane are shown. On the right side, there is a single line-of-response that goes through the center of the top plane.

For "3D' imaging, the sensitivity is very high in the center and falls off linearly toward the edge. In order to compensate for this sensitivity profile, it is necessary to have considerable overlap between adjacent bed positions. For "2D" imaging, the very top and bottom plane will be less sensitive than the other planes, but otherwise the sensitivity is relatively constant in the axial direction. In "2D" imaging, only a small amount of overlap between bed positions is needed.

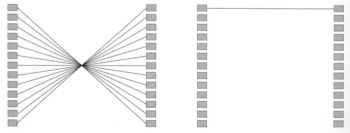

Figure 21: Sensitivity Profile. On the left, a point at the center of the middle ring can be detected by a large number of lines-of-response between each of the planes. On the right, a point at the center of the top ring can only be detected by lines-of-response within that plane.

Scatter Fraction: The decrease in axial collimation with the septa removed for "3D" imaging means that both the true and scattered coincidence events will increase. As described above the scattered coincidences will increase on the order of the square of the acceptance angle. The true coincidences will increase only linearly with the acceptance angle. Thus, the scattered fraction will increase as the axial collimation is reduced.

This increase in the scatter fraction reduces the effective benefit from increased sensitivity. The noise-equivalent-counts (NEC) will not increase as rapidly as the true coincidence count rate (see below). The exact relation between the noise-equivalent-count rate and the axial collimation will depend on the amount of scatter. If there is less scatter, e.g., in a thin patient, "3D" imaging will be more advantageous. If there is more scatter, e.g., in a large patients, there may actually be a disadvantage to "3D" imaging.

Random Fraction: The increase in sensitivity in "3D" mode means that there will be an increase in the singles rate. Like the Compton rate, the randoms rate will increase on the order of the square of the singles rate (see below), so the randoms fraction will also increase in "3D" imaging. The randoms rate also depends on the amount of activity in the field-of-view and on the coincidence time of the scanner (see below). Thus, low administered dose, fast coincidence time, and "3D" imaging tend to go together, and higher administered dose, slower coincidence time, and "2D" imaging tend to go together.

Degree of Axial Collimation: PET scanners without septa can only collect data in "3D" mode. Scanners with fixed septa can only collect data in "2D" mode. Scanners with retractable septa can collect data in either "3D" or "2D" mode.

However, the design of PET scanners is actually more complicated than just deciding between "2D" and "3D." Depending on the dimensions of the septa, the amount of axial collimation can vary. Scanners with relatively long septa have more axial collimation. Scanners with shorter septa have less axial collimation. PET cameras with panel designs like that of the Dual Anger camera PET scanners can be equipped with axial collimators that are more complicated in design. Thus, there is a range of possible axial collimation options.

The general principal is that decreasing the axial collimation increases the sensitivity of the PET scanner, but it also increases the scatter fraction and the randoms fraction. In circumstances where the scatter and randoms fractions are low, reducing the axial collimation can lead to improve image quality. However, the amount of improvement will depend on all these factors.

IMAGE RECONSTRUCTION

Lines-of-Response. **Line Integrals:** The primary PET data are the lines-of-response between crystals that are placed in coincidence. True coincidences between crystals come from annihilations that occurred in a tube connecting the crystal pair. After correction for attenuation, the count rate in each line-of-response is equal to the integral of the activity in the tube connecting the crystals. The count rate for each crystal pair can be modeled mathematically as a line integral through the activity distribution. These line integrals are analogous to the data obtained in SPECT and CT.

These lines-of-response crisscross the field of view of the PET scanner. It is natural when thinking about the coincidences to think about each crystal with a fan of lines-of-response to crystals on the other side of the scanner. However, this organization of the data is not the easiest when it comes to understanding reconstruction.

Stacks of Planes of Data: The data are easier to understand in the case where there is heavy axial collimation, "2D" mode. In that case, the data are confined to a single crystal ring or two adjacent crystal rings. A data plane, which is located in the center of each ring of crystals, is used for coincidences within that ring (see Figure 22). The lines-of-response that cross to adjacent planes are placed on additional planes located between each ring of crystals. Thus, the number of data planes is equal to two times the number of crystal rings minus one.

The lines-of-response from a single plane can be reorganized into "projections," where all the lines are parallel. Different "projections" represent lines-of-response at different angles. This same reorganization is often used with CT data. Once reorganized into a set of "projections" at different angles, the data are even more analogous to data from SPECT.

Tilted Stacks: Without axial collimation ("3D" mode), there are not only the lines-of-response that are nearly in the axial planes, but also there are lines-of-response at a considerable angle to these planes. These high-angle lines-of-response can be organized into tilted a stacks of tilted planes. There is a whole stack of planes for each angle of tilt (see Figure 22), and for each angle there is an entire stack of planes.

The data for the tilted stack of planes is not complete. Some tilted planes in the stack may lie completely within the scanner. However, other planes will come out of the scanner and have an incomplete set of lines-of-response. At first glance, one might worry that this incomplete data would make reconstruction impossible, but that is not the case.

Four-Dimensional Data: The data from the untilted stack of planes is sufficient to reconstruct the three-dimensional structure of the patient being

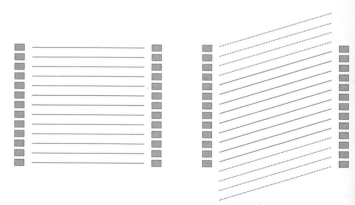

Figure 22: Stack of Planes. The diagram on the left shows the stack of planes that correspond to the in-plane coincidences. The diagram on the right shows one set of tilted planes. Coincidence data is only obtained from the center planes. No data are obtained from the dashed planes although a portion of the dashed planes is within the axial field-of-view of the PET scanner.

imaged. Each plane of data is sufficient to reconstruct that plane. The stack of planes provides the third dimension. The tilted stacks represent a fourth dimension parameterized by the tilt angle. Although the fourth dimension is incomplete, there is actually more than enough data to reconstruct the third dimension. Mathematically, one says that the problem is over-determined.

It may seem strange that the data is four-dimensional when the object and the image are only three-dimensional. The reason is that there are more lines through the data than points in the data. There is another way to identify the four-dimensional nature of the data. Each crystal can be defined using two parameters, the plane on which it is located and its position around the ring. To identify two crystals four parameters are required. These four parameters define a four-dimensional space.

Converting Four-Dimensional Data to Three Dimensions. The number of lines-of-response without axial collimation is very large. There are more than 10,000 crystals, which means there are more than 100,000,000 crystal pairs. (Not all of the crystal pairs have lines-of-response that cross the field-of-view of the scanner, but the number of crystal pairs is still enormous.) Even with current computer power, iterative reconstruction of the full four-dimensional data set can be very time-consuming. Thus, many of the reconstruction algorithms convert the four-dimensional data to three-dimensional data, and then reconstruct this data using methods similar to CT or SPECT reconstruction.

The easiest method of converting data to three dimensions is to assign each tilted lines-of-response to an untilted plane. This process is called **rebinning**. A tilted lines-of-response can be assigned to the center plane (**single-slice rebinning**) or to all the planes that it crosses (**multi-slice rebinning**). There are other, more complicated, methods perform a function similar to rebinning, e.g., **Fourier rebinning** (**FORE**). The details of these operations are beyond the scope of this book.

Pre-Filtering. Prior to reconstruction, the data may be pre-filtered. In "2D" mode or when the data have been rebinned into planes, pre-filtering can be used to smooth the data in the axial direction. This operation tends to reduce the noise, but it may also reduce the resolution in the axial direction. Pre-filtering may not be identified as a separate step, but rather be included in the overall reconstruction process.

Reconstruction Methods. The two main categories of reconstruction are Fourier reconstruction and iterative reconstruction. Filtered back-projection is a method that is often used to implement Fourier reconstruction. Fourier reconstruction assumes that the PET scan process has two mathematical properties, linearity and shift invariance. Iterative reconstruction is more general; it only assumes that the PET scan process is linear. Thus, iterative reconstruction can model many more effects than Fourier reconstruction.

The major advantage of Fourier reconstruction is much faster than a full iterative reconstruction. However, a relatively new iterative algorithm **ordered subset estimation maximization** (**OSEM**) ameliorates much of the time penalty of iterative versus Fourier reconstruction. The results produced by the ordered subset method produce results similar to the full estimation maximization algorithm in the domain of medical image reconstruction.

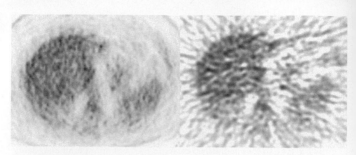

Figure 23: Reconstruction Noise. On the left is an axial FDG-PET slice through the liver that has been reconstructed with the order subset, estimation maximization (OSEM) algorithm. On the right is the same slice reconstructed with the filtered back-projection algorithm. The noise in the OSEM reconstruction tends to appear as focal areas of increased activity; the noise in the filtered back-projection reconstruction tends to appear "wormy". At the edge of the field-of-view, streaks are more prominent with the filtered back-projection method.

Noise Texture: The reconstruction algorithm may have important effects on speed of reconstruction and image quality, but these factors don't impact interpretation. One factor that is relatively more important to understand is the noise texture of the two reconstruction methods. Fourier reconstruction tends to produce streaks in areas of high activity, whereas iterative reconstruction will tend to produce blobs in areas of uniform activity (see Figure 23). The noise in Fourier reconstruction is high-pass filtered. The noise tends to have a "wormy" appearance.

In some tasks, such as trying to identify hot spots in the liver, the blobby noise from iterative reconstruction can be more confusing than the streak artifacts from Fourier reconstruction. In other tasks, such as trying to evaluate structures next to a hot bladder, the streak artifacts from Fourier reconstruction can be more confusing than the blobby artifacts from iterative reconstruction.

Generally, iterative reconstruction produces better results than Fourier reconstruction, but when the noise texture of iterative reconstruction is confusing, it may be appropriate to reconstruct the data a second time with a Fourier algorithm. The key is to understand the noise texture and to adjust the algorithm as necessary.

DETECTORS

Scintillation Crystals.   The 511-keV annihilation photons are converted to a burst of light in a scintillation crystal. Most PET scanners use a very large number of small columnar scintillation crystals. The crystals are often 4–6 mm in the axial and transaxial directions, and much longer, 20–30 mm, in the radial direction. The axial dimension of the crystal affects slice thickness. The transaxial dimension affects the in-plane resolution. The radial depth of the crystal affects the fraction of photons stopped by the crystal. In some designs a single scintillation crystal is used in the place of a large number of individual crystals.

Interaction of the Annihilation Photons in the Detector. The 511-keV annihilation photons have the same types of interactions in the detector as they do in the patient. The major interactions are the photoelectric effect and Compton scatter. Rayleigh scattering is more frequent in the detector, but it still plays a relatively minor role.

1

The photoelectric effect is the most desirable interaction in the crystal. The energy of the incoming photon less the binding energy is converted to kinetic energy of an electron. The path of the electron in the crystal is relatively short. It gives up its energy to heat and to ionization within the crystal. The ionized atoms return to the ground state by giving off light photons. The atom from which the photoelectron was ejected will have a hole in one of its shells, usually the k-shell. This atom can emit a characteristic x-ray, but often this x-ray will be stopped within a fairly short distance in the crystal.

Compton scatter is less desirable, and unfortunately, it is the most likely event at 511 keV in all the scintillation crystals used in PET. The scattered photon many travel in any direction within the crystal, or it may travel into another crystal, or it may escape altogether from the crystal. Part of the energy will be deposited at the location of the Compton interaction, and part of the energy will be deposited where the Compton scattered photon is absorbed. The measured event will be at the center of the mass of the deposited energy. Compton photons that escape the crystal will result in loss of sensitivity. Compton photons that are absorbed at a distance result in a loss of resolution.

Photomultiplier Tubes. A group of photomultiplier tubes views the flash of light from the scintillation in the crystal(s). From the relative amount of light distributed to each phototube, the position of the scintillation can be determined. With a small number of tubes, e.g., four, it is possible to distinguish a large number of positions.

Each scintillation produces a large number of light photons, say, 10,000. As the scintillation moves from crystals on one side of a block to crystals on the other side, the ratio of photons in the tubes varies. This ratio can be used to determine in which crystal the scintillation occurred. This process of identifying the position of the scintillation by detecting the relative amount of light in a small group of photomultiplier tubes was invented by Hal Anger, and it is often called **Anger logic**.

Photomultiplier tubes are quite remarkable devices. They convert the exceptionally low energy of a single light photon, 2–3 eV, into a measurable electric pulse. Compare this feat with magnetic resonance imaging. The signal from a whole ensemble of hydrogen atoms is needed to overcome the thermal noise in the receiver. (Note, however, that the dark-adapted human eye is also able to detect a single light photon.)

Photomultiplier tubes are one of the few vacuum tubes still used (another example is CRTs). There are solid-state devices, e.g., avalanche photodiodes, which are used in some applications, but so far photomultiplier tubes have been dominant in PET scanners.

Pulse Height Analyzer. The number of light photons produced by a scintillation is proportional to the energy of the incoming high-energy photon, and the charge in the photomultiplier tubes is proportional to the number of light photons. Thus, the electrical signal that comes out of the detector is proportional to the energy of the incoming gamma ray. This signal is then passed through a pulse height analyzer, which allows only signals of the proper energy to be recorded. The most important part of this discrimination is eliminating the many low-energy photons that are produced during scattering.

It is less common to have a signal that is greater than 511 keV, and often a higher energy signal may be produced by the combination of a 511-keV photon and a low-energy scattered photon. In that case, it may be desirable to establish that there was a 511-keV event and ignore the simultaneous lower energy signal. Thus, the pulse height analyzer often has only a **lower-level discriminator** and no upper level. It is possible to envision a design with simultaneous emission and transmission collection using a higher-energy photon, say, the 662-keV photon of cesium-137. In that case a pulse height analyzer with both upper- and lower-level discriminators would be useful.

Raising the lower-level discriminator will reduce the number of scattered photons that are counted as photopeak events. If the lower-level discriminator is raised too high, then true coincidence events will be lost. The energy resolution of most current PET scanners is relatively poor. Improvements in energy resolution will improve performance by allowing better separation of scattered and photopeak events.

Selection of an ideal lower-level discriminator value can be even more complicated. An annihilation photon may make it to the crystal, scatter in the crystal, and the secondary photon may escape. Since the photon did not scatter in the patient, these events represent true events; however, they deposit less energy in the crystal. A photon that undergoes a high angle scattered within the crystal may result in a pulse with a similar height to that from scatter in the patient. Thus, lowering the lower-level discriminator may both increase the number of true coincidences (those that scatter in the crystal) and bad coincidences (those that scatter in the patient).

Electronics. The electronics in a PET scanner are quite impressive, even by today's standards. One of the most difficult tasks is checking for coincidence events. This task needs to be performed in parallel very rapidly using special purpose electronics.

A crystal on one side needs to be placed in coincidence with a large number of crystals on the other side. In order to make this a manageable task, a moderate-sized group of crystals is often placed in coincidence with a group on the other side. In this fashion the number of coincidence circuits can be kept manageable, while at the same time allowing a number of independent coincidences to be processed at the same time. The details are often specific to a particular design; the important features are that the electronics are quite complicated and that the design of the electronics can have consequences on the performance of the scanner.

Coincidence Window. The coincidence window is the maximum amount of time allowed between the pulses from two detectors for a coincidence event to be recorded. This time is often on the order of about 10 ns. The speed of light is 3×10^8 m/se. In 10 ns (10^{-8} s) light will travel 3 m. The speed of electric signals in wires is only a fraction of this speed. Issues that one normally doesn't consider, like the length of the connecting wires, need to be carefully addressed in the design.

Time-of-Flight. If an annihilation event occurs toward one edge of the body, the photon will arrive at the detector on the near side of the body slightly sooner than the other photon reaches the detector on the far side of the body. If the near detector is 30 cm closer to the annihilation than the far detector, the difference in arrival times will be 1 ns. If the PET scanner were able to measure differences in arrival of less than 1 ns, then it could distinguish between annihilation positions along a single line-of-response. This type of a PET scanner is called a time-of-flight PET scanner. With this type of scanner each event is more informative. The key limitation to building a time-of-flight scanner is the time taken by the scintillation process within the crystals.

Depth-of-Interaction. The annihilation photons are attenuated according to the same relation as the photons traveling through tissue:

$$I(x) = I_0 \cdot e^{-\mu x}$$

The difference is that the linear attenuation coefficient, μ, is different in the crystal than in tissue. The radial depth of the crystal is selected so that the crystal stops most of the photons. Weight, cost, and optical properties are considerations that limit the radial depth of the crystals. It would seem that a crystal with low linear attenuation coefficient could be used so long as the radial depth of the crystal were increased appropriately. However, the depth-of-interaction of the photon in the detector can affect resolution.

If a photon goes through the center of the field-of-view, then depth-of-interaction has no effect on resolution (see Figure 24). However at the edge of the field-of-view, the depth-of-interaction can have a measurable effect. In Figure 24, the position of a scintillation is taken as the center of the front face of the crystal. As can be seen, the real annihilation does not lie along the calculated the line-of-response. Depth-of-interaction effects are one reason why the resolution of a PET scanner is higher at the center of the field-of-view and lower toward the edge of the field of view.

Schemes have been devised to measure the depth-of-interaction so that the lines of response can be adjusted accordingly. If photodetectors are placed at

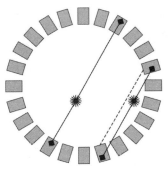

Figure 24: Depth of Interaction. For a line-of-response that goes through the center of the ring of crystals, there is no depth-of-interaction effect. For a line-of-response near the edged of the field-of-view, there can be a large depth of interaction affect. The solid line shows the real line-of-response; the dashed line shows the apparent line-of-response.

both ends of the scintillation crystal, then the ratio of the light coming out of each end can be used to measure the depth of interaction. Crystals have been constructed as a combination of crystals. If the crystals have different decay times, then it is possible to detect in which crystal the photon was stopped.

Measurement of depth-of-interaction has been difficult. Thus, use of crystals with high linear attenuation coefficients has been emphasized in PET scanners.

Properties of Scintillation Crystals. Table 2 shows the properties of several scintillation crystals that have been used in or proposed for PET scanners. Scintillation crystals are often relatively simple crystalline compounds. At times a low percentage of an impurity, called a dopant, is added to the crystal in order to alter the properties of the crystal. The dopant may increase the decay rate of the crystal. It may also change the electronic band structure of the crystal so that the light output of the crystal is at a wavelength that is more optimal for a photomultiplier tube. In addition to crystals, some ceramics have been used as scintillators.

Transparency: After a flash of light is produced it must be able to reach the photomultiplier tube. Therefore, scintillation crystals must be transparent to the light produced by the scintillation.

Stopping Power: The stopping power of a crystal depends on the elemental composition of the crystal and its density. The likelihood of an event is dependent on the Z-number, the number of protons in the nucleus. Heavier nuclei will stop photons better than light nuclei. Furthermore, the likelihood of a photon electric event goes up with the Z-number as well. Crystals are often made from a few different elements. An **effective atomic number** is the atomic number that a material made from a single element with the same stopping power would have. The second key factor is the density of the material. Denser materials have higher stopping power since they have more elements packed in the same amount of space.

There is also a higher ratio of photoelectric to Compton interaction in crystals with higher atomic number. Since photoelectric events are preferred, this is another advantage to high-Z materials.

Table 2: Properties of Scintillation Crystals

	Decay-time (ns)	μ (1/cm)	FWHM (%)	Light (%)
NaI(Tl)	230	0.35	6.6	100
BGO	300	0.95	10.2	15
LSO(Ce)	40	0.86	10.0	75
LuAp	18	0.95	~15	30
GSO(Ce)	60	0.70	8.5	25
CsF	3	0.39	18.0	5
BaF$_2$	2	0.45	11.4	5
LaCl$_3$	26	0.36	3.3	120
LaBr$_3$	35	0.47	2.6	160

μ is the linear attenuation coefficient; FWHM is the full width at half-maximum of the photopeak expressed as a percentage of the photopeak; Light is the amount of light output relative to NaI(Tl). After Surti et al.

Light Output: The efficiency of conversion of the energy of the incoming photon to the scintillation light photons varies between crystals. One of the most efficient is sodium iodide doped with thallium, NaI(Tl). It takes about 30 eV of incoming energy to produce each 3-eV light photon. Thus, a 511-keV photon produces about 17,000 light photons. NaI(Tl) is often taken as the standard, and its light output is set to 100. The light output of other crystals is given by comparison to that of NaI(Tl).

Light output puts a limit on the energy resolution that can be achieved by a crystal. The energy resolution of NaI(Tl) at the 140-keV energy of Tc-99m is largely determined by the number of scintillation photons. (The key factor is the Poisson statistics of the number of electrons reaching the first dynode in the photomultiplier tubes. This number is in turn proportional to the number of light photons.) The energy resolution may be less than this statistical limit if other factors also cause variability in light. Thus, it is common to list both light output and energy resolution when characterizing crystals.

Light output may also affect spatial resolution. The ratio of light in nearby phototubes determines the localization of the crystal. If there are too few photons, this ratio becomes noisy. High light output also improves coincidence timing as described in the next section.

Decay Time: The decay time is important in determining the coincidence window. The coincidence circuits must wait for enough light to be emitted from the crystal so that an event is reliably identified. The coincidence window is typically considerably shorter than the decay time since the start of a scintillation can be detected using only the leading edge of the light output.

After a potential coincidence is identified using the leading edge of the light output, the light output is integrated for a longer period of time. The integrated light output is used to determine the energy of the incoming photons and decide if the potential coincidence event is due to photopeak events.

If a crystal has low light output, then to get a statistically valid signal, it may be necessary to wait for most of the light to be emitted to determine reliably that an event has occurred. If there is a large amount of light, an event can be recognized earlier in the decay process. Thus, both light output and decay time are important parameters in determining the coincidence window. The coincidence window is directly related to the random fraction (see below).

The scintillation decay time is also a major determinant of dead-time. A detector cannot detect another annihilation photon until it has largely recovered from the prior scintillation.

Physical properties: Crystals like NaI(Tl) that absorb water from the atmosphere are called hygroscopic. Hygroscopic crystals must be completely sealed. Some crystals are fragile, and can be easily damaged by either physical or thermal trauma. Crystals that are non-hygroscopic and rugged are easier to work with.

Many high-density crystals have a very high index of refraction. To prevent a high amount of internal reflection, it is necessary to pay attention to the optical properties when matching the crystals to the photomultiplier tubes.

Scintillation Crystal Examples. Table 2 shows some of the key properties of a few scintillation crystals that can be used for PET scanners.

Sodium Iodide Doped with Thallium, NaI(Tl): NaI(Tl) is the workhorse for single photon imaging. The key property of NaI(Tl) is its high light output, yielding good energy and spatial resolution. The limitation of NaI(Tl) for PET scanning is its relatively poor stopping power.

Bismuth Germinate, BGO: For a long time BGO was used widely for PET scanning. The key property of BGO is its high stopping power. Its low light output is a disadvantage for single-photon imaging, and its relatively slow decay time is its major limitation for PET imaging.

Lutetium Oxyorthosilicate Doped with Cerium, LSO(Ce): LSO(Ce) is used in some PET scanners. It has good stopping power, although less than BGO. It has high light output, but the light output is variable. The key advantage of LSO(Ce) is a fast decay time. In addition to LSO(Ce), several other lutetium compounds have been investigated. For example, lutetium orthoaluminate, $LuAlO_3$(Ce) or LuAp, is notable for its high stopping power.

Germanium Oxyorthosilicate Doped with Cerium, GSO(Ce): GSO(Ce) is also used in some PET scanners. It is similar to LSO(Ce). It has lower light output, but the light output is not variable. Again, the key advantage of GSO(Ce) is the fast decay time.

Cesium Fluoride, CsF, and Barium Fluoride, BaF_2: These crystals with very fast decay times made possible the construction of time-of-flight PET scanners in the past. However, low light output and poor stopping power have kept them from being used recently.

Lanthanum Halides ($LaCl_3$, $LaBr_3$): These crystals have not been used for PET scanners; however, they have very good decay times and high light output. Sub-nanosecond coincidence times have been reported, raising the possibility of a time-of-flight scanner. The major disadvantage of these crystals is their relatively poor stopping power.

COUNT RATE

One's first impression is that the count rate of a PET scanner should be a simple concept. In fact the count rate of a PET scanner is quite complicated. Someone who has a good understanding of count rate has mastered much of the physics and instrumentation associated with PET imaging.

Types. Singles: Each detector records events when the energy deposited in a crystal is greater than the setting of the lower-level discriminator. The rate at which these events occur is called the singles count rate. Although there are usually a very large number of individual scintillation crystals in a PET camera, in order to reduce the number of components, many individual crystals are typically grouped together in a block. While the block is processing one scintillation, it is "dead" for further detection. PET scanners are constructed to process many events at the same time, but **dead-time** can become an issue at very high levels of activity. The singles count rate increases linearly with activity at low count rates; at very high count rates, the dead-time may make this relation more complicated.

Total Coincidence: If two detectors placed in coincidence both record events within the coincidence time window, then a coincident event occurs. The rate at which these events happen is the total coincidence count rate.

When one of the pair of photons is detected, it is unlikely that the other photon will be detected. Due to geometry, only one of the two photons may be directed at a detector. One of the photons may be attenuated in the tissue. One of the photons may be absorbed by a septum or by a non-sensitive portion of the detectors. One of the photons may pass through the detector without being stopped. These various factors mean that it is much more likely to have a singles event than a coincident event. Often the coincidence count rate is only one or two percent of the singles count rate.

True Coincidence: The most desirable event that a PET scanner can detect is a true coincidence event. This event occurs when both annihilation photons reach detectors without being scattered in the patient, and both photons are successfully detected. This type of event is called a true coincidence and the rate of these events is called the true coincidence count rate. When the dead-time is negligible, the true coincidence count rate is proportional to the amount of activity in the field-of-view. The true coincidence count rate will increase less rapidly and finally decrease as the dead-time becomes more important.

Scattered Coincidence: One or both of the annihilation photons may be scattered in the tissue. For low-angle scatter, there is relatively little loss of energy between the incoming and outgoing photon. Thus, the scattered photon may fall within the photopeak window of the detector. The scattered photon is thus counted as a coincidence event. The scattered and the true coincidence event are not distinguishable by the PET scanner. The scattered photon gives false positional information, leading to loss of resolution. The ratio of the scattered coincidence count rate to the true coincidence count rate is the **scatter fraction**. The scatter fraction will depend on the patient, being greater for patients with large cross sections.

Random Coincidence: It is possible just by chance that two photons from different decays will be detected by two crystals within the coincidence time window. This type of event is called a random coincidence. The chance that there will be an event within the coincidence time window is proportional to the count rates in both of the detectors. Thus, the random coincidence rate is proportional to the square of the singles count rate. The ratio of the random coincidence count rate to the true coincidence count rate is the **randoms fraction**. Since the random coincidence count rate is proportional to the square of the singles count rate and the true coincidence count rate is proportional to the singles count rate, randoms fraction will be proportional to the singles rate.

Random coincidence can be made negligible by reducing the singles count rate. However, PET scans are count-limited. Thus, the administered dose or the imaging conditions are often selected to maximize the singles count rate. Often the limit is the rate at which the random coincidence becomes a significant problem. Consequently, random coincidence is often an important consideration under clinical scanning conditions.

Scatter and Randoms Correction.   Both scatter and randoms are an important source of inaccuracy under clinical PET scan conditions. Thus, modern PET scanners include corrections for both of these effects.

Randoms Correction: There is a relatively simple method or measuring the randoms. If the signal from one side of the coincidence circuit is delayed an amount of time greater than the time it takes for a scintillation to completely decay, then no true or scattered coincidence events will be recorded. This procedure will, however, have no effect on the random coincidence rate. Thus, the only coincidences that will be recorded using a delayed window will be the random coincidences. This measurement could be used to correct the total coincidences for randoms; however, this measurement has noise associated with it. In some instances, the randoms are spatially smooth. In this case the measured values can be spatially smoothed, reducing the noise. More often, it turns out that better signal-to-noise ratios can be achieved by calculating the random count rate from the singles count rates in each of the crystals.

Scatter Correction: After correcting for randoms, an image will contain true and scatter coincidence data. Outside of the patient, there should be no true coincidence data. Thus, regions outside of the patient can be used to estimate the scatter. Scatter varies slowly from position to position in the image. Thus, the data from outside the patient can be used to predict the scatter within the patient. Alternately, the scatter can be calculated from the knowledge of the attenuation map and the activity distribution. However, iteratively calculating the scatter correction is quite time-consuming and is not typically done. The algorithms that are implemented in current scanners use some combination of approximate methods. The scatter correction is often more challenging than the random correction.

Noise Equivalent Count Rate.   Image quality in PET is heavily dependent on the total number of counts used to make the image. The number of counts in the image will be equal to the scan time times the count rate. However, the difficult question is which count rate should be used when considering image quality.

The singles count rate is easily measured, but it is a poor indicator of image quality. The total coincidence count rate is also easily measured, and it has somewhat better correlation with image quality. However, the total coincidence count rate includes scattered and random coincidence events. In a large patient, there will be a high scatter fraction. When the singles count rate is very high there will be a high randoms fraction. Thus, there may be a high total coincidence count rate and relatively poor image quality.

The desired events are the true coincidence events. After the image is corrected for the scattered and random coincidence events, it might seem that the true coincidence count rate would be the rate that should be used. However, even the true coincidence count rate is not perfect indicator of image quality. An image with a given true coincidence count rate, which started with no scatter or randoms, will be better than an image, in which there were large corrections for of scatter and randoms. In order to better reflect image quality, the true coincidence count rate needs to be adjusted for the noise caused by the scatter and randoms correction.

The corrected count rate is called the noise equivalent count rate. The noise equivalent count rate is supposed to be the true count rate of a theoretical image without any scatter or random events, which would give the same statistical quality image as a real image, which includes scatter and randoms. The noise equivalent count rate (NEC) is given by

$$NEC = T/(T + S + f \cdot R)$$

where T is the true coincidence count rate, S is the scattered coincidence count rate, R is the random coincidence count rate, and f is a factor ranging from 1 to 2.

The random count rate can be measure directly (see above). If it is directly measured, then there will be measurement noise. Thus, the random coincidence may cause noise both by being included in the original measurement and from the inaccuracy of its measurement. In that case, the factor f is equal to 2. In some PET scan situations, the random coincidences are very smooth or can be made very smooth. In that case, a very large number of measurements can be used in the estimation of each random value and the measurement of the random coincidence rate is nearly noiseless. Or, the random count rate can be calculated using the singles count rates in different crystals. In both of these later cases, the factor f is nearly equal to 1. The details of exactly what value of f to use can be complicated, but the most important concept is that the noise equivalent count attempt to capture these effects.

The noise equivalent count rate is not the only factor in image quality. Other issues like the pattern of the noise can have an effect on lesion detectability. However, the noise equivalent count rate provides a very good indication of image quality. It is a considerably better parameter than true coincidence count rate, and far superior to the total coincidence count rate. Measurement of noise equivalent count rate is not trivial. Total coincidence count rate and estimates of the random and scattered count rate are needed. However, there are NEMA specifications for the measurement, which are reasonably simple, reasonably simple at least for a physicist.

Often the noise equivalent count rate is plotted as a function of activity. Initially the noise equivalent count rate increases linearly with activity. As random coincidences become more important the noise equivalent count rate increases less rapidly, and eventually decreases. These types of curves can be very useful for comparing different scan conditions, e.g., "2D" versus "3D" mode, large patient versus small patient, different low-level discriminator settings, etc.

The noise equivalent count rate versus activity curve is also useful for comparing different PET scanners as long as the curves are collected under the same conditions. One number from this curve that is quite informative is the maximum noise equivalent count rate obtained using the conditions described in the NEMA 2001 standard. This number is most important for high activity and/or low axial collimation, when the count rate may be limited by the random rate. With lower activity or with high axial collimation, the slope of the initial portion of the curve is a more important parameter.

STANDARDIZED UPTAKE VALUE, SUV

PET scan data is complicated. It is affected by attenuation, by scatter, and by randoms. However, each of these effects can be accurately corrected. The final PET scan image is an accurate representation of the relative distribution of activity. In order to obtain an absolute measure of activity it is also necessary to measure a known source of activity. Given the value of this known source, it is possible to translate a measure count rate into an activity level.

Once the the machine has been calibrated with a known source of activity, an attenuation corrected image can be converted into activity per volume (MBq/cm^3). However, this value depends on how much activity was injected, how much decay has occurred, and how much the patient weighs. A number called the standardized uptake value (SUV) is used to try to normalize for these other effects.

The equation for calculating the standardized uptake value is

$$SUV = \text{voxel-value} \cdot \text{weight} / \text{decay-corrected-dose}$$

where the voxel-value has been normalized so that it represents MBq/cm^3, the weight is the patient weight in grams, and the decay-corrected dose is the injected dose which is decay corrected from the time of measurement to the time of scan. If the PET scanner has been calibrated, then the technologist only needs to enter the patient's weight, the administered dose, and the time the dose was measured.

The basic idea is that if the activity were uniformly distributed over the whole patient and there were no excretion, then the voxel-value would just be the decay-corrected dose/weight. Thus, the SUV would be one if the activity were uniformly distributed over the whole body. An SUV of three means that there is three times the average activity at that location. An SUV of ten means that there is ten times the average activity at that location.

There are several modifications that can be made to this SUV formula. The voxel-value from the scanner is in terms of cm^3, whereas the size of the patient is given in terms of weight in grams. This assumes that the density of the patient is 1. Instead, an actual density could be added to the formula. The idea of the SUV is that it can be used to compare different patients. There is relatively little distribution of many pharmaceuticals to the fat. In a patient with a lot of fat, the activity in the major organs might be greater on a per gram basis. Thus, it might be more reasonable to normalize for lean body mass than for total weight. Many process are more closely related to body surface area than to weight. Given that consideration, it might be more reasonable to normalize to the body surface area. To distinguish these various methods, the SUV sometimes is written with a subscript, SUV_{wt} or SUV_{lean} or SUV_{BSA}.

The SUV is particularly useful when comparing between different experimental study results. It provides a quantitative number, which can easily be compared. In clinical practice, it is used less commonly. Generally, clinicians use the internal control of image intensities, e.g., comparing pulmonary nodules to the mediastinal blood pool. However, even in clinical practice when it is readily available it can be useful to help consistency from day to day.

CONCLUSIONS

This short introduction is meant to provide a general understanding of the principles of positron physics and PET imaging instrumentation. Emphasis has been placed on the features of the physics and instrumentation that help in understanding clinical images. Much of the physics is the same for SPECT and PET; however, there are a several important differences. Someone who is familiar with the clinically important aspects of SPECT physics and instrumentation will be surprised by some aspects of PET physics and instrumentation, e.g., the relative independence of resolution and the distance between the patient and detector. Coincidence is a key new concept as is the importance of random and scattered coincidence. The importance of attenuation correction and the artifacts that can be produced during attenuation correction are other key concepts. Hopefully, this brief chapter will provide enough background to understand how PET physics and instrumentation impact clinical imaging.

BIBLIOGRAPHY

1. Cherry SR, Sorenson JA, Phelps ME. *Physics in Nuclear Medicine.* third edition ed. Philadelphia: Saunders, 2003.
2. Hill DL, Batchelor PG, Holden M, Hawkes DJ. Medical image registration. *Phys Med Biol* 2001; 46(3):R1–45.
3. Lardinois D, Weder W, Hany TF, Kamel EM, Korom S, Seifert B, et al. Staging of non-small-cell lung cancer with integrated positron-emission tomography and computed tomography. *N Engl J Med* 2003; 348(25):2500–7.
4. Osman MM, Cohade C, Nakamoto Y, Marshall LT, Leal JP, Wahl RL. Clinically significant inaccurate localization of lesions with PET/CT: frequency in 300 patients. *J Nucl Med* 2003; 44(2):240–3.
5. Surti S, Karp, J.S., Muehllehner, G., Raby, P.S. Investigation of Lanthanum Scintillators for 3-D PET. *IEEE Trans Nucl Sci* 2003; 50(3):348–354.

PET Radiotracers

RADIOISOTOPES

There are several positron-emitting radioisotopes that have been used for PET imaging. The first four isotopes in Table 1 are of particular note with regard to imaging biological systems. Carbon, nitrogen, and oxygen are key elements for biological systems. Each of them has a pure positron-emitting radioisotope, and none of them has an appropriate single-photon-emitting radioisotope. Fluorine, the fourth entry in the table, is not a normal element in biological systems, but fluorine can often replace either a hydrogen atom or a hyroxyl moiety. It also is a pure positron emitter and does not have a useful single-photon-emitting isotope.

Early in the development of nuclear medicine, the biological significance of these radioisotopes was realized, and positron emitters were viewed with great promise. The availability of these biological radioisotopes has made a major impact on PET research. A vast array of biological radiotracers has been used to help understand kinetics and function. There has been a rich PET literature over nearly half a century.

However, the great promise of these isotopes was not realized in clinical nuclear medicine until recently. The second column in Table 1 may help to explain why. The half-lives of these four isotopes are very short. Oxygen's two-minute half-life means that it needs to be pumped directly from a cyclotron to the scan room. Nitrogen's ten-minute half-life and carbon's twenty-minute half-life are a bit easier to work with, but these half-lives mean that there is little

Table 1: Radioisotopes

Isotope	Half-life	β^+ Energy (MeV)	γ Energy (MeV)
C-11	20.4 m	0.385 (99.8%)	
N-13	9.97 m	0.492 (99.8%)	
O-15	122 s	0.735 (99.9%)	
F-18	110 m	0.250 (100%)	
K-38	7.64 m	1.216 (99.3%)	2.167 (99.8%)
Cu-62	9.74 m	1.315 (97.6%)	
Cu-64	12.7 h	0.278 (17.9%)	
Ga-68	68.1 h	0.836 (8.79%), 0.352 (1.12%)	1.077 (3.0%)
Rb-82	75 s	1.523 (83.3%), 1.157 (10.2%)	0.776 (13.4%)
I-124	4.18 d	0.686 (11.3%), 0.974 (11.3%)	1.691 (10.4%), 7.228(10.0%), 1.509 (3.0%), 1.376 (1.7%), 1.325 (1.43%)

The average energy of the β^+ is given along with the percentage of decays in which the β^+ is emitted. The energy of gamma rays that occur in more than 1% of decays is given along with the percentage of decays in which that gamma ray is emitted.

time for radiopharmaceutical preparation and delivery to the imaging suite. Carbon-11 radiopharmaceuticals that require syntheses that take several half-lives have been used, but long synthesis times rapidly run into practical limits. During the early phase of PET development an on-site cyclotron was typically required.

Even with an on-site cyclotron, these short half-lives limit the biochemical and physiological processes that can be imaged. Single-photon nuclear medicine studies often allow hours or even days for radiopharmaceutical localization. Carbon-11, nitrogen-13, and oxygen-15 can only be used to study processes that have rapid uptake. Fluorine-18 with an approximately two-hour half-life allows more time for synthesis and for imaging somewhat longer physiologic processes.

Decay Schemes. The decay schemes for carbon-11, nitrogen-13, oxygen-15, and fluorine-18 are very simple. Nearly all decays emit a single positron, and there are essentially no photons emitted. The decay schemes for some of the other positron-emitting radioisotopes are more complicated. There may be several transitions that emit positrons of different energies (the most common are listed in Table 1). The progeny nuclei are often produced in an excited state, and several different prompt gamma rays may be emitted.

During the decay of a single iodine-124 atom, both a positron and one or more gamma rays may be emitted. Prompt gamma rays may cause problems with positron cameras. It is possible for one of the gamma rays to be recorded as a photopeak event. If this occurs, then there can be false coincidences between the gamma ray and one of the annihilation photons. Since the directions of the gamma ray and the annihilation photons are not related, these false coincidences will not give valid position information. This interesting problem does not, however, affect the radioisotopes that are the focus of this book.

Radioisotope Production. There are three principal methods that are used for production of radioisotopes in nuclear medicine. Radioisotopes can be produced by separation of the by-product produced during fission; they can be produced from neutron irradiation in a reactor; or they can be produced from bombardment of a target material by charged particles from accelerator.

The low-molecular-weight PET radioisotopes (C-11, N-13, O-15, and F-18) are all produced by charged particle bombardment. Typically, the radioisotopes are produced in a cyclotron, although other charged particle accelerators can be used. The charged particles that are used are usually the nuclei of very low weight isotopes, hydrogen, deuterium, or helium. The hydrogen nucleus is a single proton; the deuterium nucleus is one proton and one neutron; and the helium nucleus is two protons and two neutrons.

These very low molecular weight elements are converted to ions before injection into a cyclotron. Stripping an electron from the atom can produce a positive ion. There has been an increasing use of negative ion sources, where an electron is added to a neutral atom. Although it is somewhat harder to produce negative ions, it turns out that negative ions make it easier to in extract the beam from a cyclotron. Two electrons can be stripped from a negative ion by passing it through a carbon foil producing a positive ion that then turns in a different direction in the magnetic field of the cyclotron, allowing the beam to be extracted.

Nuclear Reactions: When accelerated to high energies, these charged particles can be smashed into nuclei of other elements. The high energy is used to overcome the electrical forces which keep the positively charge nuclei apart. After overcoming these forces, the nucleons can interact using nuclear forces to form new isotopes. Typically, a high-energy particle smashes into an isotope of an element and some other high-energy particle is emitted.

The nuclear reactions are written with the target isotope on the left, the product isotope on the right, and the incoming and outgoing particles separated by a comma within parentheses in the middle. An example, of a typical reaction for producing fluorine-18 is

$$O\text{-}18(p,n)F\text{-}18$$

where p is a proton, and n is a neutron. The high-energy proton interacts with the oxygen-18 nucleus. A high-energy neutron is emitted, leaving a fluorine-18 isotope. Since the incoming and outgoing particles each represent one nucleon, the **mass number** (N) of the product, fluorine-18, is the same as the target, oxygen-18. However, a proton replaces a neutron, thus the **atomic number** (Z) of the isotope increase and the chemical species changes from oxygen to fluorine. Some common reactions are shown in Table 2.

Some of the stable isotopes needed for the targets are easily obtained. Nitrogen-14 represents 99.6% of natural nitrogen. Oxygen-16 represents 99.8% of natural oxygen. The target for these reactions can be made from the naturally occurring element. However, oxygen-18 has a natural abundance of only 0.2%. Thus, the oxygen-18 needs to be separated from the much more common oxygen-16. In the mid-1990s the supply of oxygen-18-enriched water was somewhat tenuous. More recently, there has been a more abundant supply of oxygen-18-enriched water.

Production Yield: The nuclear reaction rate varies depending up the energy of the incoming charged particle. The dependence of this rate on energy is different for each nuclear reaction. Fortunately, there are practical reaction rates for production of all the low-weight positron emitters at relatively low energies. That means that these isotopes can be produced with relatively inexpensive cyclotrons. For example, a "medical" cyclotron which can accelerate protons to 10–15 MeV and deuterons to 5–7.5 MeV can be used to produce C-11, N-13, O-15, and F-18.

The production yield depends on how likely a particle of a certain energy is to react with a particular nucleus. This probability is given in terms of the apparent cross-sectional size of the nucleus. A convenient unit of measurement is the barn, which is 10^{-24} cm^2. The nuclear physicist who created it whimsically named this unit a barn, because is "as big as a barn". It also depends on how many particles there are in the accelerator beam. The number of particles in the beam is given in terms of current, typically in units of microamps.

Table 2: Isotope Production Reactions

N-14(p,α)C-11
O-16(p,α)N-13
N-14(d,n)O-15
O-18(p,n)F-18

Targets: Although cyclotron currents are quite low, the energy of each particle is quite high. Thus, the amount of energy in the beam is quite high. This high energy poses several problems for cyclotron targets. The targets must be able to dissipate the heat from the beam. The beam must pass through a "window" to reach the target material. In order to minimize loss of energy in the window, it is desirable to have a thin window. But the window must also be able to withstand the high energy in the beam.

Various target materials are used. In the case of FDG, the target material is water that has been enriched in the oxygen-18 isotope. Like fluorine-18, nitrogen-13 is also produced from a water target. The nitrogen is scavenged as ammonia by using a small amount of ethanol in the target. Carbon-11 and oxygen-15 are produced from nitrogen gas targets.

FDG Synthesis: Flourine-18 is produced in the target water as HF. The target water usually has a small amount of potassium carbonate, so the F-18 is recovered in the target water as the KF. Tetraacetylmannose triflate is reacted with the fluoride ion and the acetyl protection groups are removed basic hydrolysis. By starting with mannose, the desired optical isomer, D-glucose, is produced.

The FDG synthesis process is automated in a "black box," which can be purchased from the cyclotron manufacturers. Target irradiation, transfer to the "black box," and synthesis of the labeled FDG all takes place under remote control. Automation reduces radiation exposure and improves reproducibility.

RADIOPHARMACEUTICALS FOR CLINICAL PET

From the earliest development of PET scanning in the 1950s until the mid-1990s, PET remained an important research tool. However, because of the complexity of radiopharmaceutical development on-site, the clinical impact of PET was small. FDG (fluorine-18 labeled 2-flouro-2-deoxy-D-glucose) made clinical PET scanning possible. The large number of common clinical indications for FDG means that PET scanning has now reached a critical volume, so that pure clinical PET facilities are reasonable. A moderately sized hospital can support full-time operation of a PET scanner using FDG.

The critical volume of FDG imaging has allowed development of an industry to supply FDG throughout the United States and much of the world. Isotope production, radiopharmaceutical synthesis, and regional delivery of a product with a half-life less than two hours are impressive technological feats. But, these technological hurdles have been overcome, and a supply industry is now in place.

In addition to FDG, rubidium-82 is commercially available. Rubidium-82, a positron-emitting analog of potassium, has a very short half-life, 75 seconds. However, it can be obtained from a strontium-82/rubidium-82 generator as a sterile bolus for injection. The strontium-82 parent has a 25-day half-life. Although the strontium-82 parent is expensive to produce, the cost can be spread over a large number of patients given an active myocardial imaging practice. Commercial services allow sharing a generator between more than one facility.

The infrastructure that has made FDG and rubidium-82 a clinical reality should facilitate the introduction of new radiopharmaceuticals. The isotope production, the delivery system, and the clinical scanners are already in place.

All that needs to be added is new hot chemistry boxes to produce different radiopharmaceuticals. Since the development of radiopharmaceutical will be much easier now that clinical PET is firmly in place, it is reasonable to expect to see an accelerated expansion in the development of new radiopharmaceuticals.

GLUCOSE METABOLISM

Most Cancer Has a High Glucose Metabolic Rate.
In the fasting state, most tissues use free fatty acids to supply their energy needs. The brain always uses glucose as a substrate, and many other cells occasionally use glucose. After a meal that includes glucose, insulin rises and several tissues will switch from free fatty acid to glucose metabolism. FDG imaging for malignancy is performed in the fasting state where the uptake by non-malignant tissues is low.

In general, malignant cells tend to use glucose in preference to free fatty acids. Otto Warburg noticed this general principle early in the last century. In addition, if the malignant cells are hypoxic, they will use anaerobic metabolism. Anaerobic metabolism requires much more glucose than aerobic metabolism. Even when malignant cells are not hypoxic, malignant cells tend use anaerobic metabolism. Thus it is common for malignant cells to use glucose and to use a large amount of glucose.

Many cancers are associated with a high metabolic rate. It is common parlance to refer to FDG imaging as metabolic imaging with the implication that tumors are detected because of their higher rate of metabolism than surrounding tissues. This is certainly one mechanism, but in addition FDG imaging takes advantage of reduced background by studying patients during the fasting state and it takes advantage of the frequent use of anaerobic use of glucose by the cancer. More accurately, one should say that FDG imaging reflects <u>glucose</u> metabolic rate.

Tracing Glucose Metabolism.
It would seem that radioactive glucose would be the best chemical to use to trace glucose metabolism. Although this seems like the obvious choice, there are problems using radioactive glucose. Most of the glucose that is taken up by cells is promptly metabolized into water and carbon dioxide, both of which rapidly return to the general circulation. Rapid washout makes measuring glucose metabolism difficult under any circumstances; however, it is particularly difficult for imaging.

Sokoloff et al. used 2-deoxy-D-glucose instead of glucose itself to measure glucose metabolism. The missing hydroxyl group in the 2-position had relatively little effect on uptake or phosphorylation, but inhibited the transformation of deoxy-glucose-6-phosphate to deoxy-fructose-6-phosphate, thus preventing further stages in glucose metabolism. Thus, the deoxyglucose accumulated in cells in proportion to its uptake and phosphorylation. Since these steps are rate limiting, the accumulation of deoxyglucose was in proportion to glucose metabolism.

Wolf et al. found that the same mechanism worked when the hydroxyl in the 2-position is replaced by fluorine. 2-fluoro-2-deoxy-D-glucose (FDG) is shown in Figure 1. FDG like deoxyglucose accumulates in cells in proportion to glucose metabolism. With FDG it is possible to take a static image where the relative distribution of FDG will reflect the dynamic metabolic process.

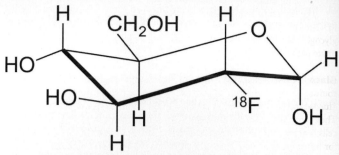

Figure 1: 2-Fluoro-2-Deoxy-D-Glucose. 2-fluoro-2-deoxy-D-glucose (FDG) is an analog of D-glucose where the hydroxyl in the 2 position is replace by fluorine-18.

COMPARTMENTAL MODEL OF FDG UPTAKE

Figure 2 shows a compartmental model of the uptake of FDG. The compartment on the left represents the FDG in the blood. The middle compartment represents the FDG inside a cell. The compartment on the right represents FDG-6-phosphate. Glucose transporters in the cell membrane facilitate the transport of glucose and FDG across the cell membrane. Glucose and FDG are phosphorylated in the 6 position by hexokinase. Phosphorylation reduces the glucose concentration in the cell, so less glucose diffuses back out of the cell than enters the cell.

The conversion of glucose-6-phospate or FDG-6-phosphate back to glucose of FDG respectively, is performed by phosphatase. In most tissues including cancer, there is little phosphatase activity. A notable exception is the liver and some hepatocellular carcinomas. One of the functions of the liver is to maintain the blood glucose level during fasting, and it uses phosphatase to return glucose-6-phosphate to glucose.

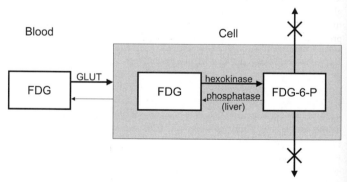

Figure 2: FDG Compartmental Model. Uptake of 2-fluoro-2-deoxy-D-glucose (FDG) from the blood into the cells is facilitated by the glucose transporters (GLUT). Since the blood glucose concentration is typically higher than the intracellular concentration, the inward rate is higher than diffusion out of the cells. Hexokinase converts FDG to FDG-6-phospate (FDG-6-P). Most cells with the notable exception of the liver have little phosphatase. FDG-6-P is not a substrate for further metabolism.

Clinical PET and PET/CT

The enzymes that further metabolize glucose-6-phosphate cannot use FDG-6-phosphate as a substrate. Thus, FDG-6-phosphate is not made into glycogen, and it is not metabolized in either the glycolytic or hexose monophosphate paths. Instead the FDG-6-phosphate accumulates in the cell.

Glucose Transporters.   There are two families of glucose transporters, the sodium-glucose transporters and the facilitative transporters. The **facilitative glucose transporters** (**GLUT**) are most important for glucose uptake into cells. They transport glucose down a concentration gradient from the blood into the cells. There are at least 12 different glucose transporters. GLUT1 is responsible for transport of glucose into the erythrocytes and across the blood—brain barrier. It is also very important for FDG imaging in oncology, because it is often expressed heavily in malignant cells. Serum insulin levels do not affect GLUT1 expression. By contrast, GLUT4, which is found in muscle, is-up regulated by insulin.

The second family of glucose transporters, the **sodium-glucose transporters** (**SGLT**), co-transport sodium down a concentration gradient and glucose up a concentration gradient. The sodium concentration gradient is maintained by the sodium-potassium ATPase, which ultimately provides the energy for glucose transportation against a gradient. Sodium-glucose transporters are used in the intestine for absorption of glucose and in the kidney for reuptake of glucose from the glomerular filtrate.

Excretion of FDG.   Glucose and FDG are freely filtered by the glomerulus. Glucose is then reabsorbed by the nephron. When the serum concentration of glucose is very high, the glucose in the glomerular filtrate can overwhelm the ability of the nephron to reabsorb the glucose and glucose is "spilled" in the urine.

The sodium-glucose transporter in the early portions of the proximal convoluted tubule (SGLT2) co-transports one glucose molecule with one sodium ion. Farther down the proximal convoluted tubule, (SGLT1) co-transports one glucose with two sodium ions. In the initial part of the proximal convoluted tubule, glucose is transported with a lower energy cost; in the later part of the proximal convoluted tubule, the concentration in the urine is reduced at higher energy cost so that almost no glucose escapes into the urine. Within the tubular cells, facilitative glucose transport returns glucose to the plasma.

FDG is a poor substrate for the sodium-glucose co-transporters. Only about half of the FDG undergoes reuptake in the nephron. Much of the FDG is excreted in the urine. In a normal patient there will be intense activity within the urinary system that is normal. It is important not to interpret this normal finding as indicating "spillage" of glucose.

The excretion of FDG is a problem for imaging the urinary system or structures close to the urinary system. However, overall, the excretion of FDG may be beneficial for imaging. Urinary excretion means that the plasma level of FDG decreases more rapidly than radioactive glucose would. This allows earlier imaging than would be feasible with glucose.

Renal excretion of FDG could be added to the compartmental model. However, FDG is removed from the blood by processes other than excretion. It is taken up into other tissues, and it is re-released into the plasma, especially by the liver. Thus, many compartments would be needed to model the blood-time activity curve. Instead, the blood-time activity curve can be used as the input to the simple three-compartment model shown in Figure 2.

Lumped Constant.   FDG metabolism is analogous to the first stages of glucose metabolism. Glucose and FDG are transported into the cells by the glucose transporters, and both are converted to phosphates by hexokinase. However, since they are different molecules, the rate constants for uptake, phosphorylation, dephosphorylation, and diffusion out of the cell are different. From a clinical imaging point of view, these differences are negligible. Physiologists who are interested in the fine details of glucose metabolism cannot ignore these differences. What is generally done when using a compartmental model is that the differences in the kinetic factors between glucose and FDG are lumped together into one constant that is called the lumped constant.

Effect of Plasma Glucose in Oncological Imaging.   Plasma glucose competes with FDG for transport into the cells and phosphorylation by hexokinase. The FDG uptake will be inversely related to the plasma glucose concentration. Thus, it is useful to measure the serum glucose concentration at the time of FDG injection. If the serum glucose is high, there may be an increase in false-negative findings for oncological imaging. It is desirable for the serum glucose to be below 140 mg/dL, but diagnostic images can often be obtained with glucose levels up to 200 mg/dL and above.

Standardized uptake value (SUV) measurement will be altered by the serum glucose. The standardized uptake value varies inversely with the serum glucose. One way to adjust for the variability in serum glucose is to multiply the standardized—uptake value by 100 divided by the serum glucose level in mg/dL. Even when this mathematical correction is not used, it is important to take the serum glucose level into account any time the standardized-uptake-value is used.

FDG IMAGING PROTOCOLS

Oncology Protocol.   In oncological imaging, the goal is to reduce uptake of FDG in normal cells. General patient instructions for oncological imaging are to fast prior to scanning. Some laboratories recommend fasting for as little as four hours. Most laboratories recommend fasting to at least six hours or longer. If a patient arrives with a high serum glucose level, it is typical to proceed with imaging. It is possible that adequate diagnostic information can be obtained, and otherwise the FDG will decay, the scanner time will not be used, and if rescheduled the patient may again present with a high serum glucose. It is useful to note the glucose value in the report and to note the potential for a false negative study in the report.

Diabetic patients pose a particular problem. It is desirable to have the serum insulin low to minimize the uptake of glucose into normal cells, but it is also desirable to have a low serum glucose level. If a patient has a high glucose level, insulin will lower the glucose and hence increase the uptake in normal cells. Unfortunately, it will also increase uptake in normal cells. What is often done is to schedule diabetic patients for the early afternoon. They are instructed to follow their normal schedule in the morning and then to skip lunch. This simple schedule will work for many diabetic patients.

Cardiology Protocol.   In cardiac imaging, the goal generally is to increase cardiac uptake of FDG. The heart can use either glucose or free fatty acids to supply its energy needs. There are two strategies for increasing uptake in cardiac cells: increase the serum insulin level or decrease the free fatty acid level. In non-diabetic patients, the equivalent of a glucose tolerance test can be performed. After fasting, 50 g of glucose is given orally. FDG is injected one hour after the glucose at a time when the insulin is high and the serum glucose has returned to normal.

Unfortunately, many cardiac patients are diabetic. In diabetic patients, exogenous insulin must be administered. The most reliable method is to perform a glucose-clamp. Glucose and insulin are infused simultaneously, and the rate of infusion is adjusted to keep the serum glucose in the normal range while the insulin is at a high level. Because insulin drives potassium into the cells, it is also necessary to infuse potassium during the glucose-clamp procedure. There are also several simplified methods for achieving a high insulin level with a normal glucose.

The heart can be made to switch from free fatty acid to glucose metabolism by lowering the serum free fatty acids. One of insulin's effects is to lower serum free fatty acids, so the methods above also have the effect of lowering free fatty acids. However, free fatty acids can be more effectively lowered using nicotinic acid derivatives. Acipomox, a nicotinic acid derivative, has been used successfully for cardiac imaging particularly in Europe.

Delayed Imaging.   In most tissues, the model shown in Figure 2 is adequate for understanding clinical imaging. While there is appreciable activity of FDG in the blood, there is continuing uptake of FDG by the tissues. Once inside the cell, the FDG is promptly converted to FDG-6-phosphate. The FDG-6-phosphate is then trapped in the cell. After a reasonable amount of time for uptake (45 minutes to one hour), there is little change in activity in the tissue. Consequently, washout of FDG uptake is often not considered when choosing an imaging time.

FDG washout is, however, important in a few instances. There is often intense FDG activity in the urinary system at the time of imaging. Because FDG is concentrated in the urine, there will continue to be an important amount of FDG extracted until the blood levels of FDG are very low. Furthermore, even after it is extracted from the blood, it takes time for the FDG to be eliminated from the urinary system. Thus, to get an unobstructed view of the urinary system or of structures that lie near the urinary system, delayed imaging can be used.

In most tissues, there is little phosphatase activity. However, phosphatase activity can be important. The liver has considerable uptake of FDG, even in the fasting state. However, one of the functions of the liver is to supply glucose to the circulation during fasting. Thus, phosphatase is important in the kinetics of FDG in the liver. At the usual time of imaging (about one hour) there is moderate liver uptake. This uptake can mask small or low-uptake FDG-avid lesions. With time there is a decrease in the normal background FDG activity, so that these types of lesions may become more conspicuous.

There tends to be very low washout of FDG from tumor cells. There is evidence that inflammatory tissue, which is a major source of false-positive findings in oncological imaging, may have appreciable washout. Thus, some investigators have found that comparison of uptake on early (say, one-hour) images with uptake on delayed (say, three-hour) images can help to distinguish inflammation from cancer.

Maximal FDG Activity.   In most tissues, FDG continues to accumulate with time. There is a relatively rapid decrease in the blood activity, so the majority of the uptake takes place early, during the first half-hour, with some uptake during the second half-hour. The rate of FDG accumulation decreases considerably after the first hour. Fluorine-18 has a short half-life, 110 minutes. The decay of fluorine-18 competes with the continued uptake of FDG in terms of the total activity of FDG in the tissues. The maximal signal-to-noise given these two considerations often occurs at somewhat less than one hour. For this reason, clinical scan times starting at 45 minutes to one hour are often used.

The previous section noted that the contrast between two tissues may improve with a greater delay time. This improvement also needs to be balanced against the decrease in activity due to decay. Even if the contrast improves, the increased noise may make an FDG-avid lesion less visible.

Instrumentation considerations also need to be considered when selecting an imaging time. Dual-use Anger camera PET scanners have a very low maximum count rate. Consequently, it is common to use a low administered dose of FDG with these machines. An alternate is to use a standard administered dose and image at a more delayed time. The low peak noise-equivalent-count rate of these machines is ameliorated in part by better contrast obtained with delayed scanning.

Dedicated PET scanners with little axial collimation, e.g., "3D" mode, may suffer from a high randoms rate at early scan times. The reduction in randoms rate as the activity decreases will slow the decrease in noise-equivalent-count rate. This effect may also tend to favor somewhat later scan times.

Picking an imaging time is a fairly complex tradeoff that involves several factors. Fast coincidence time, low random rate, high axial collimation, and fixed tissue contrast ratios will tend to favor imaging at earlier times. Slow coincidence time, high randoms rate, little axial collimation, and tissue contrast ratios that increase over time will favor imaging at later times.

ALTERED FDG BIODISTRIBUTION

Muscle Uptake.   Localized Muscle Uptake: Exercising muscle or muscle post-exercise uses glucose as an energy substrate. Resting muscle predominantly uses free fatty acids. Thus, part of the instructions for patients is to avoid strenuous exercise for at least one day prior to imaging. In addition to intentional exercise, muscles may be used inadvertently. For example, a patient may swing his/her leg or tap his/her finger. Chewing gum can increase uptake in the muscles of mastication. Talking can increase uptake in the vocal chords. In patients with recurrent laryngeal nerve palsy, there is often intense unilateral uptake in the vocal cord region. If a patient is tense, there can be uptake in the neck muscles, torticollis being an extreme example. Latissimus dorsi uptake, either unilateral or bilateral, is seen often. A small dose of a muscle relaxant, e.g., 5–10 mg of diazepam (Valium), can markedly reduce muscle uptake as well as uptake in brown fat (see below).

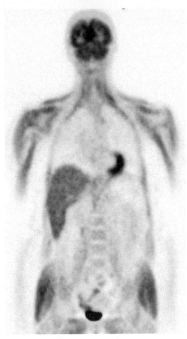

Figure 3: Diffuse Muscle Uptake. This image is a thick coronal section of a patient who reported having a large meal just prior to FDG injection. Note the prominent skeletal muscle uptake due to the postprandial, endogenous insulin release.

Diffuse Muscle Uptake: Diffuse muscle uptake can be seen when there is an elevated serum insulin level (see Figure 3). Insulin translocates the GLUT3 to the surface of the cell, thereby increasing the uptake of FDG.

Myocardial Uptake: Myocardial uptake is quite variable. There is high myocardial uptake in the presence of either high insulin or low free fatty acid in the plasma. Patient preparation to increase the myocardial uptake of FDG is described in the chapter on myocardial imaging. In fasting patients, there may be no uptake in the myocardium; there may be uniform uptake in the myocardium; or there may be non-uniform uptake. The lateral wall most often shows FDG uptake. The septum least often shows uptake. An important point is that a defect in uptake of FDG in a fasting patient should not be interpreted as myocardial disease.

Brown Fat. Brown fat has recently been recognized as an important cause of altered FDG biodistribution. Brown fat is involved in thermoregulation prior to the point of shivering. It is found abundantly in rodents. It used to be thought that brown fat did not occur in the adult human, but recently it has been found that brown fat can be seen in adults. Brown fat is often found in the neck, along the spine, and occasionally in the abdomen (see Figure 4). Brown fat is richly supplied with vessels and with sympathetic nerves. Patients who are nervous or

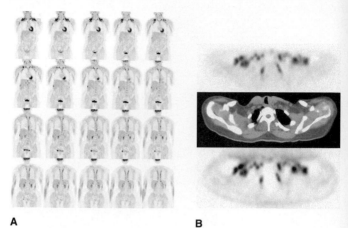

A   **B**

Figure 4: Brown Fat Uptake. Coronal FDG-PET images in a patient with brown fat uptake are shown in part A. Note the typical spotty appearance in the neck and the paravertebral uptake. This patient also has some uptake in brown fat in the abdomen. Part B shows registered attenuation corrected FDG, CT, and uncorrected FDG slices which show the location of the uptake corresponds to fat on the CT.

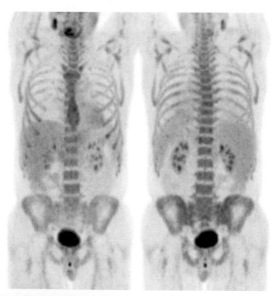

Figure 5: Diffuse Bone Marrow Uptake. Anterior (left) and posterior (right) maximum intensity renderings show diffuse bone marrow uptake in a patient treated with bone marrow stimulants.

cold may show spotty uptake in the neck and along the spine due to the brown fat.

Brown fat can be confused with neck muscle uptake, although neck muscle uptake is more linear and brown fat uptake is more spotty in distribution. Originally, brown fat uptake was confused with muscle uptake. Brown fat uptake can also be abolished by low does of diazepam (Valium). And this response to muscle relaxants reinforced this confusion. However, with the introduction of PET/CT, it became apparent that the spotty type of uptake was located in fat not muscle. In children, uptake of meta-iodo-benzyl-guanidine (MIBG) and tetrofosmin in brown fat has also been recognized.

Bone Marrow.   There is normally uptake in the bone marrow on FDG. The uptake may be intense in patients treated with stimulating factors or in patients rebounding from chemotherapy (see Figure 5).

Areola.   The uptake in the areola is variable, but prominent uptake may be seen (see Figure 6).

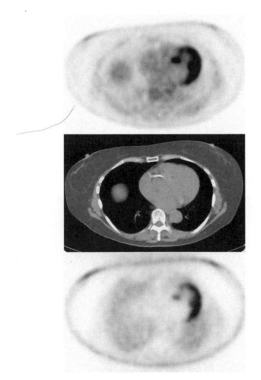

Figure 6: Areolar Uptake. This patient has mild increase uptake in the areolar area. Top is the attenuation corrected FDG; middle is the CT; and bottom is non-corrected FDG.

Thyroid. Uptake of FDG in the thyroid is a relatively frequent variant. Homogeneous intense uptake can be seen in Graves' disease and in subacute thyroiditis. Diffuse uptake is also seen in patients with Hashimoto's thyroiditis. In patients without the clinical diagnosis of Hashimoto's thyroiditis, diffuse uptake is often associated with elevated antithyroid antibody levels. Focal uptake can be seen in thyroid nodules, and increases the chance that thyroid nodules are malignant. Focal thyroid uptake can be further evaluated with fine needle aspiration.

Thymus. The thymus gland may take up FDG in children and young adults. After chemotherapy there can be an increase in the size of the thymus with intense uptake of FDG. This benign finding is called thymic rebound.

GI Tract. There is variable uptake of FDG in the GI tract. It is common to see uptake at the gastroesophageal junction. Diffuse or segmental uptake is often seen in the stomach or the colon. Generally, this uptake is incidental, although some pathological conditions such as lymphoma can cause diffuse or segmental uptake. Focal, intense (greater than the liver) uptake in the colon can be incidental, but it is associated with colon cancer or adenomatous polyps about one-half of the time. Focal colonic uptake can be further evaluated with colonoscopy

Sarcoidosis. There is variable uptake in sarcoidosis, but the uptake can be intense. The pattern of uptake may suggest sarcoidosis, but the patterns of uptake overlap with lymphoma.

Inflammation. Inflammatory cells, particularly macrophages, utilize glucose metabolism. This fact is the basis of imaging infection. In addition,

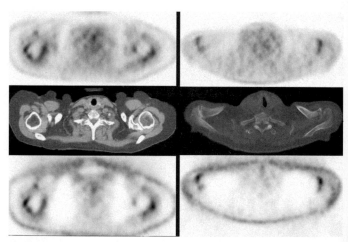

Figure 7: Periarticular Inflammation. The patient shown on the left shows increased uptake around the humeral heads. The patient shown on the right shows uptake at the acromioclavicular joint. Top is the attenuation corrected FDG; middle is the CT; and bottom is the non-corrected FDG.

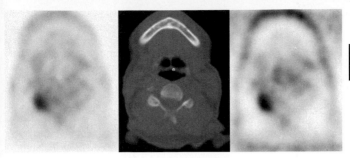

Figure 8: Facet Joint Inflammation. There is intense uptake at the location of facet joint inflammation. Left is the attenuation corrected FDG; in the center is the CT; and on the right is the non-corrected FDG.

inflammatory/infectious conditions can lead to false-positive diagnoses. Reactive lymph nodes, particularly those draining the limbs, frequently show a mild increase in uptake, and occasionally show intense uptake.

Periarticular Inflammation: It is common to see increased uptake of FDG around joints, particularly in association with periarticular inflammation. Close anatomic localization can be useful in distinguishing facet joint inflammatory disease from bone marrow metastatic disease (see Figures 7 and 8).

Granulomatous Disease: Granulomatous lesions particularly fungal disease can cause intense FDG uptake. Fugal granulomatous lesions are a particular problem in the lung. They are a frequent cause of false-positive single pulmonary nodule in regions that have endemic fungal disease.

Silicon: Silicon can cause an inflammatory reaction. It can be a cause of false-positive lymph node uptake. Figure 9 shows an FDG-PET/CT in a patient 12 years post-mastectomy for breast cancer and one year post-saline implant

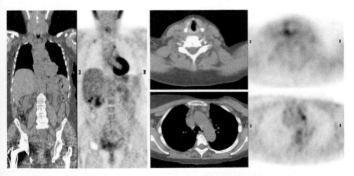

Figure 9: Inflammatory Node Secondary to Silicon. On the left are CT and FDG coronal images, which show focal uptake in the left mediastinum and in the right vocal chord. Also note the right hip prosthesis. On the upper right, CT and FDG axial images through the vocal chord region show uptake on the right. On the lower right, CT and FDG axial images through the chest show uptake in a prevascular lymph node. The larger more anterior lymph node is not FDG-avid.

replacement of a ruptured silicone breast implant. She presented with hoarseness and was found to have left recurrent nerve palsy. The FDG uptake in the region of the right vocal chord is secondary to increased work of the muscles on the right side in compensation for the paralysis on the left side. The moderate uptake in the prevascular lymph node was found on biopsy to correspond to inflammatory reaction compatible with silicone.

MYOCARDIAL PERFUSION AGENTS

First Pass Extraction.   There are three conditions that are sufficient for a tracer to be distributed in tissue in accordance with blood flow. 1) The tracer must be mixed across the cross section of blood flow. Streaming of a tracer in the blood after intraarterial injection violates this condition. Agents that are injected intravenously are generally well mixed by the time they get to the pulmonary circuit. 2) The tracer must be completely extracted by the tissue. Particles such as microspheres are the prototype of an agent that is completely extracted in one pass. 3) The tracer must have a stable distribution over the time on sampling. Thallium-201 is an example of a tracer where the washout can be important over the time of imaging.

It is possible to relax the second condition from complete extraction to uniform extraction. The advantage of complete extraction is that it is easy to confirm that all tissues have equal extraction. However, as long as the tracer has the same fractional extraction in all of the tissues of interest, then the distribution will still be according to blood flow. It may take several passes through the tissue to extract all of the tracer, but as long as the same fraction is extracted in each pass, the final distribution will be according to blood flow.

Rubidium-82.   Potassium Analogs: Rubidium is in the position just below potassium on the periodic table. Both are monovalent cations. The radii are similar enough that both are good substrates for the sodium-potassium ATPase in the cell membrane. Cesium, the element below rubidium, is a less good substrate for the sodium-potassium ATPase. (Although thallium-201 is in a much different location on the periodic table, it is also a monovalent cation with high affinity for the sodium-potassium ATPase.)

There is a marked concentration gradient between the intra- and extracellular fluid for potassium and its analogs. The ATP-dependent sodium potassium pump maintains the gradient. All viable cells are able to maintain the gradients for sodium and potassium. In theory, dead cells would have reduced fractional extraction of rubidium. In practice it is unusual for there to be blood flow to areas where there are no viable cells.

Potassium and its analogs are taken up efficiently after a single pass through tissue. In the myocardium, the first pass extraction of the potassium analogs is about 85%. Furthermore, the extraction of the potassium analogs is fairly uniform in the myocardium. At very high flow rates, particularly after pharmacological vasodilation, there is a small decrease in fractional extraction. At very low flow rates, there is a small increase in fractional extraction. However, in general, the potassium analogs follow the requirement for uniform extraction.

Because of the transmembrane gradient, most of the potassium is within the cell. Relatively little potassium is in the blood or extracellular fluid.

Consequently, the rate of washout of potassium from tissue is relatively slow. From the point of view of the potassium space, the cell is a very large volume, and the blood flow is very low. In terms of potassium space, the blood is a trickle going by a large cell.

In terms of washout rate, it is necessary to distinguish between the one-way washout and the net washout. The one-way washout is what happens to a tracer that starts within the cell. The net washout includes both the washout from within the cell and the wash-in from the blood. Although there is little potassium in the blood, the continued wash-in over long times cannot be ignored. The one-way washout of potassium in man probably has a half-life somewhat over an hour. The net washout half-life is on the order of 6–8 hours.

The very short half-life of rubidium-82 means that washout is never a consideration in its distribution. (This is not true for longer-lived isotopes such as thallium-201.) Thus, rubidium also meets the blood flow tracer requirement for no washout.

Strontium-82/Rubidium-82 Generator: Rubidium-82 has a very short half-life, 75 s. Fortunately, rubidium-82 has a parent, strontium-82, from which a convenient generator system can be produced. Strontium-82 has a half-life of 25.36 days and decays by electron capture to the ground state of rubidium-82. (The energy difference between the strontium-82 and rubidium-82 ground states is too low for positron emission.) Rubidium-82 decays 96% of the time by positron emission, and 4% of the time by electron capture. There are several different beta energies, but the most abundant has an energy of 1.523 MeV. This high energy means that the beta particle may travel far enough in tissue to result in some loss in resolution. In addition to the 511 keV annihilation photons, rubidium-82 decay results in several prompt gamma rays. The most common, 13.4% of decays, is a 776 keV gamma ray. Rubidum-82 decays to krypton-82, which is stable.

Strontium-82 is usually produced in an accelerator by a spallation reaction using high-energy proton bombardment of rubidium-85, Rb-85(p,4n)Sr-82. This (p,4n) reaction requires at least 60 MeV, and it is commercially produced using protons of about 500 MeV. (A **spallation reaction** is where many nucleons are ejected from a nucleus by bombardment with a single very-high-energy incident particle.) Most of the other isotopes produced during bombardment can be efficiently separated; however, some strontium-85, which can't be chemically separated from strontium-82, will also be produced (see radionuclide purity below). Because this reaction requires a high-energy incident proton, the cost of the strontium-82 parent is high. Fortunately, the generator can be used repeatedly and the cost can be distributed over a large number of patients, making use of the generator system feasible.

The strontium-82/rubidium-82 generator is made from hydrous stannic oxide. It is eluted with 50 mL of normal saline over one minute. The generators are usually loaded with 3.33–5.55 GBq (90–150) mCi of strontium-82. A typical dose is 1.5 GBq (40 mCi) with a range of 0.37–2.22 GBq (10–60 mCi).

Ammonia.   Nitrogen-13-labeled ammonia is another agent that is approved for myocardial perfusion. Although ammonium, NH_4, is a monovalent cation with about the same ionic radius as potassium, ammonia uptake is by a different mechanism. Ammonia, NH_3, is highly lipid soluble and can cross the cell membrane easily. Ammonia and ammonium are in equilibrium in the blood with ammonium being the predominant species. Although ammonium is the predominant species, the equilibrium is fast enough that the transfer into the cell is rapid. Once in the cell, ammonia rapidly undergoes ammonia fixation. This whole process—the equilibrium between ammonia and ammonium, diffusion across the membrane, and ammonia fixation within the cell—is fast enough that ammonia has a high first-pass extraction.

Nitrogen-13 has a short half-life, 10 min, and there is no generator system; therefore, N-13-labeled ammonia is only available in facilities with an on-site cyclotron. The N-13 can be produced using the O-16(p,α)N-13 reaction.

OTHER PET AGENTS

Tumor Proliferation.   C-11-Thymidine: One hallmark of cancer is rapid cell proliferation. Several positron-emitting radiopharmaceuticals which are correlated with tumor proliferation have been developed. One of the most extensively studied has been C-11-thymidine. Thymidine is a nucleoside that is incorporated into DNA, especially during the synthetic (S) phase of the cell cycle. However, the short half-life of carbon-11 is not well suited to the relatively slow incorporation of thymidine into DNA. The necessity of an on-site cyclotron and radiopharmaceutical synthesis will restrict the use of this agent to academic PET centers.

F-18-FLT: 3′-deoxy-3′-fluorothymidine (FLT) is a thymidine analog with fluorine substituted for the hydroxyl in the 3′ position (see Figure 10). The uptake of FLT has considerable analogy with the uptake of FDG. The phosphorylation of FLT by thymidine kinase 1 is not affected by the presence of the fluorine substitution. The subsequent step in DNA synthesis is, however, prevented by this substitution. Thus, FLT is trapped in the cell. The thymidine kinase 1 activity is a measure of DNA synthesis and hence of cell proliferation.

Buck et al. investigated 26 patients with lung nodules using both FDG and FLT PET. They compared the SUV values in the lesion with a histological marker of proliferation, Ki-67 immunostaining of the specimen obtained at surgery. They found a better correlation between the proliferative activity and the

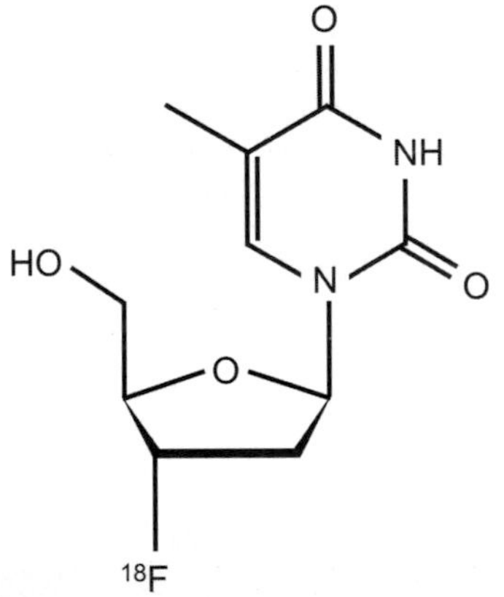

Figure 10: 3′-Deoxy-3′Fluorothymidine (FLT). The chemical structure of FLT is shown.

uptake of FLT (r = 0.92) than the uptake of FDG (r = 0.59). The average uptake of FDG (4.1) was, however, greater with FDG than FLT.

This study is very interesting. FDG uptake reflects glucose metabolism; FLT reflects thymidine metabolism, which reflects DNA synthesis. This study shows that these two different markers are able to reflect different aspects of these pulmonary nodules.

Metabolism. The major PET metabolic tracer is FDG. As already described in some detail FDG reflects glucose metabolism. It is also the only commercially available PET tracer of metabolism. However, there are several other metabolic tracers that have been used and may become commercially available in the future.

C-11-Acetate: C-11-acetate is a very interesting tracer of metabolism since it reflects the activity of the tricarboxylic acid cycle. Glucose and free fatty acids, which are the major sources of energy for cells, undergo oxidative metabolism in the tricarboxylic acid cycle. C-11-acetate gives a measure of the overall oxidative metabolism. Acetate is rapidly converted into carbon dioxide and water. Therefore, it is necessary to perform dynamic imaging and model the metabolic process.

C-11-Fatty Acids: C-11-labeled free fatty acids, such as C-11-palmitate, can be used to measure fatty acid metabolism. Because of metabolism, the C-11-palmitate information must also be collected with dynamic imaging and be analyzed with a compartmental model.

C-11-Methoionine: C-11-methionine can be used as a measure of protein synthesis.

Blood Flow. Rubidium-82 from a strontium-82/rubidium-82 generator is the only commercially available PET radiopharmaceutical for measurement of blood flow. Nitrogen-13-labeled ammonia can be made in an on-site cyclotron and myocardial perfusion studies using this agent are reimbursable. In addition, many other PET tracers have been used for blood flow measurement.

Pre-capillary Arteriolar Blockade: Relative blood flow can be measured using small particles analogously to single-photon lung scintigraphy. A wide range of positron-emitting isotopes can be labeled to microspheres, to be used for measuring relative blood flow.

First-Pass Extraction: In addition to rubidium-82 and nitrogen-13 ammonia, there are several PET radiopharmaceuticals that can be used to measure relative blood flow using first-pass extraction. Copper-62-labeled pyruvaldehyde bis(N-methylthiosemicarbazone (PTSM), is rapidly taken up inside cells and then trapped by being metabolically altered.

The requirements to be distributed according to blood flow–mixing in the blood flow, uniform extraction in the tissue, and stable distribution–are met at least partially by many radiopharmaceuticals.

When trying to measure another physiologic paramater, say, receptor distribution, first-pass extraction according to blood flow can present a problem. A tracer that has a high affinity for a receptor is often highly extracted and stable in distribution. Thus, instead of measuring the receptor density, the tracer ends up largely reflecting blood flow.

Washout: Absolute blood flow can be measured from the rate of washout of a diffusible tracer from a tissue. After bolus injection the rate of washout depends on the partition of the tracer between the blood and tissue, and on the blood flow per volume of tissue. In more complicated systems, a compartment model can be used to model the uptake and washout. Often blood flow is one of the parameters that is derived by fitting the data to the compartmental model.

Water is generally freely diffusible in tissue. (Butanol may be more diffusible in the brain.) Water is one of the products of C-11-acetate metabolism. It is also readily available from O-18-labeled carbon dioxide. Carbonic anhydrase catalyses the conversion of carbon dioxide and water to the bicarbonate ion:

$$CO_2 + H_2O \leftrightarrow HCO_3^- + H^+$$

In blood, this reaction proceeds rapidly. The bicarbonate ion is a tetrahedral molecule, where all of the oxygen atoms are equivalent. Thus, a radioactive oxygen element on the bicarbonate will be distributed to the carbon dioxide or water molecule irrespective of which molecule it originated from. With the rapid conversion back and forth between these species, a labeled oxygen molecule will tend to be distributed between carbon dioxide, water, and bicarbonate in proportion to the amount of each species. Since the water pool is many orders of magnitude larger than the carbon dioxide or bicarbonate pools, almost all of the labeled oxygen will rapidly be transferred to the water. In the biological context, it is common PET slang to refer to O-18-labeled carbon dioxide as O-18 water.

RADIOPHARMACEUTICAL PROPERTIES

Radioactivity.   Radioactivity is given in terms of becquerels, Bq, where one Bq is equal to one disintegration per second. The unit is named after Henri Becquerel. Typical units used in nuclear medicine are megabecquerels, MBq, or gigabecquerels, GBq, where a megabequerel, MBq, is a million (10^6) becquerels, and a gigabecquerels is a billion (a US billion equal to a thousand million, 10^9) becquerels. In the United States, radioactivity is still given in terms of the older unit, the Curie, Ci, where one Ci is equal to 3.7×10^{10} disintegrations per second. The Curie is named after Pierre Curie. Pierre and Marie Curie shared the Nobel Prize in Physics with Henri Becquerel in 1903 for the discovery of radioactivity. Typical units used in nuclear medicine are microcuries, µCi, or millicuries, mCi, where a microcurie is one-millionth (10^{-6}) of a curie, and a millicurie is one-thousandth (10^{-3}) of a curie. Conversion between units in Becquerels and units in curies can be derived from these definitions, but a convenient conversion for the activities typically used is

$$37 \text{ MBq} = 1 \text{ mCi}$$

Note that the units of radioactivity are given in terms of disintegrations per second. "Disintegrations" refers to the number of atomic nuclei that undergo decay. It does not refer directly to the number of particles or photons that are emitted. The details of the decay process are not important in calculating the radioactivity. For example, flourine-18 almost always emits a positron when it decays, and each positron gives rise to two 511-keV annihilation photons. If one fluorine-18 atom decays each second there are nearly two 511-keV photons produced per second. Even though there are almost two photons per second, the radioactivity is equal to 1 Bq because that is the number of atoms that are decaying.

Specific Activity.   Specific activity is equal to the activity per unit of material. Often it is given in terms of the activity per gram or moles of tracer. The first step is to calculate the number of atoms in a sample from the activity. All of the atoms eventually decay, so the number of atoms is equal to the area under the time activity curve (see Chapter 1, Figure 2). The area under the time activity curve is:

$$N = A_0 \cdot T_{1/2}/\ln(2)$$

where N is the number of atoms. Dividing by Avogadro's number gives the moles. For 370 MBq (10 mCi) of fluorine-18, this number is $370 \cdot 10^6 \cdot 110 \cdot 60/0.693/6.02 \cdot 10^{23} = 5.85 \cdot 10^{-12}$, where $370 \cdot 10^6$ is A_0 in disintegrations/second, 110 is the fluorine-18 half-life, 60 is the number of seconds per minute, 0.693 is $\ln(2)$, and $6.02 \cdot 10^{23}$ is Avogadro's number. Note that 370 MBq (10 mCi) of fluorine-18 is an incredibly small amount of fluorine, 5.85 pmole.

FDG, which has a composition given by $FC_6H_{11}O_5$, has a weight of $18 + 6 \cdot 12 + 11 \cdot 1 + 5 \cdot 16 = 181$ g/mole. Multiplying the number of moles by this number gives $1059 \cdot 10^{-12}$ g. Therefore, 370 MBq (10 mCi) of FDG represents about $1.05 \cdot 10^{-9}$ ng of FDG. A typical dose of FDG corresponds to about a nanogram of radioactive material. The specific activity is given as the ratio of the activity to the number of moles or the number of grams of material. In the case of FDG these numbers are 63.3 MBq/pmole (1.71 mCi/pmole) and 349 MBq/ng (9.44 mCi/ng).

These calculations are fairly straightforward, but the number of steps required makes them difficult to perform. There is an ImageJ (http://rsb.info.nih.gov/ij/) plugin (htpp://www.med.Harvard.edu/JPNM/ij/plugins/AtoNTP.html) which does these calculations automatically.

This calculation assumes that all of the FDG is radioactive, that there is no stable FDG. If there is stable FDG, then there will be more grams of chemical FDG for the same amount of radioactive FDG. The specific activity of the FDG will be lower than the specific activity that is calculated above. Fluorine-18-labeled FDG is produced without any bulk excess of FDG, but as is often true with tracer chemistry, there may be some non-radioactive fluorine available. Consequently, the actual specific activities are lower than this completely carrier-free calculation. However, the total chemical quantity of FDG is insignificant from a clinical point of view.

Purity.   Radionuclide Purity: Radionuclide purity is defined as the fraction of radioactive species that is the desired isotope. Radionuclide purity is usually most important because of radiation dose. If the radiopharmaceutical is contaminated with an unwanted isotope, this isotope will deliver some radiation absorbed dose to the patient without providing any useful information. Radionuclide purity will vary with time after production depending on the half-lives of the desired and contaminant isotopes. If the contaminant isotope has a long half-life, then with time the fraction of the unwanted isotope will increase.

For several PET radioisotopes, there is relatively little problem with radionuclide purity. For example, fluorine-18 is generally produced with very little contamination by other isotopes. Contamination is more of a problem with the strontium-82/rubidium-82 generator. The high-energy spallation reaction used to produce strontium-82 can result in production of other isotopes as well. Often other isotopes can be separated chemically with high efficiency. However, in the case of strontium-82, one of the other products is strontium-85.

Generator systems usually allow for high-efficiency elution of the progeny isotope with high retention of the parent. Breakthrough of strontium-82 and strontium-85 should be tested for when using a strontium-82/rubidium-82 generator. The rubidium-82 can be measured shortly after elution of the generator. Because of rubidium-82's very short half-life, a correction needs to be made for decay between the time of elution and the time of measurement. The sample can then be allowed to decay until the rubidium-82 is completely decayed. One hour is a convenient time. Then the sample can be measured again. The strontium-85/strontium-82 ratio is provided with the generator. Since strontium-85's half-life, 64.8 days, is longer than strontium-82's half-life, 25 days, this ratio needs to be adjusted using the time since analysis.

Radiochemical Purity: Radiochemical purity is defined as the fraction of the radioactive species that isin the desired chemical form. During synthesis of the radiopharmaceutical, other radioactive species may be produced. After production, the desired radiochemical can be changed to another radiochemical. The special consideration for radiopharmaceuticals is radiolysis. The radiopharmaceutical is often contained in a very small volume. A good deal of energy is deposited in this volume by radioactive decay, often with the production of free radicals. This environment often has deleterious affects on the radiopharmaceutical itself. Fortunately FDG is a very stable compound and undergoes relatively little breakdown after production. However, radiochemical purity, especially when there is an extended time between production and use, can be a problem with other PET radiopharmaceuticals.

CONCLUSIONS

The utility of FDG imaging for a vast number of tumors has made the long-recognized potential of PET a clinical reality. An infrastructure has developed, including a radiopharmaceutical supply network and widely available dedicated PET cameras. Other applications are emerging, e.g., inflammation/infection imaging, neurological imaging, and cardiac imaging. Now that this infrastructure has been developed, it is possible that many other lower-volume studies will flow from development of new PET radiopharmaceuticals, resulting in a flourishing of PET imaging in the near term.

BIBLIOGRAPHY

1. Buck AK, Halter G, Schirrmeister H, et al. Imaging Proliferation in Lung Tumors with PET: (18)F-FLT Versus (18)F-FDG. *J Nucl Med* 2003; 44(9):1426–31.
2. Cohade C, Osman M, Pannu HK, Wahl RL. Uptake in supraclavicular area fat ("USA-Fat"): description on 18F-FDG PET/CT. *J Nucl Med* 2003; 44(2):170–6.
3. Fukuchi K, Ono Y, Nakahata Y, et al. Visualization of interscapular brown adipose tissue using (99m)tc-tetrofosmin in pediatric patients. *J Nucl Med* 2003; 44(10):1582–5.
4. Gatley SJ. Labeled glucose analogs in the genomic era. *J Nucl Med* 2003;44(7):1082–6

5. Okuyama C, Ushijima Y, Kubota T, et al. 123I-Metaiodobenzylguanidine uptake in the nape of the neck of children: likely visualization of brown adipose tissue. *J Nucl Med* 2003; 44(9):1421–5.

6. Sapirstein LA. Fractionation of the cardiac output of rats with isotopic potassium. *Circ Res* 1956; 4:689–92.

7. Sapirstein LA. Regional blood flow by fractional distribution of indicators. *Am J Physiol* 1958; 193:161–8.

8. Sokoloff L, Reivich M, Kennedy C, et al. The [14C]deoxyglucose method for the measurement of local cerebral glucose utilization: theory, procedure, and normal values in the conscious and anesthetized albino rat. *J Neurochem* 1977; 28(5):897–916.

9. Warburg O, Wind F, Neglers E. On the metabolism of tumors in the body. In: Warburg O, editor. *Metabolism of tumours*. London: Constabel, 1930:254–70.

10. Warburg O. *Biochem Zeitschrift* 1924; 152:479.

11. Wolf M. Labeled 2-deoxy-D-glucose analogs. 18F-labeled 2-deoxy-2-fluoro-D-glucose, 2-deoxy-2-fluoro-D-manose and C-14-2-deoxy-2-fluoro-D-glucose. *J Labeled Compounds Radiopharmaceuticals* 1978; 14:175–182.

Cardiology

Positron emission tomography has been important in cardiovascular research for nearly half a century. A number of isotopes and numerous radiopharmaceuticals have been used to obtain physiological, biochemical, and clinical information. In addition, PET has become a clinically useful tool. Fluorodeoxyglucose imaging is one of the principal methods for identification of jeopardized but viable myocardium, myocardium that can be salvaged with revascularization.

Myocardial perfusion imaging using PET agents provides higher resolution than with SPECT agents, and PET agents can be use to determine absolute blood flow. Rubidium-82, used for myocardial perfusion imaging, was the first PET agent approved by the United States Food and Drug Administration. PET myocardial perfusion imaging, especially quantitative myocardial perfusion imaging, has proven clinical value. Yet, imaging using SPECT is likely to remain the dominant method for myocardial perfusion imaging in most circumstances since it is less expensive to perform.

CORONARY ARTERY EVALUATION

Myocardial perfusion imaging was first used for the detection of coronary artery disease. It is still used for this purpose, but now it is often used in the evaluation of patients with known coronary artery disease. It can help evaluate the significance of individual stenoses, and provide valuable prognostic information.

Quantitative myocardial perfusion imaging can also be used to provide information about the microvasculature and with appropriate stress, endothelial-dependent changes in the microvasculature. There is considerable interest in the physiology of the microvasculature, both in coronary artery disease and in a number of diseases that affect myocardial perfusion in patients without obstructive epicardial coronary artery disease. Both SPECT and PET imaging can be used to evaluate epicardial coronary stenoses, but PET has a unique advantage in being able to evaluate coronary flow reserve using quantitative myocardial perfusion imaging.

Radiopharmaceuticals. Although rubidium-82 is the only FDA-approved radiopharmaceutical for myocardial perfusion imaging, a number of other radiopharmaceuticals are worth mentioning. (The myocardial perfusion radiopharmaceuticals are described more fully in Chapter 2, "PET Radiopharmaceuticals.") In facilities with a cyclotron, **nitrogen-13-labeled ammonia** is a readily available radiopharmaceutical with a half-life of 10 min. In the blood, the predominant species is ammonium, NH_4^+, but ammonium is in equilibrium with ammonia, NH_3, which can rapidly cross the cell membrane. Ammonia fixation is prompt and efficient within the cell, so that ammonia a good first-pass extraction agent. **Potassium-38-labeled potassium chloride**, with a 7.6-min half-life, can be used as a first-pass extraction agent similarly to thallous chloride.

A number of radiopharmaceuticals can be used to measure myocardial perfusion using the rate of washout if the radiopharmaceutical is rapidly diffusible compared to the washout rate. The most commonly used agent is **oxygen-15-labeled water**. Absolute myocardial blood flow can be calculated directly using a simple washout model. Oxygen's short half-life, 2 min, makes the coordination between production, on-line delivery, and administration challenging. **Carbon-11-labeled butanol** has a longer half-life, 20 min, and a better patrician coefficient than water, although it has been used less often for myocardial blood flow imaging. With the washout agents, the large blood pools within the ventricular cavities require correction for blood pool activity.

Carbon-11, nitrogen-13, oxygen-15, and potassium-38 all require an on-site cyclotron. Rubidium-82 and copper-62 are available from generator systems. Copper-62 comes from a Zinc-62/Copper-62 generator. Zinc-62 is relatively easy to produce with a medium-energy cyclotron; however, its short half-life, 9.3 h, means that a new generator is needed each day. Copper-62, which has a 9.7-min half-life, can be labeled to pyruvaldehyde-bis(N4-methylthiosemicarbazone) (PTSM). Because **copper-62-labeled PTSM** is lipid soluble; it rapidly crosses the cell membrane, where it is rapidly degraded trapping the copper inside the cell. Thus, Cu-62-PTSM is another first-pass extraction agent.

The most commonly used positron-emitting myocardial perfusion agent is **rubidium-82-labeled rubidium chloride**. The rubidium ion is taken up by the sodium-potassium ATPase in a fashion similar to potassium and thallium. Rubidium-82 comes from a strontium-82/rubidium-82 generator. The parent half-life is 25 days. Thus, the generator only needs to be replaced every 4–6 weeks. Rubidium-82 has a 76-s half-life, thus the generator is eluted directly into the patient.

Strontium-82 requires a high-energy cyclotron for production; therefore, it is relatively expensive. Several patients each day are required for commercially successful operation. However, it is not necessary to fill the schedule with myocardial perfusion patients. It is possible to share a camera economically between oncology and cardiology patients, and this strategy may allow a facility to start up before the volume of either application by itself would allow.

The commercial generator is mounted in a cart with appropriate shielding. The desired administered dose is entered as well as an injected volume limit. The generator is eluted automatically with normal saline. An on-board radiation detector monitors the activity in the eluate and delivers the desired administered dose to the connected tubing. The administered dose is often 1.5–2.25 GBq (40–60 mCi), but this dose depends on the PET camera and imaging mode. The volume of the connecting tubing should be kept small to assure that the desired dose reaches the patient's circulation.

The half-life of rubidium-82, 76 s, is shorter than is desirable. Ideally, imaging should be delayed until nearly all of the rubidium is out of circulation. However, since half of the total counts are gone after just 76 s, better counting statistics can be obtained by starting imaging as soon as possible. There is a tradeoff between obtaining more counts and having the low blood activity at the start of imaging. For patients with slow transit times, e.g., patients with congestive heart failure, it is best to delay the start of imaging to allow for clearance of blood activity. Because of the limited time for image acquisition, a high count-rate PET camera is preferable for rubidium-82 imaging.

Rubidium-82 has a relatively high energy positron. Thus, the positron will travel for a considerable distance in tissue before it undergoes an annihilation interaction (see Chapter 1, PET Physics and Instrumentation). The mean positron range is 2.6 mm; the 90% range is 13.2 mm. The high-energy positron causes a noticeable loss in resolution compared to isotopes with low-energy positrons like fluorine-18.

The limited counting statistics due to the short half-life means that reconstruction at lower resolution is needed to avoid excessive noise. That effect combined with the effect of the high-energy positron means that rubidium-82 images are lower resolution than images with many other PET isotopes. The final resolution is well below what is needed to distinguish sub-endocardium from the sub-epicardium. However, the final resolution is noticeably better than the resolution obtained with SPECT imaging.

Attenuation Correction.   Although annihilation radiation is much higher energy, 511 keV, than typical single photon agents, e.g., 140 keV, both of the photons from the annihilation need to escape the body and be detected in order to record an event. Further, attenuation does not decrease linearly with energy. The result is that attenuation is a larger factor for PET myocardial imaging than it is for SPECT imaging. The attenuation of the chest is considerably different from the attenuation of the abdomen, and within the chest the attenuation varies from location to location. Typically the inferior wall indents the diaphragm and has considerably more attenuation than the anterior wall. However, each patient is different.

The increased sensitivity of "3D" imaging can be used to ameliorate the poor counting statistics due to the short half-life of rubidium-82. However, the non-axial lines-of-response tend to have more varied attenuation. The net effect of these factors is that accurate attenuation correction is very important in myocardial perfusion imaging.

Breathing causes considerable motion of the diaphragm. The best solution is to collect the attenuation information at the same time as the perfusion information. Simultaneous collection of emission and transmission data has been very successful for SPECT imaging. So far, simultaneous emission and transmission scanning has not been introduced on a commercial PET scanner. The transmission and emission scans are obtained sequentially.

There can be differences in the diaphragmatic position, differences in cardiac motion, and differences in patient position between emission and transmission. This difference in position is especially a problem with CT attenuation correction, where the attenuation information is collected for a single diaphragmatic position compared to an average diaphragmatic position for the perfusion imaging. For CT attenuation correction, it may be wise to obtain a scan both before and after the perfusion imaging, and then use the scan that results in the least artifacts in the final corrected image. This quick summary of the problems associated with attenuation correction is expanded upon in Chapter 1.

Quantization of Myocardial Blood Flow.   Relative myocardial blood flow compares the perfusion of one portion of the heart to another portion. Relative myocardial blood flow and the differences in relative myocardial blood flow between stress and rest provide valuable information in a number of diseases, including coronary artery disease. Both SPECT and PET imaging can obtain relative myocardial blood flow. PET imaging is higher resolution, but SPECT imaging, which can be performed less expensively, is generally adequate to evaluate relative perfusion.

Absolute myocardial blood flow, measured in units of flow per gram of tissue ((mL/min)/g), provides additional information compared to relative perfusion. Absolute myocardial blood flow is especially important when comparing stress and rest perfusion studies. The ratio of the maximum flow to the resting flow gives the coronary flow reserve. The coronary flow reserve is important both for evaluating individual coronary artery lesions and for evaluating the overall coronary vasculature.

Absolute myocardial blood flow is obtained directly from the washout of diffusible tracers. The mean transit time (min) of a diffusible tracer through tissue is equal to the amount of tissue (g) divided by the product of the density (g/mL) and the blood flow (mL/min). This calculation is simple to perform when a bolus of activity is injected into an isolated tissue. It is a bit more complicated when there is a more prolong input. And, it is made even more complicated in the myocardium, where there is an important contribution of the blood pool to the pixels in the myocardium. Generally, a compartmental model is used to model the components, and the absolute blood flow is one of the parameters that are derived.

Tracers that are uniformly distributed in the blood flow, that have uniform first-pass extraction, and that do not wash out, will have a distribution that is proportional to relative blood flow. Absolute blood flow can also be obtained from these first-pass extraction agents if the input function can be measured quantitatively. The input function is equal to the concentration of tracer in the arterial blood (MBq/mL) as a function of time. The final activity in the tissue (MBq/mL) will be equal to the integral of the input function (min-MBq/mL) times the blood flow ((mL/min)/g) times the tissue density (g/mL).

Quantization of myocardial blood flow with rubidium-82 is less well established than with diffusible tracers or with the first-pass extraction agent, ammonia. Quantization is made difficult both by the proximity of the blood pool to the myocardium, but also the short half-life of rubidium-82. However, dynamic data can be fit to an appropriate model and absolute blood flow ((mL/min)/g) can be obtained. By comparing maximal vasodilation to rest, myocardial flow reserve can be calculated.

Clinical Applications. Coronary Artery Disease Evaluation with Myocardial Perfusion Imaging: Myocardial perfusion imaging with PET has been used for detection of coronary artery disease for more than two decades.[1] Tamaki et al.[2] reviewed the reported literature and found an average sensitivity 94% and a specificity of 95%. In this somewhat limited literature, PET imaging of myocardial perfusion performs well with respect to SPECT imaging.

Because of the short half-life of rubidium-82, the patient needs to be in position in the camera before infusion. Performance of supine leg exercise is possible, but from a practical point of view, stress imaging is limited to pharmacological stress. Other radiopharmaceuticals are less available at the present time, but when they become available, they may allow more flexibility in the choice of stress.

The residual activity from a rest study decays rapidly with the 76-second half-life of rubidium-82. Further, the activity in the generator also rebuilds with

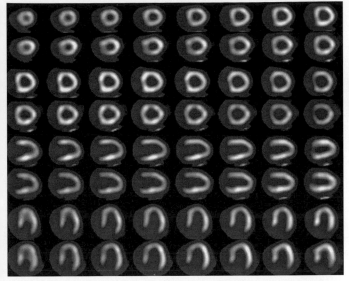

Figure 1: Normal Perfusion. A normal myocardial dipyridamole stress/rest rubidium-82 myocardial perfusion scan. The top four rows are short axis from apex to base; the next two rows are vertical long axis from septum to lateral; the bottom two rows are horizontal long axis from inferior to anterior. The odd rows show stress images, which are directly above the corresponding rest images. Note the high resolution by comparison to SPECT imaging. (From color images courtesy of Marcelo F. Di Carli, MD, FACC.)

the short half-life of the rubidium-82 progeny. Thus, after 10 min, there is minimal residual activity in the patient and nearly complete buildup of isotope in the generator. Imaging can be repeated every 10 min without contamination from prior imaging. Although the imaging time and the repeat interval are short, the stress procedure needs to be performed in the camera room. Adequate space should be allotted for personnel and adequate scan room time for the stress procedure.

Figure 1 shows a normal rubidium-82 dipyridamole stress/rest myocardial perfusion scan. The image resolution is good compared to SPECT imaging, but lower than FDG imaging. Figure 2 shows a rubidium-82 dipyridamole stress/rest myocardial perfusion scan with a fixed inferior wall defect.

Perfusion in Combination with Other Studies: Another utility of myocardial perfusion imaging is in combination with other studies. In the next section, myocardial perfusion imaging is combined with FDG imaging to detect jeopardized, but viable myocardium. The CT component of a PET/CT scanner can be a multi-slice CT capable of doing CT coronary angiography. Rubidium-82 myocardial perfusion imaging can be fused with anatomic coronary imaging to provide more accurate regional evaluation of the significance of coronary artery lesions.

Coronary Perfusion Reserve: An exciting, emerging area for PET is quantitative myocardial perfusion imaging. There is a rich literature on the

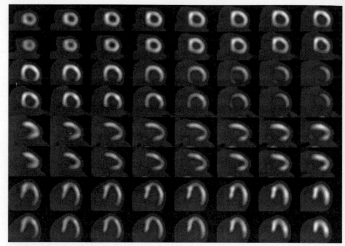

Figure 2: Fixed Inferior Perfusion Defect. This dipyridamole stress/rest myocardial rubidium-82 perfusion scan shows a fixed inferior wall defect. The top four rows are short axis from apex to base; the next two rows are vertical long axis from septum to lateral; the bottom two rows are horizontal long axis from inferior to anterior. The odd rows show stress images, which are directly above the corresponding rest images. (From color images courtesy of Marcelo F. Di Carli, MD, FACC.)

physiology of impaired coronary perfusion reserve. Impaired flow reserve is thought to relate to dysfunction of the endothelial control of the microvasculature. Coronary perfusion reserve is important not only in evaluating individual epicardial coronary stenoses, but also in the evaluation of a number of disease processes which affect the heart.

Coronary flow reserve can be measured invasively at the time of cardiac catheterization. PET offers the advantage of making this measurement non-invasively. Schindler et al. have recently shown a close correlation between invasively measured luminal area and PET measurements of blood flow in response to the cold pressor test. Changes in forearm vascular resistance, which also provide information about microvascular responsiveness, are more easily measured than coronary perfusion reserve. However, in idiopathic dilated cardiomyopathy, forearm vascular resistance was shown not to be a good surrogate of coronary flow reserve. The valuable information provided by PET measurement of coronary perfusion reserve may become integrated into clinical algorithms in the near future.

VIABLE JEOPARDIZED MYOCARDIUM

Revascularization is one of the most effective cardiovascular therapies. The goal of revascularization is to provide an improved blood supply to living myocardial tissue. Reversible perfusion defects on myocardial perfusion imaging identify many of the locations that are appropriate for revascularization. However, it became apparent shortly after the introduction of angioplasty that there were territories with fixed defects that improved after revascularization. Often these territories had abnormal resting wall motion, and the wall motion would improve after revascularization. These areas have a jeopardized vascular supply, but the myocardial cells remain viable.

After an acute episode of ischemia has resolved, the vascular supply may return to normal, but there may be persistent dysfunction—hypokinesis or akinesis. Postischemic dysfunction after an acute episode of ischemia is called **myocardial stunning**. There can also be more chronic problems with the vascular supply to a myocardial territory. An area where there is chronic long-term insufficiency of blood supply will also show abnormal contraction. In such an area, the myocardial function is said to be down-regulated; the function is more appropriately matched to the supply. This process of chronically insufficient blood supply with associated decreased function is called **myocardial hibernation**.

Both the demand on the myocardium and the supply of blood to the myocardium are dynamic processes. The vessel walls change dynamically, and plaque-associated palette aggregation also change dynamically. At one end of the spectrum, a hibernating area with chronically jeopardized vascular supply may have relatively stable demand and blood supply. At the other end of the spectrum, a stunned area may have one or two or three episodes of acute ischemia. The distinction between a single episode of ischemia and chronically decrease blood flow should be viewed more of as a continuum of states,[11] Stunning implies a relatively more acute scenario, and hibernation implies a relatively more chronic scenario.

There is also a continuum in the physiological and the histological response of the myocardium. After an acute episode of ischemia, the myocardial cells appear entirely normal. Although the territory may by dysfunctional at rest, with simulation the territory can be made to contract. Typically, low-dose dobutamine is used to simulate the myocardium and the wall motion is seen to improve. The classic response to dobutamine infusion is a biphasic response where at low doses, the dobutamine recruits the myocardium to contract. At a higher doses, the jeopardizing lesion limits flow and results in frank ischemia and decreased function. Revascularization at this point results in prompt (days to weeks) return of function to normal.

As the limited supply becomes more chronic, there are ultrastructural changes in the myocardium with influx of glycogen.[12–15] Eventually, the myocardium will no longer respond to acute stimulation. However, the cells may still return to normal function with revascularization. The greater the changes and the more fibrosis, the longer the return of function may take, and the function may not return completely.[14,16,17]

Stress Myocardial Perfusion Scintigraphy.
Stress myocardial perfusion scintigraphy is important in the evaluation of patients with jeopardized but viable myocardium. Most territories that will benefit from revascularization will be detected as reversible defects on stress myocardial perfusion scintigraphy. Even in patients with viable territories that show fixed defects, stress myocardial perfusion scintigraphy may provide enough information about other territories to proceed without further study. Thallium-201 redistribution imaging may demonstrate viable territories as fixed at rest but redistributing on delayed imaging.

The level of resting blood flow to a region helps to distinguish territories that may be viable from territories that are not viable. Areas with little blood flow (less than 20% of maximum) will rarely show improvement with revascularization. Areas with moderate blood flow (50% of maximum) can represent a combination of scar and normal tissue, but they may represent areas of viable jeopardized myocardium.

In the group of patients with moderate fixed defects, determination of the amount of jeopardized but viable myocardium will be important in deciding about revascularization. In addition, areas of normal resting blood flow and impaired myocardial contraction have more recently become emphasized as another important pattern seen in jeopardized but viable myocardium.

Dobutamine Echocardiography. Dobutamine echocardiography evaluates regional myocardial wall motion at rest and then at several levels of dobutamine stimulation. The classic response of jeopardized but viable myocardium is a biphasic response. The resting wall motion abnormalities improves with low-dose dobutamine and then worsens at high-dose. The myocardium initially is stimulated to contract and then becomes ischemic as the blood flow demand outstrips the available supply. This pattern of response is very specific for jeopardized but viable myocardium. A high fraction of segments with this response will show a prompt return of function with revascularization.

Territories that show improvement with stimulation but then do no show any worsening at high-dose infusion are viable. However, the etiology of the abnormal wall motion at rest may not be a jeopardized vascular supply. Thus, this pattern implies viability, but it is a little less specific about the mechanism than the biphasic response.

Dobutamine echocardiography is less sensitive in detection of viable myocardium in territories with more prolong and severe changes. These territories tend not to show any improvement in contraction with stimulation. These territories also tend to respond more slowly after revascularization. To detect late improvement after revascularization it is important to wait 6 months or longer after revascularization.

FDG/Perfusion PET Imaging. FDG/Perfusion imaging can be used to identify regions that will improve with revascularization. The myocardium tends to use free fatty acids for the majority of its metabolic needs, especially in the fasting state. There is considerable variability in the amount of uptake of FDG or glucose during the fasting state between individuals and in different regions of the myocardium. The lateral wall tends to have the most fasting FDG uptake and the septum tends to have the least FDG uptake.

When the myocardium is subjected to ischemic injury, one of the first things that happen is that it switches from free fatty acid metabolism to glucose metabolism. The tricarboxylic acid cycle is very efficient at extracting energy from glucose. If the cell is using anaerobic metabolism, then the uptake of glucose will be even higher. When initially described for detecting jeopardized but viable myocardium, FDG was administered in the fasting state. In the fasting state, regions of jeopardized but viable myocardium appear as hot spots.

The considerable variability of FDG uptake in normal myocardium in the fasting state complicates interpretation for jeopardized but viable areas.

Furthermore, an FDG-PET study with a single region of FDG uptake can be difficult to align with a perfusion image because of the few landmarks present. (This second limitation can be overcome when using dual-isotope SPECT.) Consequently, FDG-PET studies are usually performed using a protocol where the myocardium is using glucose.

The regional FDG uptake is compared with regional blood flow. Two main patterns of uptake are described. In areas of scar, there is both reduced perfusion and reduced FDG uptake. This **FDG/perfusion matched pattern** indicates nonviable tissue. In areas of hibernating myocardium, there is reduced perfusion. About 80% of perfusion normally is used to support the energy needed for contraction. When the wall is not contracting, the blood flow requirements are considerably reduced. These areas preferentially use glucose, so the FDG uptake will be out of proportion to the perfusion. The **FDG/perfusion mismatched pattern**, normal or increased FDG in an area with decrease perfusion, indicates hibernation.

Areas with normal perfusion were initially considered to represent normal tissue. However, some of these areas correspond to regions with abnormal wall motion. An area with abnormal wall motion, normal perfusion, and normal or increased FDG uptake often indicates an area of jeopardized but viable myocardium. Often these regions are on the stunned end of the stunned/hibernating spectrum.

Schinkel et al. defined hibernating myocardium as regions of dysfunctional myocardium with decrease perfusion and mismatched FDG uptake. Stunned myocardium was defined as regions of dysfunctional myocardium with normal perfusion. Wall motion improvement with dobutamine was seen on echocardiography more frequently in stunned than in hibernating myocardium (61% of segments versus 51% of segments). Dysfunctional regions with matched decrease in perfusion and FDG were defined as scared segments. Only 14% of scared segments showed improvement in function, with non-transmural scars being more likely to show improvement in function.

Simulation of FDG Uptake. The goal for FDG imaging of the myocardium is to prepare the patient so that there is good uptake throughout the myocardium. Insulin stimulates the translocation of GLUT4, one of the glucose transporters, to the cell membrane. Insulin stimulates uptake of glucose not only in normal, but also in the hibernating myocardium. Thus, one method of stimulating FDG uptake is to increase plasma insulin levels. At the same time, it is desirable to have low serum glucose levels, since serum glucose will compete directly with FDG for uptake by the myocardium.

In non-diabetic patients, a procedure similar to a glucose tolerance test can be performed. In the fasting state, the patient is given an oral glucose load, about 50 g of glucose. Initially the serum glucose goes up followed by a surge in insulin. By about one hour the glucose has returned to near normal, and the serum insulin levels are still high. FDG can be administered once the glucose has fallen below about 140 mg/dL.

One problem with this protocol is that there is considerable variability between patients in their response to a glucose load. Within the coronary artery disease population there is a considerable amount of diabetes, and even among the patients not known to be diabetic, some glucose intolerance is frequently encountered. Therefore it is important to measure the glucose before administering the FDG. If the glucose is high, then a low dose of intravenous insulin can be used to lower the glucose and facilitate the uptake of FDG.

Some investigators have used this ad hoc protocol successfully. Others note that the problem with this ad hoc method is that scheduling is complicated because FDG injection may have to be delayed in some patients, and the actual levels of insulin and glucose are not well controlled.

An alternate procedure is to perform a hyperinsulinemic euglycemic clamp. During hyperinsulinemic euglycemic clamp, both insulin and glucose are infused continuously. Since insulin lowers the serum potassium, potassium is also part of the infusate. The rate of glucose infusion is adjusted to obtain a fixed level of serum glucose. In non-diabetic patients it is possible to simplify the procedure.

An alternate to raising the serum glucose is to lower the serum free fatty acids. Nicotinic acid derivatives (niacin in the United States, acipimox in Europe) lower free fatty acids by inhibiting release of free fatty acids by the fat cells. Lowering the free fatty acids increases myocardial uptake of glucose and FDG.

Bax et al. compared oral glucose loading hyperinsulinemic euglycemic clamp, and acipimox. The myocardium to blood activity and the FDG clearance was better with either the clamp method or acipimox than with oral glucose loading.

Imaging Technique. There are a number of protocols for performing FDG/perfusion imaging. Any of the myocardial imaging agents may be used. The perfusion images are generally obtained in the resting state; however, some investigators have combined stress myocardial perfusion imaging with FDG imaging.

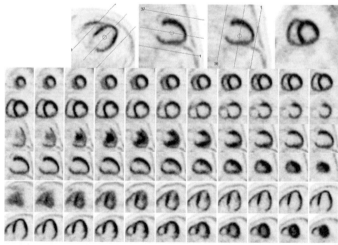

Figure 3: FDG-PET Dilated Ventricle. FDG images from a patient with a dilated ventricle due to coronary cardiomyopathy are shown. The papillary muscles are clearly visible. The top row shows the slice selection procedure. The next two rows show the short axis from apex to base; the next two rows are vertical long axis from septum to lateral; the bottom two rows are horizontal long axis from inferior to anterior.

It is typical to perform both the FDG and the perfusion imaging on a dedicated PET camera (see Figure 3). Attenuation information can be obtained from a transmission source or with a PET/CT scanner (see Figure 4). However, the FDG images can be obtained using Anger-camera based PET imaging. FDG-PET images from either a dedicated PET scanner or an Anger-camera based PET can be registered with SPECT perfusion images. And finally, both the FDG and perfusion images can be obtained using a SPECT camera equipped with 511-keV collimators. Although SPECT scanners have considerably lower resolution than dedicated PET scanners, the advantage of SPECT imaging is that the FDG and perfusion images can be obtained simultaneously with dual-energy imaging, resulting in perfectly aligned images (see Figure 5).

Clinical Applications. Patients with reversible myocardial perfusion defects have improved function after revascularization. In patients with fixed myocardial perfusion defects, the degree of improvement in ventricular function after

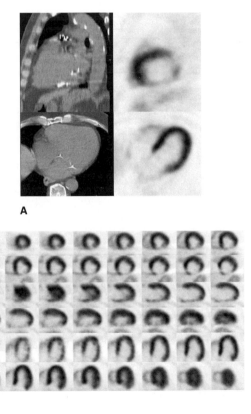

Figure 4: PET/CT Imaging. The CT data from the PET/CT provides measured attenuation and it can be used to help in orientation. **A.** FDG-PET and CT images are shown in the sagittal and axial planes. **B.** Slices from the same study are shown in the short axis, the vertical long axis, and the horizontal long axis.

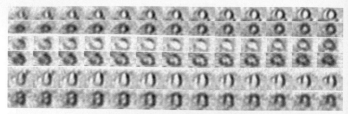

Figure 5: FDG/sestamibi SPECT. This FDG/sestamibi SPECT scan was performed in a 63-year-old diabetic man with three-vessel coronary artery disease and a left ventricular ejection fraction of 18% who presented with congestive heart failure. The sestamibi images are shown in the odd rows, which are directly above the corresponding FDG images. There is better FDG uptake than perfusion in the anteroseptal territory. The top two rows are short axis from apex to base; the middle two rows are vertical long axis from septum to lateral; and the bottom two rows are horizontal long axis from inferior to anterior.

myocardial revascularization depends on the amount of jeopardized but viable myocardium that is revascularized. Patients with large amounts of jeopardized but viable myocardium have marked improvement in both global and regional ventricular function, whereas patients with little or no jeopardized but viable myocardium receive little benefit from revascularization.

Eitzman et al. compared cardiac events (cardiac death, nonfatal myocardial infarction, cardiac arrest, or late revascularization) in 82 patients after PET imaging of FDG uptake and myocardial perfusion imaging with nitrogen-13-labeled ammonia or rubidium-82. Events occurred in nine of 18 patients (50%) with a mismatch pattern treated medically and in 3 of 26 patients (12%) treated with revascularization. By comparison, medical and revascularization had similar outcomes in patients with matched patterns. Events occurred in 3 of 24 (13%) of patients with a matched pattern treated medically and in 1 of 14 (7%) of patients treated with revascularization (Figure 6). A similar important difference in outcome has been seen in several other studies.

The amount of viable but jeopardized myocardium can be estimated in several ways. On perfusion scintigraphy, regions with moderately reduced perfusion are more likely to be viable. However, these regions can also represent regions with a mixture of infarct and normal tissue. On stress echocardiography, regions with a biphasic response are very likely to be viable. Wall motion in response to low-dose dobutamine can similarly be assessed on gated perfusion SPECT imaging or with MRI. On FDG/perfusion-PET imaging, regions that show a mismatch pattern are very likely to be viable.

The gold standard for jeopardized but viable myocardium is a change in wall motion from pre- to post-revascularization. Improvement in the most severely effected segments may require follow-up of 6 months or longer.[14,16,17] Although studies comparing different methods of assessing viable myocardium are very difficult to perform, several studies have compared these methods.

Hernandez-Pamaploni et al. compared thallium-201 rest-redistribution SPECT, FDG PET, and dobutamine echocardiography in 109 revascularized segments using echocardiography at 6 weeks after surgery to detect improvement in wall motion. There was improvement in the left ventricular ejection fraction from 30 ± 10% to 42 ± 13%, and improvement in wall motion 62 of

FDG / Perfusion

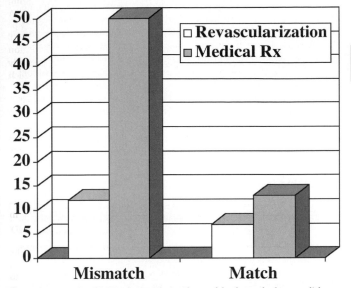

Figure 6: Prognosis—FDG/Perfusion. The incidence of death, nonfatal myocardial infarction, cardiac arrest, or late revascularization an average of 12 months after imaging is shown as a function of therapy and FDG/perfusion pattern. Patients with a mismatch pattern who were treated medically had a significantly worse prognosis than the other groups. (These results are from Eitzman et al.)

segments 109 (57%). The thallium prediction of wall motion improvement was as sensitive as both biphasic dobutamine echocardiography response and FDG PET, but it was less specific than either.

Barrington et al. compared stress/rest sestamibi scans, redistribution thallium scan, dobutamine echocardiography, and FDG/ammonia-PET scans in the evaluation of hibernating myocardium in 25 patients with left ventricular ejection fractions (LVEF) less than 40% scheduled to undergo myocardial revascularization by coronary artery bypass graft (CABG). Hibernating myocardium was defined as improvement 6–12 months after CABG in two segments within one vascular territory. There were relatively few vascular territories that showed functional recovery, 6 of 75 vascular territories that were assessed. Univariate predictors of hibernating myocardium were sestamibi, ammonia, and FDG uptake. FDG uptake was the only multivariate predictor.

In order to improve the specificity of thallium-201 imaging and the sensitivity of dobutamine echocardiography, Bax et al. compared two strategies using thallium-201 and dobutamine echocardiography to FDG-PET for predicting left ventricular function improvement six months after revascularization. Strategy 1 used thatlium-201 imaging with dobutamine echocardiography for indeterminate thallium-201 scans. Strategy 2 used dobutamine echocardiography with thallium-201 for "uncertain" segments. Both strategies had high sensitivities (89% and 89%) and specificities (89% and 86%), and both strategies were comparable to FDG-SPECT sensitivity (89%) and specificity (86%).

These recent as well as several older studies[20] suggest that perfusion imaging, dobutamine stress wall motion, and FDG metabolic imaging all provide information about jeopardized but viable myocardium. A severe fixed perfusion defect is a strong indicator of non-viable myocardium. Moderate fixed perfusion defects are sensitive, but not specific, indicators of viable myocardium; however, there are also some jeopardized regions with normal perfusion. A biphasic response in wall motion to dobutamine is a specific indicator of jeopardized but viable myocardium with somewhat lower sensitivity. FDG-PET imaging has similar sensitivity and specificity as stress dobutamine wall motion imaging. The strength of FDG-PET is in identifying the more chronically down-regulated segments, which may not respond to dobutamine, but which may over time regain function after revascularization.

VULNERABLE PLAQUE

Some patients with coronary artery disease show slow steady progression of their stenotic lesions. They develop slowly progressive chest pain, and show orderly progression of their disease on myocardial perfusion imaging. They have progressive narrowing of stenotic lesions on coronary arteriography. Unfortunately, many patients have sudden death as their first symptom of coronary artery disease, or they suddenly develop a myocardial infarction in a vascular territory with an "insignificant" coronary artery stenosis. What happens in these cases is that there is rupture of a non-obstructive plaque with secondary occlusion of the vessel by a thrombus.

The difference between these two extremes in presentation has lead to the idea of the importance of the vulnerable plaque. The vulnerable plaque is a plaque that is subject to rupture. Patients with vulnerable plaques are apt to develop symptoms unexpectedly, whereas patients with stable plaques develop an orderly progression of symptoms. Developing methods for imaging the vulnerable plaque may be important in better understand of the pathophysiology of the vulnerable plaque, and may be important in developing therapies directed at the vulnerable plaque.

Macrophages show avid FDG uptake especially under acidic and hypoxic conditions found in an atheroma, and they are important in the pathophysiology of atheromatous plaque. For example, there is more FDG uptake in carotid arteries associated with a recent transient ischemic attack than in the contralateral carotid artery. In some arterial locations, the uptake of FDG has been shown to be correlated with atherogenic risk factors. The location of uptake of FDG in the aorta is not well correlated with the location of aortic calcifications. Calcified plaque may be an indicator of old, burned-out disease, and FDG uptake may be telling use about more acute metabolic changes. Thus, FDG is likely providing a different window on the atheromatous process than calcification.

Imaging of the coronary arteries is a very difficult task for PET both because of their small size and the cardiac motion. An agent with very high relative uptake could be imaged with current methods. Or, the atherosclerotic process in other vessels could be useful in evaluation the coronary arteries or anti-atherogenic therapies. In any event, the molecular imaging capability of PET is may be important for this new area.

CONCLUSIONS

PET imaging of myocardial perfusion and metabolism is a valuable tool in identifying and monitoring coronary artery disease. It provides powerful prognostic information. It helps to select patients who will benefit most from revascularization. Clinical utility has so far depended on evaluation of coronary artery disease and the detection of viable but jeopardized myocardium. There is emerging interest in coronary perfusion reserve both in epicardial coronary artery disease as well as in many other conditions. An exciting new area for future development is better understanding and hopefully treatment of the atheromatous process.

3

BIBLIOGRAPHY

1. Barrington SF, Chambers J, Hallett WA, et al. Comparison of sestamibi, thallium, echocardiography and PET for the detection of hibernating myocardium. *Eur J Nucl Med Mol Imaging* 2004; 31(3):355–61.
2. Bax JJ, Maddahi J, Poldermans D, et al. Preoperative comparison of different non-invasive strategies for predicting improvement in left ventricular function after coronary artery bypass grafting. *Am J Cardiol* 2003; 92(1):1–4.
3. Bax JJ, Veening MA, Visser FC, et al. Optimal metabolic conditions during fluorine-18 fluorodeoxyglucose imaging; a comparative study using different protocols. *Eur J Nucl Med* 1997; 24(1):35–41.
4. Chin BB, Esposito G, Kraitchman DL. Myocardial contractile reserve and perfusion defect severity with rest and stress dobutamine (99m)Tc-sestamibi SPECT in canine stunning and subendocardial infarction. *J Nucl Med* 2002; 43(4):540–50.
5. Depre C, Vanoverschelde JL, Gerber B, et al. Correlation of functional recovery with myocardial blood flow, glucose uptake, and morphologic features in patients with chronic left ventricular ischemic dysfunction undergoing coronary artery bypass grafting. *J Thorac Cardiovasc Surg* 1997; 113(2):371–8.
6. Depre C, Vanoverschelde JL, Melin JA, et al. Structural and metabolic correlates of the reversibility of chronic left ventricular ischemic dysfunction in humans. *Am J Physiol* 1995; 268(3 Pt 2):H1265–75.
7. Depre C, Vanoverschelde JL, Taegtmeyer H. Glucose for the heart. *Circulation* 1999; 99(4):578–88.
8. Eitzman D, al-Aouar Z, Kanter HL, et al. Clinical outcome of patients with advanced coronary artery disease after viability studies with positron emission tomography [see comments]. *J Am Coll Cardiol* 1992; 20(3):559–65.
9. Gibson RS, Watson DD, Taylor GJ, et al. Prospective assessment of regional myocardial perfusion before and after coronary revascularization surgery by quantitative thallium-201 scintigraphy. *J Am Coll Cardiol* 1983; 1(3):804–15.
10. Haas F, Augustin N, Holper K, et al. Time course and extent of improvement of dysfunctioning myocardium in patients with coronary artery disease and severely depressed left ventricular function after revascularization: correlation with positron emission tomographic findings. *J Am Coll Cardiol* 2000; 36(6):1927–34.
11. Hashimoto A, Fischman AJ, Gold HK, et al. "Functional" viability assessment by dual isotope F18-FDG and Tc99m-sestamibi in acute myocardial infarction. *J Nucl Med* 1999; 40(5):48P.
12. Hauser M, Bengel F, Kuehn A, et al. Myocardial Blood Flow and Coronary Flow Reserve in Children with "Normal" Epicardial Coronary Arteries After the Onset of Kawasaki Disease Assessed by Positron Emission Tomography. *Pediatr Cardiol* 2003.
13. Heiba SI, Abdel-Dayem HM, Gould R, et al. Value of low-dose dobutamine addition to routine dual isotope gated SPECT myocardial imaging in patients with healed

myocardial infarction or abnormal wall thickening by echocardiogram. *Am J Cardiol* 2004; 93(3):300–6.

14. Hernandez-Pampaloni M, Peral V, Carreras JL, et al. Biphasic response to dobutamine predicts improvement of left ventricular dysfunction after revascularization: correlation with positron emission and rest-redistribution 201Tl tomographies. *Int J Cardiovasc Imaging* 2003; 19(6):519–28.

15. Hesse B, Meyer C, et al. Myocardial perfusion in type 2 diabetes with left ventricular hypertrophy: normalisation by acute angiotensin-converting enzyme inhibition. *Eur J Nucl Med Mol Imaging* 2004; 31(3):362–8.

16. Jadvar H, Strauss HW, Segall GM. SPECT and PET in the evaluation of coronary artery disease. Radiographics 1999; 19(4):915–26.

17. Knuuti MJ, Nuutila P, Ruotsalainen U, et al. Euglycemic hyperinsulinemic clamp and oral glucose load in stimulating myocardial glucose utilization during positron emission tomography [see comments]. *J Nucl Med* 1992; 33(7):1255–62.

18. Liu P, Kiess MC, Okada RD, et al. The persistent defect on exercise thallium imaging and its fate after myocardial revascularization: does it represent scar or ischemia? *Am Heart J* 1985; 110(5):996–1001.

19. Maki M, Luotolahti M, Nuutila P, et al. Glucose uptake in the chronically dysfunctional but viable myocardium. *Circulation* 1996; 93(9):1658–66.

20. Martin WH, Jones RC, Delbeke D, Sandler MP. A simplified intravenous glucose loading protocol for fluorine-18 fluorodeoxyglucose cardiac single-photon emission tomography. *Eur J Nucl Med* 1997; 24(10):1291–7.

21. Mazzadi AN, Janier MF, Brossier B, et al. Dobutamine-tagged MRI for inotropic reserve assessment in severe CAD: relationship with PET findings. *Am J Physiol Heart Circ Physiol* 2004.

22. Nienaber CA, Brunken RC, Sherman CT, et al. Metabolic and functional recovery of ischemic human myocardium after coronary angioplasty [see comments]. *J Am Coll Cardiol* 1991; 18(4):966–78.

23. Parker JA. Cardiac nuclear medicine in monitoring patients with coronary heart disease. *Semin Nucl Med* 2001; 31(3):223–37.

24. Pirich C, Leber A, Knez A, et al. Relation of coronary vasoreactivity and coronary calcification in asymptomatic subjects with a family history of premature coronary artery disease. *Eur J Nucl Med Mol Imaging* 2004.

25. Rudd JH, Warburton EA, Fryer TD, et al. Imaging atherosclerotic plaque inflammation with [18F]-fluorodeoxyglucose positron emission tomography. *Circulation* 2002; 105(23):2708–11.

26. Sandler MP, Bax JJ, Patton JA, et al. Fluorine-18-fluorodeoxyglucose cardiac imaging using a modified scintillation camera. *J Nucl Med* 1998; 39(12):2035–43.

27. Sandler MP, Videlefsky S, Delbeke D, et al. Evaluation of myocardial ischemia using a rest metabolism/stress perfusion protocol with fluorine-18 deoxyglucose/technetium-99m MIBI and dual-isotope simultaneous-acquisition single-photon emission computed tomography. *J Am Coll Cardiol* 1995; 26(4):870–8.

28. Schelbert HR, Phelps ME, Huang SC, et al. N-13 ammonia as an indicator of myocardial blood flow. *Circulation* 1981; 63(6):1259–72.

29. Schindler TH, Nitzsche EU, Olschewski M, et al. PET-measured responses of MBF to cold pressor testing correlate with indices of coronary vasomotion on quantitative coronary angiography. *J Nucl Med* 2004; 45(3):419–428.

30. Schinkel AF, Bax JJ, van Domburg R, et al. Dobutamine-induced contractile reserve in stunned, hibernating, and scarred myocardium in patients with ischemic cardiomyopathy. *J Nucl Med* 2003; 44(2):127–33.

31. Stolen KQ, Kemppainen J, Kalliokoski KK, et al. Myocardial perfusion reserve and peripheral endothelial function in patients with idiopathic dilated cardiomyopathy. *Am J Cardiol* 2004; 93(1):64–8.

32. Strauss HW, Grewal RK, Pandit-Taskar N. Molecular imaging in nuclear cardiology. *Semin Nucl Med* 2004; 34(1):47–55.

33. Tamaki N, Ruddy TD, deKemp R, Beanlands RSB. Myocardial Perfusion. In: Buchanan JW, editor. *Principles and practice of positron emission tomography.* Philadelphia: Lippincott Williams & Wilkins, 2002:320–33.

34. Tillisch J, Brunken R, Marshall R, et al. Reversibility of cardiac wall-motion abnormalities predicted by positron tomography. *N Engl J Med* 1986; 314(14):884–8.

35. Vallabhajosula S, Fuster V. Atherosclerosis: imaging techniques and the evolving role of nuclear medicine. *J Nucl Med* 1997; 38(11):1788–96.

36. Vanoverschelde JL, Depre C, Gerber BL, et al. Time course of functional recovery after coronary artery bypass graft surgery in patients with chronic left ventricular ischemic dysfunction. *Am J Cardiol* 2000; 85(12):1432–9.

37. Vanoverschelde JL, Wijns W, Borgers M, et al. Chronic myocardial hibernation in humans. From bedside to bench. *Circulation* 1997; 95(7):1961–71.

38. Wijns W, Vatner SF, Camici PG. Hibernating myocardium. *N Engl J Med* 1998; 339(3):173–81.

39. Wyss CA, Koepfli P, Mikolajczyk K, et al. Bicycle exercise stress in PET for assessment of coronary flow reserve: repeatability and comparison with adenosine stress. *J Nucl Med* 2003; 44(2):146–54.

40. Yokoyama I, Yonekura K, Ohtake T, et al. Role of insulin resistance in heart and skeletal muscle F-18 fluorodeoxyglucose uptake in patients with non-insulin-dependent diabetes mellitus. *J Nucl Cardiol* 2000; 7(3):242–8.

41. Yun M, Jang S, Cucchiara A, et al. 18F FDG uptake in the large arteries: a correlation study with the atherogenic risk factors. *Semin Nucl Med* 2002; 32(1):70–6.

3

4

Neurology and Psychiatry

An early application of PET was in neurochemical imaging of the brain for assessing the regional distributions of blood flow, glucose metabolism, neurotransmitters, enzymes, and receptors. Despite the early and the current broad PET applications in brain research, however, the clinical applications of PET in neurology and psychiatry are limited to a few clinical conditions. In this chapter, we will first briefly review normal variants and the effect of aging and drugs on the imaging pattern on PET. We will then review in relatively greater depth the more common applications of PET in epilepsy, stroke, Alzheimer's disease, and Parkinson's disease. We will discuss briefly the other applications in Huntington's disease, schizophrenia, and depression. However, one must note that PET has been employed as an imaging research tool in many other conditions, including, but not limited to, movement disorders, dementia, autism, attention deficit hyperactivity disorder, bipolar disorders, anxiety disorders, personality disorders, substance abuse, and eating disorders. The discussion of the potential diagnostic utility of PET in these neuropsychiatric disorders is beyond the scope of this book. The exact role of PET in these clinical settings remains undefined, but further experience may result in expanded role of PET in the diagnostic imaging evaluation of these and many other neuropsychiatric diseases.

NORMAL VARIANTS AND EFFECTS OF AGING AND DRUGS

Normal gray matter displays much higher (about four times) glucose metabolism than the white matter. More prominent gray matter metabolism and blood flow is seen in the frontal eye fields (anterior to the primary motor cortex), posterior cingulate cortex (anterosuperior to the occipital cortex), the Wernicke region (posterosuperior temporal lobe), the visual cortex, the posterior parietal lobes, and the basal ganglia.

Brain blood flow increases to adult values during adolescence. However, whether there is decline in cerebral perfusion with healthy aging is controversial. The reports of regional decline may be explained by the lack of partial volume correction for the age-related cerebral volume loss and the possibility of the effect of pre-clinical dementia on blood flow.

In neonates, glucose metabolism is highest in the cerebellar vermis, brainstem, thalamus, and the sensorimotor cortex. By three months, the metabolic activity increases in the cerebellar cortex, basal ganglia, and the occipital, temporal, and parietal cortices. By six to eight months, there is an additional increase in the metabolism of the frontal and the dorsolateral occipital cortices. The brain glucometabolism reaches adult values by two years and then exceeds the adult values until the age of nine years, at which point the metabolic activity declines and reach the adult values again by the late 20s. The greatest age-associated metabolic changes occur in the thalamus and the anterior cingulate cortex. Cortical glucose metabolism declines with advancing age, particularly in the frontal lobes with either variable or no significant change in the other areas of the brain.

Hyperglycemia impairs cortical FDG uptake by the competition of glucose with FDG for the glucose receptors. Many drugs (e.g., benzodiazepines, antiepileptics) tend to decrease regional or global cerebral blood flow and glucose metabolism, which will need to be taken into account for proper image interpretation. Some drugs such as haloperidol may have mixed effects with increase in the cortical metabolic activity in some areas (cerebellum, putamen) and decrease in cortical metabolism in the other areas (frontal, occipital).

An imaging variant related to remote functional effect of a brain lesion is diaschisis. Diaschisis is referred to as the coupled reduction in both the cortical perfusion and the metabolism in an area of brain due to a remote brain lesion. This phenomenon usually involves the cerebellum (crossed cerebellar diaschisis) in relation to a contralateral supratentorial cerebral lesion. However, ipsilateral and contralateral subcortico-cortical (thalamocortical) diaschisis may also be observed.

EPILEPSY

Epilepsy is a relatively common and potentially devastating neurologic condition. Seizures can be classified as either partial or generalized. The generalized epilepsy is associated with diffuse epileptiform discharges and no focal brain lesions. In contrast, an epileptogenic focus causes the partial seizure. The 1990 National Institutes of Health Consensus Conference on Surgery for Epilepsy estimated that 10–20% of epilepsy cases prove medically intractable and that 2,000–5,000 epilepsy patients per year can benefit from surgical resection of the seizure focus.

Accurate preoperative localization of the epileptogenic region is a crucial task, which is best accomplished by combining the findings of clinical examination, electroencephalography (EEG), neuropsychological evaluation, and imaging studies. Computed tomography (CT) and magnetic resonance imaging (MRI) are used to detect structural lesions which may be the epileptogenic regions. Ictal or interictal single-photon emission tomography (SPECT) evaluation of regional cerebral blood flow (rCBF) can also localize the epileptogenic region even in the absence of discernable structural abnormalities on anatomic imaging studies. The characteristic appearance of an epileptogenic region is relative zonal hyperperfusion on ictal SPECT and relative zonal hypoperfusion on interictal SPECT. The sensitivity of ictal rCBF tracer SPECT may approach 90%, while that of interictal SPECT is in the range of 50%.

FDG PET has proven useful in preoperative localization of the epileptogenic region (Fig. 1). The best results have been obtained in epilepsy of temporal lobe origin corresponding to mesial temporal sclerosis, for which CT and MRI have relatively low sensitivity, but metabolic abnormalities may be evident in as many as 90% of surgical candidates. Surgical excision of this focus usually results in the elimination of epilepsy or marked clinical improvement. Extratemporal epileptogenic regions may be regional or diffuse and are more difficult to identify on PET due to limited sensitivity.

FDG PET is generally performed following an interictal injection due to the relatively short half-life of F-18, which limits the window of opportunity during which it can be administered ictally. Also due to the brain-uptake time of FDG, the ictal FDG studies may show not only the seizure focus but also the

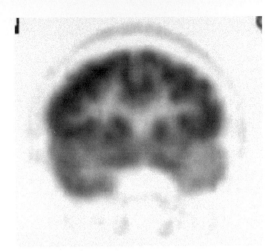

Figure 1: A 25-year-old woman with medically intractable epilepsy. An interictal PET scan shows asymmetric left temporal lobe hypometabolism corresponding to the epileptogenic area.

areas of seizure propagation. For interictal PET, FDG should be administered in a setting, such as a quiet room and dim lights, where environmental stimuli are minimal during the 30 min following FDG administration. Pharamacologic sedation is best withheld during the tracer uptake phase, since sedation may affect FDG distribution in the brain. The characteristic appearance of interictal FDG PET is regional hypometabolism at the location of the epileptogenic lesion. In order to avoid false lateralization from subclinical seizure, which results in spurious depression of tracer localization in the contralateral temporal lobe, concurrent EEG recording would be helpful. Additionally, the normal asymmetric metabolism of the temporal lobes (up to 15%) should be considered. The sensitivity of interictal FDG PET approaches that of ictal rCBF SPECT in localizing the epileptogenic region.

In addition to FDG, PET tracers that assess altered abundance or function of receptors, enzymes, and neurotransmitters in epileptogenic regions have been applied to localizing the epileptogenic region.

STROKE

CT and MRI are cornerstones of the imaging evaluation of stroke. PET with various tracers, however, allows the assessment of the pathophysiology of stroke through the evaluation of several important parameters, such as cerebral blood volume, cerebral blood flow, and cerebral oxidative and glucose metabolism.

The regional cerebral blood volume (CBV) may be imaged following the inhalation of C-11- or O-15-labeled carbon monoxide (CO) through the formation of carboxyhemoglobin. Cerebral blood flow (CBF) can be imaged by using intravenous O-15 water and inhaled O-15 carbon dioxide. The gray matter CBF is about three times greater than that of the white matter. The cerebral oxidative metabolism ($CMRO_2$) is measured using O-15 oxygen. $CMRO_2$ is calculated from the following relationship, where OEF represents the oxygen extraction fraction which increases as blood flow decreases:

$$CMRO_2 = CBF \times OEF \times \text{arterial blood oxygen concentration}$$

FDG is used to determine the cerebral glucometabolism. As described above, the gray matter displays much greater FDG uptake than the white matter.

Cerebral blood flow, oxidative metabolism, and glucometabolism are all normally linked in the normal brain. In stroke, however, uncoupling may occur. Both the amount and the duration of the reduction in cerebral blood flow determine if irreversible tissue damage occurs. In acute ischemic stroke, the identification of viable tissue (penumbra) is important for potential intervention in order to restore the blood flow. These areas correspond to "misery" perfusion areas where there is preservation of CMRO2 in view of decreased flow by increasing OEF. In subacute ischemia, some patients may have postischemic reactive hyperemia ("luxury" perfusion) at the periphery of the ischemic stroke. This phenomenon may represent recanalization of the occluded artery and is associated with increased CBF and low OEF. PET imaging assessments of rCBF, CBV, and $CMRO_2$ and glucose metabolism have been shown to aid in the clinical management decision-making by demonstrating the salvageable tissue at risk. PET can also provide a quantitative estimate of the cerebrovascular reserve by comparing the rest and the vasodilatory (e.g., acetazolamide) stress cerebral perfusion patterns. Prognosis may also be evaluated by FDG PET with the preserved glucometabolism associated with reversal of the neurologic deficits and a good clinical outcome. Table 1 below summarizes the changes in the various homodynamic parameters in relation to the clinical condition.

ALZHEIMER'S DISEASE

Alzheimer disease (AD) is a progressive neurodegenerative disorder associated with gradual decline in cognition and behavior. It is estimated that 8% of people over the age of 65 years suffer from AD and the prevalence climbs with increasing age. The neuropathologic (neurofibrillary tangles and neuritic plaques) spread of the disease progresses from transentorhinal to the limbic and then to the neocortical brain regions. Association cortices are more severely involved, while the primary somatosensory and motor cortices, the basal ganglia, the thalamus, and the cerebellum are relatively spared. Accurate early diagnosis of AD is important, since early use of medications such as cholinesterase inhibitors may improve or delay the cognitive loss that occurs in mild to moderate disease. Additionally, there may be a psychosocial benefit for the individ-

Table 1

Clinical Condition	CBF	OEF	CMRO2
Acute ischemia ("Misery" perfusion)	Low	High	Low~normal
Subacute Ischemia ("Luxury" perfusion)	~High	Low	Low
Chronic infarct	Low	Low~normal	Low

ual patient if the patient becomes aware of the diagnosis before the clinical manifestation of the disease.

FDG PET demonstrates reductions in the cerebral glucometabolism, which may occur a few years before the overt clinical manifestation of disease. A classical pattern is bilateral parietotemporal hypometabolism, which may be asymmetric (Fig. 2). FDG PET is particularly useful in differentiating the Alzheimer-type glucose metabolic pattern from the pattern of the other dementias and in this sense can aid with the differential diagnosis. FDG PET also has been shown to provide important prognostic information such that a negative PET scan is indicative of unlikely progression of cognitive impairment for a mean follow-up of 3 years in patients who initially present with cognitive symptoms of dementia. Other PET radiotracers directed toward imaging the cholinergic system and the neurofibrillary tangles may also prove useful in the future imaging diagnosis of AD.

PARKINSON'S DISEASE

Parkinson's disease (PD) is a progressive neurodegenerative disorder characterized by selective death of the dopaminergic neurons in the nigrostriatal pathway. The symptoms include motor disturbances of rigidity, bradykinesia, resting tremor, and postural imbalance, which occur after a loss of approximately 70%

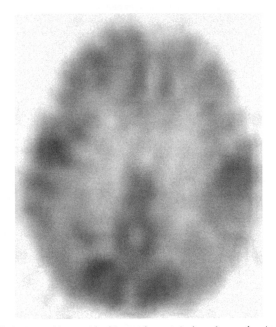

Figure 2: A 76 year old man with a history of progressive loss of comprehension and memory. CT of the brain demonstrated mild atrophy. PET scan demonstrates relatively symmetric marked hypometabolism of the frontal, parietal and temporal lobes with sparing of the sensory motor strips, occipital lobes, cerebellum (not shown), and deep gray matter (not shown) structures.

of the striatal dopaminergic neurons. Cognitive disorder may also be observed with a prevalence of dementia that can approach 40% of patients.

PET can image the presence and severity of dopaminergic neuronal loss and the terminal dysfunction in PD. Dopamine release during motor tasks can be evaluated by the changes in receptor availability to PET ligands. The functional effects of focal dopamine replacement via implantation of fetal cells into putamen can also be monitored. The loss of dopaminergic nerve terminals in the basal ganglia (putamen and caudate) can be assessed in vivo by PET imaging with [F-18]fluoro-DOPA (a radiolabeled analog of the dopamine precursor dihydroxyphenylalanine—FDOPA) to image the presynaptic dopamine metabolism, which is diminished in PD. Carbidopa, which inhibits the peripheral metabolism of the tracer by the enzyme DOPA decarboxylase, improves the brain uptake of FDOPA. Other PET radiotracers have also been investigated to assess the alterations in the D2 dopamine receptors (up-regulated in early PD) and the dopamine reuptake system. FDG PET may also demonstrate reductions in the glucometabolism of the basal ganglia (advanced PD) and the primary visual cortex in the occipital lobe with a relative preservation of the metabolic activity in the medial temporal lobe in contradistinction to AD.

HUNTINGTON'S DISEASE

Huntington's disease (HD) is a progressive autosomal dominant neurodegenerative disorder with complete penetrance characterized by chorea, psychiatric symptoms, and dementia. There is severe neuronal loss and atrophy of the caudate and putamen. FDG PET demonstrates hypometabolism in the caudate and putamen many years before the onset of the symptoms and before evidence for atrophic changes on CT or MRI. Other PET radiotracers such as C-11 raclopride (a specific marker of D2 dopamine receptor binding), have also been shown to be useful in detecting the presence and the severity of HD by demonstrating significant reductions in the striatal, frontal, and temporal tracer.

SCHIZOPHRENIA

Schizophrenia is a heterogeneous group of psychiatric disorders characterized by disturbances of thinking, mood, and behavior, which may be associated with altered concept of reality, inappropriate emotional responses, social withdrawal, delusions, and hallucinations. A commonly described finding in patients with chronic schizophrenia, especially those with paranoid features, is hypofrontality defined as hypometabolism and diminished CBF in the frontal cortex.

PET imaging of schizophrenia has also been based on the assessment of striatal dopamine transmission, including both the presynaptic and the postsynaptic functions. FDOPA PET has been studied to evaluate the presynaptic DOPA decarboxylase activity in patients with schizophrenia. It appears that in patients with paranoid symptoms there is an increase in dopamine synthesis, while conversely in patients with depressive symptoms (e.g., catatonia), there is low FDOPA accumulation. The postsynaptic striatal D2 receptor density has also been studied with PET extensively. In a recent meta-analysis, a small but significant increase in striatal D2 receptors was reported in patients with schizophrenia as demonstrated with various PET radiotracers, including C-11 raclopride and C-11-N-methyl-spiperone. C-11 raclopride PET imaging of striatal D2 receptors, however, has failed to demonstrate a relationship between the degree of D2-receptor occupancy and clinical response. The presynaptic striatal D1 receptor levels also appear to be relatively unaltered in schizophrenia. Additionally, studies with I-123-β-CIT and F-18-CFT have reported no significant difference in the striatal dopamine transporter (DAT) binding between schizophrenic patients and controls. PET imaging of the alterations in the serotoninergic and the γ-aminobutyric acid (GABA)-ergic systems may also prove important for monitoring schizophrenia in the future studies.

DEPRESSION

PET has been investigated in the evaluation of patients with depressive disorders. Radiolabeled PET tracers have been used to assess the serotoninergic system. In particular, 5-HT1A and 5-HT2A receptors and 5-HT transporters have been studied. Although overall findings suggest that there are no major alterations in the 5H2A receptor density and binding there appears to be a generalized decrease in the cortical 5-HT1A receptor binding in depression. Reductions in 5-HT transporter levels have also been observed in depression by postmortem studies, SPECT imaging with I-123-β-CIT, and PET imaging with various selective radiolabeled tracers. Additionally studies of the dopaminergic system in depression suggest that there is no consistent relationship except a potential relationship in some clinical conditions such as psychomotor retardation.

BIBLIOGRAPHY

1. Baron JC, Bonsser MG, Comar D, et al. Crossed cerebellar diaschisis in human supratentorial brain infarction. Trans Am Neurol Assoc 1980; 105:459–61.
2. Baron JC, D'Antona R, Pantano P, et al. Effects of thalamic stroke on energy metabolism of cerebral cortex. A positron tomography study in man. Brain 1986; 109:1243–59.
3. Bartlett EJ, Brodie JD, Simkowitz P, et al. Effects of haloperidol challenge on regional cerebral glucose utilization in normal human subjects. Am J Psychiatry 1994; 151:681–86.
4. Braak H, Braak E. Staging of Alzheimer's disease-related neurofibrillary changes. Neurobiol Aging 1995; 16:271–84.
5. Brooks DJ. PET studies on the function of dopamine in health and Parkinson's disease. Ann N Y Acad Sci. 2003; 991:22–35.
6. Cochen V, Ribeiro MJ, Nguyen JP, et al. Transplantation in Parkinson's disease: PET changes correlate with the amount of grafted tissue. Mov Disord. 2003; 18:928–32.
7. Cummings TJ, Chugani DC, Chugani HT. Positron emission tomography in pediatric epilepsy. Neurosurg Clin North Am 1995; 6:465–472.
8. Derdeyn CP, Grubb RLJ, Powers WJ. Cerebral hemodynamic impairment: methods of measurement and association with stroke risk. Neurology 1999; 53:251–259.
9. Engel J Jr, Kuhl DE, Phelps ME. Patterns of human local cerebral glucose metabolism during epileptogenic seizures. Science 1982; 218:64–66.
10. Feigin A, Leenders KL, Moeller JR, et al. Metabolic network abnormalities in early Huntington's disease: an [(18)F]FDG PET study. J Nucl Med 2001; 42:1591–5.
11. Heiss WD, Herholz K. Assessment of pathophysiology of stroke by positron emission tomography. Eur J Nucl Med 1994; 21:455–465.
12. Hietala J, Syvalahti E, Vickman H, et al. Depressive symptoms and presynaptic dopamine function in neuroleptic-naïve schizophrenia. Schizophr Res 1999; 35:41–50.

13. Karlsson P, Farde L, Halldin C, et al. D1-dopamine receptors in schizophrenia examined by PET. Schizophr Res 1997; 24:179.

14. Kushner M, Reivich M, Fieschi C, et al. Metabolic and clinical correlates of acute ischemic infraction. Neurology 1987; 37:1103–10.

15. Laakso A, Vilkman H, Alakare B, et al. Striatal dopamine transporter binding in neuroleptic-naïve patients with schizophrenia studied with positron emission tomography. Am J Psychiatry 2000; 157:269–71.

16. Laruell M, Abi-Dargham A, van Dyck C, et al. Dopamine and serotonin transporters in patients with schizophrenia: an imaging study with I-123-beta-CIT. Biol Psychiatry 2000; 47:371–79.

17. Lewis DA. GABAergic local circuit neurons and prefrontal cortical dysfunction in schizophrenia. Brain Res Rev 2000; 31:270–76.

18. Loessner A, Alavi A, Lewandrowski KU, et al. Regional cerebral function determined by FDG-PET in healthy volunteers: normal patterns and changes with age. J Nucl Med 1995; 36:1141–49.

19. Martinot M, Bragulat V, Artiges E, et al. Decreased presynaptic dopamine function in the left caudate of depressed patients with affective flattening and psychomotor retardation. Am J Psychiatry 2001; 158:314–16.

20. Mayeux R, Stern Y, Rosenstein R, et al. An estimate of the prevalence of dementia in idiopathic Parkinson's disease. Arch Neurol 1988; 45:260–62.

21. McMahon PM, Araki SS, Sandberg EA, et al. Cost-effectiveness of PET in the diagnosis of Alzheimer disease. Radiology. 2003; 228(2):515–22.

22. Meltzer CC, Cantwell MN, Greer PJ, et al. Does cerebral blood flow decline in healthy aging? A PET study with partial volume correction. J Nucl Med 2000; 41:1842–48.

23. Meyer JH, kapur S, Houle S, et al. Prefrontal cortex 5-HT2 receptors in depression: an [18F]septoperone PET imaging study. Am J Psychiatry 1999; 156:1029–34.

24. National Institutes of Health Consensus Development Conference Statement: surgery for epilepsy. Epilepsia. 1990; 31:806–812.

25. Ngan ET, Yatham LN, Ruth TJ, et al. Decreased serotonin 2A receptor densities in neuroleptic-naïve patients with schizophrenia: a PET study using [F-18]setoperone. Am J Psychiatry 2000; 157:1016–18.

26. Pavese N, Andrews TC, Brooks DJ, et al. Progressive striatal and cortical dopamine receptor dysfunction in Huntington's disease: a PET study. Brain. 2003; 126(Pt 5):1127–35.

27. Petrella JR, Coleman RE, Doraiswamy PM. Neuroimaging and early diagnosis of Alzheimer disease: a look to the future. Radiology 2003; 226:315–36.

28. Reith J, Benkelfat C, Sherwin A, et al. Elevated dopa decarboxylase activity in living brain of patients with psychosis. Proc Natl Acad Sci USA 1994; 91:11651–54.

29. Sargent PA, Kjaer KH, Bench CJ, et al. Brain serotonin(1A) receptor binding measured by positron emission tomography with [11C]WAY-100635: effects of depression and antidepressant treatment. Arch Gen Psychiatry 2000; 57:174–180.

30. Shinotoh H, Namba H, Fukushi K, et al. Progressive loss of cortical acetylcholinesterase activity in association with cognitive decline in Alzheimer's disease: a positron emission tomography study. Ann Neurol. 2000; 48:194–200.

31. Shoghi-Jadid K, Small GW, Agdeppa ED, et al. Localization of neurofibrillary tangles and beta-amyloid plaques in the brains of living patients with Alzheimer disease. Am J Geriatr Psychiatry. 2002; 10:24–35.

32. Silverman DH, Gambhir SS, Huang HW, et al. Evaluating early dementia with and without assessment of regional cerebral metabolism by PET: a comparison of predicted costs and benefits. J Nucl Med 2002; 43:253–66.

33. Silverman DH, Small GW, Chang CY, et al. Positron emission tomography in evaluation of dementia: Regional brain metabolism and long-term outcome. JAMA. 2001; 286:2120–7.

34. Takahashi T, Shirane R, Sato S, et al. Development changes of cerebral blood flow and oxygen metabolism in children. Am J Neuroradiol 1999; 20:917–22.

35. Tatlidil R, Luther S, West A, et al. Comparison of fluorine-18 deoxyglucose and O-15 water PET in temporal lobe epilepsy. Acta Neurol Belg 2000; 100:214–20.
36. Theodore WH. Antiepileptic drugs and cerebral glucose metabolism. Epilepsia 1988; 29[suppl 2]:S48–S55.
37. Treves ST, Connolly LP. Single photon emission computed tomography in pediatric epilepsy. Neurosurg Clin North Am 1995; 6:473–480.
38. Van Bogaert P, Wikler D, Damhaut P, et al. Regional changes in glucose metabolism during brain development from age of 6 years. Neuroimage 1998; 8:62–68.
39. Vercouillie J, Tarkiainen J, Halldin C, et al. Precursor synthesis and radiolabeling of [11C]ADAM: a potent radioligand for the serotonin transporter exploration by PET. J labeled Compounds Radiopharm 2001; 44:113–20.
40. Volkow ND, Fowler JS. Neuropsychiatric disorders: investigation of schizophrenia and substance abuse. Semin Nucl Med 1992; 22(4):254–267.
41. Weinberger DR, Laruelle M. Neurochemical and neuropharmacological imaging in schizophrenia, in neuropharmacology. In: Davis KL, Charney DS, Coyle JT, et al, eds., The fifth generation of progress. Philadelphia, Lippincott Williams & Wilkins, 2001.
42. Wolkin A, Barouche F, Wolf AP, et al. Dopamine blockade and clinical response: evidence for two biological subgroups of schizophrenia. Am J Psychiatry 1989; 146:905–8.
43. Zakzanis KK, Graham SJ, Campbell Z. A meta-analysis of structural and functional brain imaging in dementia of the Alzheimer's type: a neuroimaging profile. Neuropsychol Rev. 2003; 13(1):1–18.

4

5

Oncology—Brain

Primary brain tumors are classified according to the cell of origin (e.g., neuroepithelial, meningeal, etc.). Neuroepithelial tumors in adults compose more than 90% of primary brain tumors. These tumors are collectively called gliomas and include astrocytoma, oligodendriogliomas, and ependymomas. An increasing grade of tumor indicates an increasing degree of malignancy.

CT and MRI are commonly performed imaging procedures to delineate the location, size, and vascularity of the tumor. Gliomas are often heterogeneous with intermixed areas of low- and high-grade neoplastic cells, hemorrhage, and necrosis. Primary treatment usually involves surgical resection followed by observation, adjuvant external beam radiotherapy, radiosurgery, brachytherapy, or chemotherapy. Anatomic imaging is typically employed for follow-up and assessment of therapy response. However, there are serious limitations of anatomic imaging in differentiating residual or recurrent tumor from post-therapy anatomic alterations. Functional imaging such as PET improves on this distinction noninvasively and leads to cost-effective impact

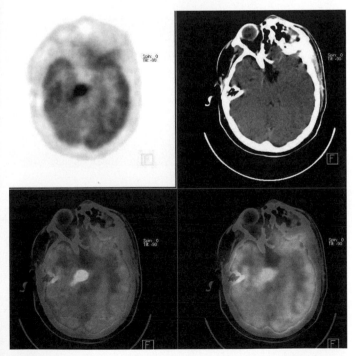

Figure 1: A 24-year-old male with brainstem glioma with subsequent radiation therapy. Intense hypermetabolism in the brainstem, right cerebral peduncle is consistent with recurrent high grade tumor.

on patient management and clinical outcome (Figs. 1–3). Many radiotracers have been employed with PET in the imaging evaluation of brain tumors. However, the bulk of the literature, similar to that for other tumors, has been with FDG.

The patient preparation for a FDG PET scan is similar regardless of the tumor type. Patients fast for at least four to six hours and should be well-hydrated. Hyperglycemia results in decreased cerebral FDG uptake and poor-quality images. For this reason, in patients with diabetes mellitus, the blood glucose level should be managed so that optimally the fasting blood glucose level is in the normal range. If the level is more than 200 mg/dl, the PET images may be degraded. Corticosteroids, which may be employed in patients with brain tumors for symptomatic relief of cerebral edema, can result in diminished brain glucose utilization independent of concurrent anticonvulsant medication, blood glucose level, cerebral atrophy, and any therapy. Sedatives may also reduce cerebral glucose metabolism.

FDG is administered intravenously while the patient rests in a quiet room with dim lights and minimal environmental stimulation during the uptake phase of 30–40 min before imaging acquisition. Cerebral cortical and subcortical gray matter and the cerebellar cortex demonstrate physiologic high glucose metabolic activity. For image interpretation, the metabolic activity of a lesion is compared relative to the physiologic low activity of the white matter with the

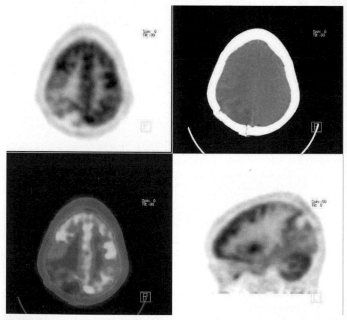

Figure 2: A 53-year-old female with glioblastoma multiforme treated with resection followed by cyber knife, gamma knife, and chemotherapy. PET-CT shows rim of moderately intense hypermetabolism surrounding an area of hypometabolism in the right posterior parietal region consistent with recurrent/residual tumor in the surgical bed.

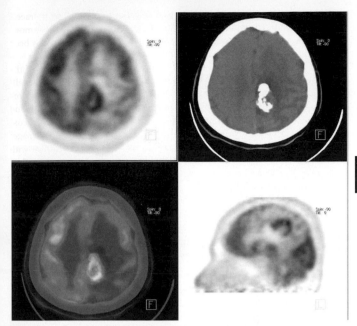

Figure 3: A 31-year-old male with a history of grade II left frontoparietal lobe oligodendroglioma that was treated with radiation therapy and gamma knife surgery. The patient now presents with aphasia and cognitive impairment. PET-CT shows an area of hypermetabolism in the left paramedian parietal lobe at the location of dense calcification seen on CT consistent with recurrent oligodendroglioma. There is decreased radiotracer activity in the left parietal cortex secondary to radiation therapy.

centrum semiovale of the contralateral cerebral hemisphere used as reference. High grade tumors (e.g., anaplastic astrocytoma, glioblastoma multiforme) demonstrate hypermetabolism while low-grade tumors show less than, equal to, or slightly higher than white matter metabolic activity.

Cerebellar diaschisis may also be seen with asymmetric cerebellar hemispheric hypometabolism contralateral to the remote primary supratentorial cerebral tumor. The mechanism of this observation is an interruption of the corticopontocerebellar pathway from the cerebral hemispheres through the ipsilateral pons to the opposite cerebellar cortex. There is no clinical correlate to the cerebellar diaschisis and it may be reversible in patients with stroke but often remains persistent in patients with brain tumors.

FDG PET has been shown to be useful in grading tumors, directing biopsy site and resection, assessing for malignant transformation of low-grade tumors, evaluating treatment response, and assessing for cerebral metastases in patients with other malignancies such as melanoma. FDG PET may also be useful in localizing hypermetabolic epileptogenic zones adjacent to the site of original tumor which are unrelated to recurrent tumor but responsible for focal or global neurologic impairment and nonconvulsive status epilepticus in patients with brain tumors.

Assessment for treatment response and detection of residual or recurrent tumor is the most common current utility of FDG PET in patients with brain tumor. Although it is not entirely clear when after therapy to perform a FDG PET scan to assess for response, reduction in lesion glucose metabolism and favorable response may be seen in as early as one week after chemotherapy. The detection of residual or recurrent tumor after high doses of local radiation with a gamma knife may occasionally be difficult due to the intense inflammatory response, which is induced as a result of the pathologic injury of radiation necrosis. However, even the histopathologic assessment may also be difficult due to heterogeneous distribution of distorted potentially viable tumor cells and necrotic cells. Further therapeutic decisions are best made in the individual clinical context.

Other PET radiotracers have also been investigated in evaluating brain tumors but none are currently used routinely. These tracers include but are not limited to [C-11]-methionine and [F-18]-fluorotyrosine (amino-acid transport), [F-18]-fluoromisonidazole (tumor hypoxia), [C-11]-thymidine (DNA incorporation), and [C-11]-choline (lipid metabolism). As PET imaging technology and PET radiochemistry evolve, these and other radiotracers may become more important in the diagnostic and prognostic imaging assessment of patients with brain tumors.

BIBLIOGRAPHY

1. Alavi JB, Alavi A, Chawluk J, et al. Positron emission tomography in patients with glioma: a predictor of prognosis. Cancer 1988; 62:1074–8.
2. Becherer A, Karanikas G, Szabo M, et al. Brain tumor imaging with PET: a comparison between [18F]fluorodopa and [11C]methionine. Eur J Nucl Med Mol Imaging 2003; 30:1561–7.
3. Blacklock JB, Oldfield EH, Di Chiro G, et al. Effect of barbiturate coma on glucose utilization in normal brain versus glioma. Positron emission tomography studies. J Neurosurg 1987; 67:71–5.
4. Coleman RE, Hoffman JM, Hanson MW, et al. Clinical application of PET for the evaluation of brain tumors. J Nucl Med 1991; 32:616–22.
5. Davis WK, Boyko OB, Hoffman JM, et al. [18F]2-fluoro-2-deoxyglucose positron emission tomography correlation of gadolinium-enhanced MR imaging of central nervous system neoplasia. AJNR 1993; 14:515–23.
6. De Witte O, Lefranc F, Levivier M, et al. FDG-PET as a prognostic factor in high-grade astrocytoma. J Neurooncol 2000; 49:157–63.
7. De Witte O, Levivier M, Violon P, et al. Prognostic value positron emission tomography with [18F]fluoro-2-deoxy-D-glucose in the low-grade glioma. Neurosurgery 1996; 39:470–6.
8. Derlon J-M, Petit-Taboue M-C, Chapon F, et al. The in vivo metabolic pattern of low-grade brain gliomas: a positron emission tomographic study using 18F-fluorodeoxyglucose and 11C-L-methylmethionine. Neurosurgery 1997; 40:276–88.
9. Di Chiro G, Brooks RA. PET-FDG of untreated and treated cerebral gliomas. J Nucl Med 1988; 29:421–22.
10. Di Chiro G, DeLaPaz R, Brooks RA, et al. Glucose utilization of cerebral gliomas measured by [18F]fluorodeoxyglucose and positron emission tomography. Neurology 1982; 32:1323–29.
11. Di Chiro G. Positron emission tomography using [F-18]fluorodeoxyglucose in brain tumors: a powerful diagnostic and prognostic too. Invest Radiol 1987; 22:360–71.
12. Di Chiro G. Which PET radiopharmaceutical for brain tumors [Editorial]. J Nucl Med 1991; 32:1346–8.

13. Di Chiro G, Oldfield E, Wright DC, et al. Cerebral necrosis after irradiation and/or intraarterial chemotherapy for brain tumors: PET and neuropathologic studies. AJNR 1987; 8:1083–9.
14. Doyle W, Budinger TF, Valk PE, et al. Differentiation of cerebral radiation necrosis from tumor recurrence by [18F]FDG and 82Rb positron emission tomography. J Comput Assisted Tomogr 1987; 11:563–70.
15. Eary JF, Mankoff DA, Spence AM, et al. 2-[C-11]thymidine imaging of malignant brain tumors. Cancer Res 1999; 59:615–21.
16. Francavilla TL, Miletich RS, Di Chiro G, et al. Positron emission tomography in the detection of malignant degeneration of low-grade gliomas. Neurosurgery 1989; 24:1–5.
17. Fulham MJ, Brunetti A, Aloj L, et al. Decreased cerebral glucose metabolism in patients with brain tumors: an effect of corticosteroids. J Neurosurg 1995; 83: 657–64.
18. Gaillard WD, Zeffiro T, Fazilat S, et al. Effect of valporate on cerebral metabolism and blood flow: an 18F-2-deoxyglucose and 15O water positron emission tomography study. Epilepsia 1996; 37:515–21.
19. Griffeth LK, Rich KM, Dehdashti F, et al. Brain metastases from non-central nervous system tumors: evaluation with PET. Radiology 1993; 186:37–44.
20. Guerin C, Laterra J, Drewes LR, et al. Vascular expression of glucose transporter in experimental brain neoplasms. Am J Pathol 1992; 140:417–25.
21. Hanson MW, Glantz MJ, Hoffman JM, et al. FDG-PET in the selection of brain lesions for biopsy. J Comput Assist Tomogr 1991; 15:796–801.
22. Hara T, Kondo T, Hara T, Kosaka N. Use of 18F-choline and 11C-choline as contrast agents in positron emission tomography imaging-guided stereotactic biopsy sampling of gliomas. J Neurosurg 2003; 99:474–9.
23. Herholz K, Holzer T, Bauer B, et al. 11C-methionine PET for differential diagnosis of low-grade gliomas. Neurology 1998; 50:1316–22.
24. Holzer T, Herholz K, Jeske J, et al. FDG PET as a prognostic indicator in radio-chemotherapy of glioblastoma. J Comput Assisted Tomogr 1993; 17:681–7.
25. Jacobs AH, Dittmar C, Winkeler A, et al. Molecular imaging of gliomas. Mol Imaging 2002; 1:309–35.
26. Kaschten B, Stevenaert A, Sadzot B, et al. Preoperative evaluation of 54 gliomas by PET with fluorine-18-fluorodeoxyglucose and/or carbon-11 methionine. J Nucl Med 1998; 39:778–85.
27. Kim CK, Alavi JB, Alavi A, et al. New grading system of cerebral gliomas using positron emission tomography with F-18 fluorodeoxyglucose. J Neurooncol 1991; 10:85–91.
28. Kleihues P, Burger PC, Scheithauer BW, et al. The new WHO classification of brain tumors. Brain Pathol 1993; 3:225–68.
29. Langleben DD, Segall GM. PET in differentiation of recurrent brain tumor from radiation injury. J Nucl Med 2000; 41:1861–7.
30. Levivier M, Goldman S, Pirotte B, et al. Diagnostic yield of stereotactic brain biopsy guided by positron emission tomography with [18F]fluorodeoxyglucose. J Neurosurg 1995; 82:445–52.
31. Lilja A, Lundqvist H, Olsson Y, et al. Positron emission tomography and computed tomography in differential diagnosis between recurrent or residual glioma and treatment-induced brain lesions. Acta Radiol 1989; 30:121–8.
32. Mirzaei S, Knoll P, Kohn H. Diagnosis of recurrent astrocytoma with fludeoxyglucose F18 PET scanning. N Engl J Med 2001; 344:2030–1.
33. Mosskin M, Ericson T, Hindmarsh T, et al. Positron emission tomography compared with magnetic resonance imaging and computed tomography in supratentorial gliomas using multiple stereotactic biopsies as reference. Acta Radiol 1989; 30:225–32.
34. Ogawa T, Shishido F, Kanno I, et al. Cerebral glioma: evaluation with methionine PET. Radiology 1993; 186:45–53.
35. Ohtani T, Kurihara H, Ishiuchi S, et al. Brain tumor imaging with carbon-11 choline: comparison with FDG PET and gadolinium-enhanced MR imaging. Eur J Nucl Med 2001; 28:1664–70.

36. Padma MV, Said S, Jacobs M, et al. Prediction of pathology and survival by FDG PET in gliomas. J Neurooncol 2003; 64:227–37.

37. Patronas NJ, Di Chiro G, Kufta C, et al. Prediction of survival in glioma patients by means of positron emission tomography. J Neurosurg 1985; 62:816–22.

38. Patronas NJ, Di Chiro G, Brooks RA, et al. Work in progress: [18F]fluorodeoxyglucose and positron emission tomography in the evaluation of radiation necrosis of the brain. Radiology 1982; 144:885–9.

39. Patronas NJ, Di Chiro G, Smith BH, et al. Depressed cerebellar glucose metabolism in supratentorial tumors. Brain Res 1984; 291:93–101.

40. Ribom D, Eriksson A, Hartman M, et al. Positron emission tomography (11)C-methionine and survival in patients with low-grade gliomas. Cancer 2001; 92:1541–9.

41. Roelcke U, Leenders KL. PET in neuro-oncology. J Cancer Res Clin Oncol 2001; 127:2–8.

42. Schifter T, Hoffman JM, Hanson MW, et al. Serial FDG PET studies in the prediction of survival in patients with primary brain tumors. J Comput Assisted Tomogr 1993; 17:509–16.

43. Thompson TP, Lunsford LD, Kondziolka D. Distinguishing recurrent tumor and radiation necrosis with positron emission tomography versus stereotactic biopsy. Stereotact Funct Neurosurg 1999; 73(1–4):9–14.

44. Tralins KS, Douglas JG, Stelzer KJ, et al. Volumetric analysis of 18F-FDG PET in glioblastoma multiforme: prognostic information and possible role in definition of target volumes in radiation dose escalation. J Nucl Med 2002; 43:1667–73.

45. Tsuyuguchi N, Sunada I, Iwai Y, et al. Methionine positron emission tomography of recurrent metastatic brain tumor and radiation necrosis after stereotactic radio-surgery: is a differential diagnosis possible? J Neurosurg 2003; 98:1056–64.

46. Tyler JL, Diksic M, Villemure J-G, et al. Metabolic and hemodynamic evaluation of gliomas using positron emission tomography. J Nucl Med 1987; 28:1123–33.

47. Valk PE, Budinger TF, Levin VA, et al. PET of malignant cerebral tumors after inter-stitial brachytherapy: demonstration of metabolic activity and clinical outcome. J Neurosurg 1988; 69:830–8.

48. Valk PE, Mathis CA, Prados MD, et al. Hypoxia in human gliomas: demonstration by PET with florine-18-fluoromisonidazole. J Nucl Med 1992; 33:2133–7.

49. Vander Borght T, Pauwels S, Lambotte L, et al. Brain tumor imaging with PET and 2-[carbon-11]thymidine. J Nucl Med 1994; 35:974–82.

50. Wong TZ, van der Westhuizen GJ, Coleman RE. Positron emission tomography imaging of brain tumors. Neuroimaging Clin N Am 2002; 12:615–26.

Oncology—Head, Neck, and Thyroid

I. HEAD AND NECK

Head and neck cancers are increasing in incidence and are associated with excess alcohol ingestion and tobacco use. The most common histology is squamous cell carcinoma. Prognosis depends on the stage of disease. Cervical lymph nodes represent the major lymph drainage of the head and neck. In 1–5% of patients with cervical lymph node metastases, the site of the head and neck primary tumor remains unknown despite thorough diagnostic evaluation.

Most primary head and neck malignancies are discernible through complete office examination. Diagnostic evaluation includes fine-needle aspiration of the neck mass, chest roentgenography, computed tomography (CT), and/or magnetic resonance imaging (MRI) of the head and neck, followed by panendoscopy and biopsies. The primary tumor will be detected in approximately 40% of patients. Approximately 80% of cancers are located in the base of the tongue or tonsillar fossa. Management options depend on the extent of disease and may be multimodal including surgery and radiation therapy for early disease and chemotherapy for advanced disease. Functional imaging with FDG PET has been shown to be useful in the detection of the primary tumor site in patients with metastatic cervical adenopathy, initial staging of disease, differentiation of post-therapy changes from residual and recurrent disease, monitoring of tumor response to therapy, detection of synchronous lung lesions, and in prognostication (Fig. 1).

Unique preparation attributes in this group of patients include potential oral administration of diazepam (5–10 mg orally) given 30 min to 1 h prior to intravenous FDG injection to reduce physiologic skeletal muscle uptake that may mimic or obscure nodal disease. Patients are also instructed not to chew, talk, and move head or dry–swallow excessively during the FDG uptake phase. Drinking a glass of water prior to imaging will diminish the retained salivary activity in the mouth and upper esophagus. Comfortable ambient temperature will reduce tracer uptake in brown fat. Dental implants and non-removable bridgework can cause artifacts in attenuation-corrected images using either the Ge-68 transmission source or the CT scan obtained with a hybrid PET/CT imaging system. Examination of the non-attenuation-corrected PET images helps in the recognition of this artifact in patients undergoing PET of the head and neck. Furthermore, one should also be aware of the physiologic distribution of FDG in the head and neck. Palatine tonsils and adenoids may display relatively high symmetric hypermetabolism, especially in children and young adults. FDG localizations in the normal laryngeal tissue and the salivary glands are symmetric and low, with benign lesions typically displaying only slight increases in FDG uptake.

Squamous cell carcinoma is highly FDG avid. PET with FDG complements anatomic imaging modalities such as CT and MRI in accurately detecting the presence and extent of primary tumor and regional nodal metastases, especially in borderline or normal-sized nodes. Unsuspected distant metastases may also be detected which may lead to significant changes in treatment options.

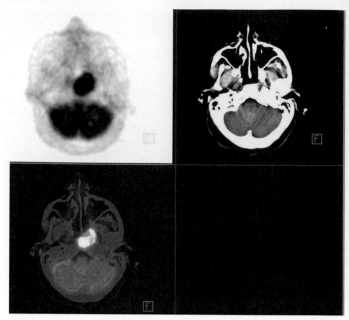

Figure 1: A 44-year-old woman with nasopharyngeal squamous cell carcinoma. PET-CT demonstrates intense hypermetabolism in the primary tumor. There was no evidence of regional and distant metastatic disease.

PET has been shown to be useful in localizing the site of unknown primary tumor in 20–35% of patients with metastatic cervical lymphadenopathy and an occult head and neck tumor leading to treatment-related implications on up to 25% of these patients. However, false-positive results may result due to inflammation or infection and small or superficial (submucosal) tumors may be missed.

The biggest advantage of PET over conventional imaging modalities is in the evaluation of patients after treatment for detection of residual or recurrent disease (Figs. 2, 3). The treatment-related anatomic alterations and edema reduce the accuracy of CT and MRI in the post-therapy setting. FDG PET has been shown to be more sensitive and specific than both CT and MRI in this clinical setting. The timing of PET scanning after therapy is an important factor to improve the specificity of PET in differentiating acute post-therapy inflammatory changes from tumor. Whole-body PET scanning approximately six weeks after completion of a combined treatment regimen with radiation and chemotherapy can reliably identify locoregional residual cancer and distant metastases or secondary tumors in patients with advanced-stage disease which may then lead to changes in clinical management. The timing is, however, more critical after head and neck radiation therapy, since this form of treatment induces an intense inflammatory reaction. PET scanning after a delay of at least 12 weeks from the completion of radiation therapy seems to be the optimal

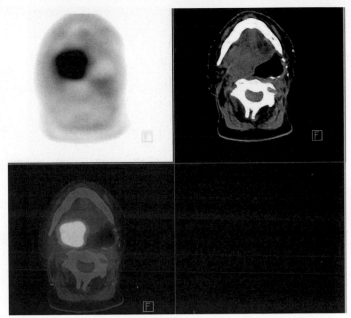

Figure 2: A 75-year-old male with recurrent squamous cell carcinoma treated initially with total laryngectomy and partial pharyngectomy followed by radiation therapy. PET-CT shows a large hypermetabolic soft tissue mass in the oropharynx which involves the right lateral and posterior oropharyngeal wall as well as the tongue base.

time as it allows early assessment for response while reducing the false-positive results.

A decline in FDG accumulation has been shown to be correlated with favorable treatment response, improved local control, and longer survival. Lesions that demonstrate persistent high FDG uptake indicate resistant disease that may require modification of the therapeutic approach. FDG PET in the early phase of treatment of HNSCC is associated with In other clinical scenarios, FDG-PET can contribute to the detection of residual/early recurrent tumors, leading to potential institution of salvage therapy and prevention of unnecessary tissue samplings which may aggravate injury.

The clinical experience with PET-CT in the imaging evaluation of patients with head and neck cancer is currently limited. However, PET-CT appears to be superior to PET, and probably also to PET and CT viewed side by side. In particular, PET-CT may be widely used for treatment planning for radiation therapy. PET-CT has the potential for reducing tissue misses, to minimize the dose of ionizing radiation applied to non-target areas, and to incorporate both anatomic and metabolic features of cancer into the three-dimensional conformal radiation therapy planning, which may then affect treatment outcome favorably. The exact clinical utility of the other PET radiotracers such as C-11 methionine, C-11 tyrosine, and Cu-62 ATSM (diacetyl-bis(N(4)-methylthiosemicarbazone) also remain to be established.

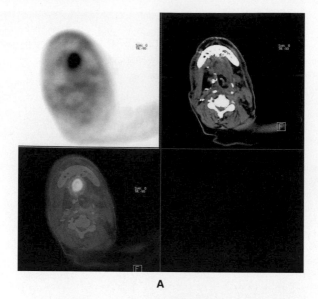

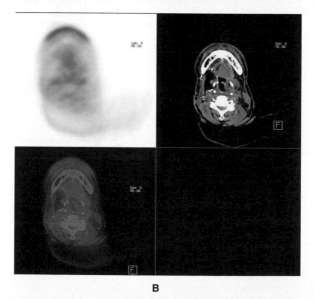

Figure 3: An 8-year-old male with tongue carcinoma treated with partial glossectomy and partial supraglottic laryngectomy followed by radiation. **A.** Pre-therapy PET-CT shows intense focal hypermetabolism in the primary at the tongue base. **B.** Post-therapy PET-CT demonstrates treatment-related anatomic changes but no evidence for residual or recurrent tumor.

II. THYROID CANCER

The usual presentation of thyroid cancer is a palpable nodule or a cervical lymph node discovered on physical examination. Dominant nodules in multinodular goiter, nodules that are increasing in size, and thyroid nodules in men convey greater risk for cancer. The prognosis of thyroid cancer is affected by many factors including gender, age, histology, and extent of disease. Thyroid carcinomas arise from follicular epithelium (papillary, follicular, anaplastic) or from parafollicular cells (medullary). Rare thyroid cancers include lymphoma and squamous cell carcinoma. Initial diagnosis is usually made by needle aspiration or biopsy.

The normal thyroid gland typically demonstrates no or low FDG accumulation. Focal hypermetabolism may indicate benign autonomous nodules or otherwise unknown malignancy (Figs. 4, 5). Overexpression of GLUT1 on the cell membrane of thyroid neoplasms has been shown to be closely related to more aggressive biological behavior. In patients with thyroid cancer, the standard therapy is thyroidectomy followed by radioiodine (I-131) ablation. Patients are followed for evidence of recurrent or metastatic disease based on serial physical examination and monitoring of serum thyroglobulin (Tg) level. It has been noted that occasionally the diagnostic radioiodine scan may be negative in view of high clinical suspicion for disease (e.g., high Tg level or abnormal physical findings). In these situations, other nuclear studies have been employed using Tc-99m tetrofosmin, Tc-99m sestamibi, In-111 octreotide, thallium-201, and FDG. While well-differentiated thyroid cancer may show low FDG uptake and good iodine avidity, poorly differentiated malignancy and

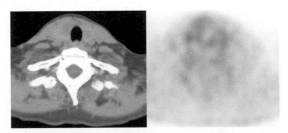

Figure 4: Multinodular Goiter. FDG-PET/CT in a patient with bilateral follicular adenomas does not show abnormal FDG uptake.

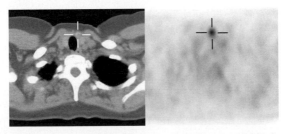

Figure 5: Papillary Cancer. FDG-PET/CT of a 0.7-cm papillary cancer of the thyroid.

tumors such as anaplastic carcinoma and Hurthle cell carcinoma tend to demonstrate high FDG accumulation and no iodine accumulation ("flip-flop" phenomenon) (Figs. 6–10).

Many studies have now documented the diagnostic utility of FDG PET in localizing the non-iodine avid metastases in up to 70% of patients and it is most

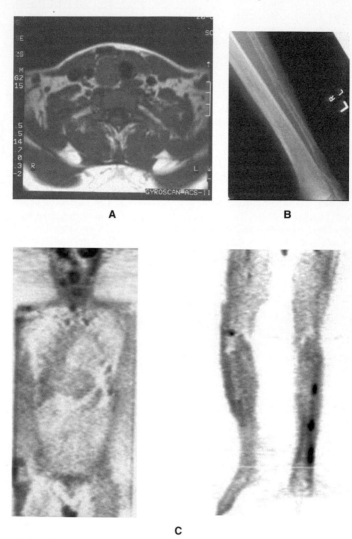

Figure 6: A 21-year-old man with thyroid cancer who presented with fracture of the left fibula. **A.** Neck MRI shows right thyroid lobe mass. **B.** Left lower extremity radiograph shows lytic lesions in the fibula. **C.** PET shows focal hypermetabolism corresponding to the primary tumor in the neck and the metastatic lesions in the left fibula with an additional unsuspected lesion in the right distal femur.

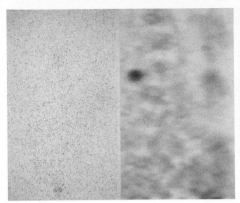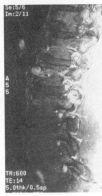

Figure 7: A male patient with history of thyroid cancer s/p total thyroidectomy who presents with elevated serum thyroglobulin level. Whole-body I-131 radioiodine scan is negative (left panel) while sagittal PET (middle panel) shows a focal hypermetabolic lesion in the lumbar spine corresponding to a paravertebral lesion on lumbar spine MRI (right panel). Excisional biopsy demonstrated recurrent thyroid cancer.

promising at Tg levels of >10 µg/L. The localization of disease may be amenable to local surgical or radiotherapeutic intervention without resort to systemic therapy. Earlier studies showed that the efficacy of FDG PET in localizing disease may not depend on the presence of high serum thyroid-stimulating hormone (TSH) level. However, recent reports indicate that endogenous TSH stimulation or exogenous recombinant TSH (rhTSH) stimulation improves the detectability of occult thyroid metastases with FDG PET in comparison with scans performed on TSH suppression. FDG PET has also been shown to have prognostic utility. Patients with positive PET studies, high rates of FDG accumulation in the lesions, and overall high volume of FDG-avid disease (>125 ml) have reduced survival in comparison to those patients without these findings. In patients with medullary thyroid cancer, FDG PET has been shown to be the most sensitive and specific single modality for localizing metastases in the clinical setting of increased serum calcitonin level. Recent studies have also demonstrated the utility of the combined PET-CT imaging systems for the diagnosis and anatomic localization of recurrent and metastatic thyroid cancer.

In summary, with the recent support of the Center for Medicare and Medicaid Services, it is expected that FDG PET will continue to have a growing role in the imaging assessment of patients with thyroid cancer, specifically in thyroidectomized patients with rising serum Tg levels and negative radioiodine scan.

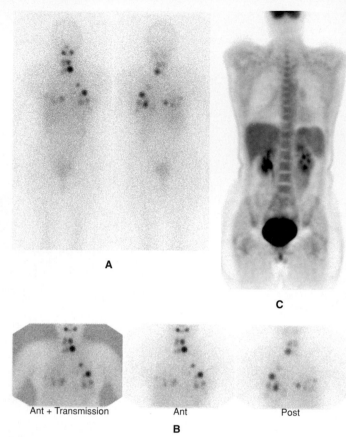

Figure 8: Papillary Cancer Pulmonary Metastases. Twenty-two years after papillary thyroid cancer, a 35-year-old woman presented for recurrent cancer in neck nodes. **A.** A whole body scan after therapy with iodine-131 showed several pulmonary metastases. **B.** Images of the chest in the anterior and posterior projection with a transmission scan to outline the chest cavity again show the pulmonary metastases. **C.** An FDG-PET scan showed no uptake in the lungs (A thick coronal section is shown.). FDG may be negative with iodine-avid metastatic thyroid cancer.

BIBLIOGRAPHY

Head and Neck Cancer

1. Anzai Y, Carroll WR, Quint DJ, et al. Recurrence of head and neck cancer after surgery or irradiation: prospective comparison of 2-deoxy-2-[F-18]fluoro-D-glucose PET and MR imaging diagnoses. Radiology 1996; 200:135–41.
2. Brun E, Kjellen E, Tennvall J, et al. FDG PET studies during treatment: prediction of therapy outcome in head and neck squamous cell carcinoma. Head Neck 2002; 24:127–35.

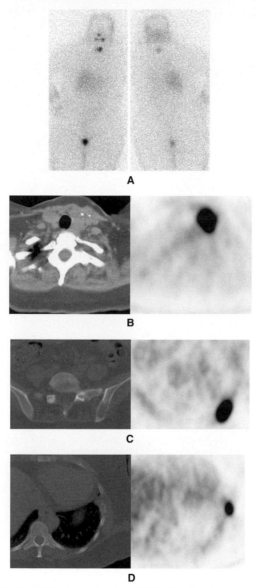

Figure 9: Hurthle Cell Carcinoma. A patient with Hurthle cell carcinoma was treated with 1.1 GBq (30 mCi) of iodine-131 for a large residual after a completion thyroidectomy. Anterior and posterior images (**A**) after therapy with 6.8 GBq (185 mCi) of I-131 show residual uptake in the thyroid bed representing residual remnant and/or cancer. There is no focal uptake in the illium or ribs. FDG-PET/CT three months later shows focal uptake in the thyroid bed (**B**), in the illium (**C**), and in a right rib (**D**). Hurthle cell carcinoma is typically not iodine-avid but shows intense FDG avidity.

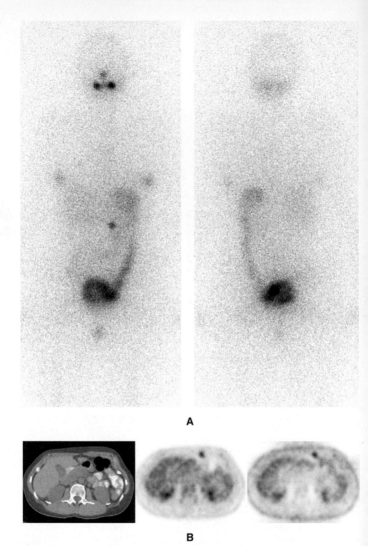

A

B

Figure 10: Abdominal Wall Thyroid Cancer Metastasis. **A.** Whole body I-131 scan seven days after therapy with 104 mCi of I-131 shows a focus of activity corresponding to an abdominal wall mass. **B.** FDG-PET/CT shows focal uptake of FDG in a mass in the rectus muscle.

3. Chisin R, Macapinlac HA. The indications of FDG-PET in neck oncology. Radiol Clin North Am 2000; 38:999–1012.
4. Ciernik IF, Dizendorf E, Baumert BG, et al. Radiation treatment planning with an integrated positron emission and computer tomography (PET/CT): a feasibility study. Int J Radiat Oncol Biol Phys 2003; 57:853–63.

5. Fukui MB, Blodgett TM, Meltzer CC. PET/CT imaging in recurrent head and neck cancer. Semin Ultrasound CT MR 2003; 24(3):157–63.

6. Goerres GW, Hany TF, Kamel E, et al. Head and neck imaging with PET and PET/CT: artifacts from dental metallic implants. Eur J Nucl Med Mol Imaging 2002; 29(3):367–70.

7. Goerres GW, Schmid DT, Bandhauer F, et al. Positron emission tomography in the early follow-up of advanced head and neck cancer. Arch Otolaryngol Head Neck Surg 2004; 130:105–9.

8. Goerres GW, Von Schulthess GK, Hany TF. Positron emission tomography and PET-CT of the head and neck: FDG uptake in normal anatomy, in benign lesions, and in changes resulting from treatment. AJR Am J Roentgenol 2002; 179:1337–43.

9. Goerres GW, von Schulthess GK, Steinert HC. Why most PET of lung and head-and-neck cancer will be PET/CT. J Nucl Med 2004; 45(Suppl 1):66S–71S.

10. Greven KM, Williams DW 3rd, McGuirt WF Sr, et al. Serial positron emission tomography scans following radiation therapy of patients with head and neck cancer. Head Neck 2001; 23:942–6.

11. Hanasono MM, Kunda LD, Segall GM, et al. Uses and limitations of FDG positron emission tomography in patients with head and neck cancer. Laryngoscope 1999; 109:880–5.

12. Hannah A, Scott AM, Tochon-Danguy H, et al. Evaluation of 18 F-fluorodeoxyglucose positron emission tomography and computed tomography with histopathologic correlation in the initial staging of head and neck cancer. Ann Surg 2002; 236:208–17.

13. Jadvar H, Segall GM, Norbash AM. Unknown head and neck primary tumors: identification with F-18 FDG PET. Radiology 1996; 201(P):239.

14. Johansen J, Eigtved A, Buchwald C, et al. Implication of 18F-fluoro-2-deoxy-D-glucose positron emission tomography on management of carcinoma of unknown primary in the head and neck: a Danish cohort study. Laryngoscope 2002; 112:2009–14.

15. Jungehulsing M, Scheidhauer K, Damm M, et al. 2[F]-fluoro-2-deoxy-D-glucose positron emission tomography is a sensitive tool for the detection of occult primary cancer (carcinoma of unknown primary syndrome) with head and neck lymph node manifestation. Otolaryngol Head Neck Surg 2000; 123:294–301.

16. Keyes JW Jr, Watson NE Jr, Williams DW 3rd, et al. FDG PET in head and neck cancer. AJR Am J Roentgenol 1997; 169:1663–9.

17. Kubota K, Yokoyama J, Yamaguchi K, et al. FDG-PET delayed imaging for the detection of head and neck cancer recurrence after radio-chemotherapy: comparison with MRI/CT. Eur J Nucl Med Mol Imaging 2004. [Epub ahead of print]

18. Lapela M, Grenman R, Kurki T, et al. Head and neck cancer: detection of recurrence with PET and 2-[F-18]fluoro-2-deoxy-D-glucose. Radiology 1995; 197:205–11.

19. Lowe VJ, Dunphy FR, Varvares M, et al. Evaluation of chemotherapy response in patients with advanced head and neck cancer using [F-18]fluorodeoxyglucose positron emission tomography. Head Neck 1997; 19:666–74.

20. McGuirt WF, Greven K, Williams D III, et al. PET scanning in head and neck oncology: a review. Head Neck 1998; 20:208–15.

21. Regelink G, Brouwer J, de Bree R, et al. Detection of unknown primary tumors and distant metastases in patients with cervical metastases: value of FDG-PET versus conventional modalities. Eur J Nucl Med Mol Imaging 2002; 29:1024–30.

22. Schechter NR, Gillenwater AM, Byers RM, et al. Can positron emission tomography improve the quality of care for head-and-neck cancer patients? Int J Radiat Oncol Biol Phys 2001; 51(1):4–9.

23. Stoeckli SJ, Mosna-Firlejczyk K, Goerres GW. Lymph node metastasis of squamous cell carcinoma from an unknown primary: impact of positron emission tomography. Eur J Nucl Med Mol Imaging 2003; 30:411–6.

24. Wax MK, Myers LL, Gabalski EC, et al. Positron emission tomography in the evaluation of synchronous lung lesions in patients with untreated head and neck cancer. Arch Otolaryngol Head Neck Surg 2002; 128:703–7.

6

25. Yen RF, Hung RL, Pan MH, et al. 18-fluoro-2-deoxyglucose positron emission tomography in detecting residual/recurrent nasopharyngeal carcinomas and comparison with magnetic resonance imaging. Cancer 2003; 98:283–7.

Thyroid Cancer

1. Bockisch A, Brandt-Mainz K, Gorges R, et al. Diagnosis in medullary thyroid cancer with [18F]FDG-PET and improvement using a combined PET/CT scanner. Acta Med Austriaca 2003; 30:22–5.

2. Chin BB, Patel P, Cohade C, et al. Recombinant human thyrotropin stimulation of fluoro-D-glucose positron emission tomography uptake in well-differentiated thyroid carcinoma. J Clin Endocrinol Metab 2004; 89:91–5.

3. Conti PS, Durski JM, Bacqai F, et al. Imaging of locally recurrent and metastatic thyroid cancer with positron emission tomography. Thyroid 1999; 9:797–804.

4. Diehl M, Risse JH, Brandt-Mainz K, et al. Fluorine-18 fluorodeoxyglucose positron emission tomography in medullary thyroid cancer: results of a multicentre study. Eur J Nucl Med 2001; 28:1671–6.

5. Frilling A, Tecklenborg K, Gorges R, et al. Preoperative diagnostic value of [(18)F] fluorodeoxyglucose positron emission tomography in patients with radioiodine-negative recurrent well-differentiated thyroid carcinoma. Ann Surg. 2001; 234:804–11.

6. Gianoukakis AG, Karam M, Cheema A, Cooper JA. Autonomous thyroid nodules visualized by positron emission tomography with 18F-fluorodeoxyglucose: a case report and review of the literature. Thyroid 2003; 13:395–9.

7. Grunwald F, Kalicke T, Feine U, et al. Fluorine-18 fluorodeoxyglucose positron emission tomography in thyroid cancer: results of a multicentre study. Eur J Nucl Med 1999; 26:1547–52.

8. Helal BO, Merlet P, Toubert ME, et al. Clinical impact of (18)F-FDG PET in thyroid carcinoma patients with elevated thyroglobulin levels and negative (131)I scanning results after therapy. J Nucl Med 2001; 42:1464–9.

9. Jadvar H, McDougall IR, Segall GM. Evaluation of suspected recurrent papillary thyroid carcinoma with [18F]fluorodeoxyglucose positron emission tomography. Nucl Med Commun 1998; 19:547–554.

10. Kang KW, Kim SK, Kang HS, et al. Prevalence and risk of cancer of focal thyroid incidentaloma identified by 18F-fluorodeoxyglucose positron emission tomography for metastasis evaluation and cancer screening in healthy subjects. J Clin Endocrinol Metab 2003; 88:4100–4.

11. Khan N, Oriuchi N, Higuchi T, et al. PET in the follow-up of differentiated thyroid cancer. Br J Radiol 2003; 76:690–5.

12. Larson SM, Robbins R. Positron emission tomography in thyroid cancer management. Semin Roentgenol 2002; 37:169–74.

13. Lind P, Kresnik E, Kumnig G, et al. 18F-FDG-PET in the follow-up of thyroid cancer. Acta Med Austriaca 2003; 30:17–21.

14. Lowe VJ, Mullan BP, Hay ID, et al. 18F-FDG PET of patients with Hurthle cell carcinoma. J Nucl Med 2003; 44:1402–6.

15. McDougall IR, Davidson J, Segall GM. Positron emission tomography of the thyroid, with an emphasis on thyroid cancer. Nucl Med Commun 2001; 22:485–92.

16. Moog F, Linke R, Manthey N, et al. Influence of thyroid-stimulating hormone levels on uptake of FDG in recurrent and metastatic differentiated thyroid carcinoma. J Nucl Med 2000; 41:1989–95.

17. Muros MA, Llamas-Elvira JM, Ramirez-Navarro A, et al. Utility of fluorine-18-fluorodeoxyglucose positron emission tomography in differentiated thyroid carcinoma with negative radioiodine scans and elevated serum thyroglobulin levels. Am J Surg 2000; 179:457–61.

18. Petrich T, Borner AR, Otto D, et al. Influence of rhTSH on [(18)F]fluorodeoxyglucose uptake by differentiated thyroid carcinoma. Eur J Nucl Med Mol Imaging 2002; 29:641–7.

19. Schluter B, Bohuslavizki KH, Beyer W, et al. Impact of FDG PET on patients with differentiated thyroid cancer who present with elevated thyroglobulin and negative 131I scan. J Nucl Med 2001; 42:71–6.
20. Schonberger J, Ruschoff J, Grimm D, et al. Glucose transporter 1 gene expression is related to thyroid neoplasms with an unfavorable prognosis: an immunohistochemical study. Thyroid 2002; 12:747–54.
21. Van den Bruel A, Maes A, De Potter T, et al. Clinical relevance of thyroid fluorodeoxyglucose-whole body positron emission tomography incidentaloma. J Clin Endocrinol Metab 2002; 87:1517–20.
22. van Tol KM, Jager PL, Piers DA, et al. Better yield of (18)fluorodeoxyglucose-positron emission tomography in patients with metastatic differentiated thyroid carcinoma during thyrotropin stimulation. Thyroid 2002; 12:381–7.
23. Wang W, Larson SM, Fazzari M, et al. Prognsotic value of [18F]fluorodeoxyglucose positron emission tomographic scanning in patients with thyroid cancer. J Clin Endocrinol Metab 2000; 85:1107–13.
24. Wang W, Macapinlac H, Larson SM, et al. [18F]-2-fluor-2-deoxy-D-glucose positron emission tomography localizes residual thyroid cancer in patients with negative diagnostic (131I) whole body scans and elevated serum thyroglobulin levels. J Clin Endocrinol Metab 1999; 84:2291–02.
25. Zimmer LA, McCook B, Meltzer C, et al. Combined positron emission tomography/computed tomography imaging of recurrent thyroid cancer. Otolaryngol Head Neck Surg 2003; 128:178–84.

6

7

Oncology—Lungs

Lung cancer is the leading cause of cancer death for both men and women in the United States. The estimated incidence of cancer of the lung and bronchus for the United States for 2003 is 91,800 men and 80,100 women, with estimated deaths of 88,400 and 68,800, respectively. Most lung cancer is related to smoking. The incidence of lung cancer increased dramatically in the twentieth century following the increase in smoking in men at about the time of the First World War. In men, lung cancer peaked in the mid to late 1980s, and has shown in a slow decline in the 1990s. This decline is correlated with a slow decline in smoking several decades earlier. Smoking in women did not increase markedly until about the time of the Second World War. Lung cancer may have peaked in women, but it is yet to have shown an important decline.

About 30% of all cancer deaths in the United States are due to cigarette smoking, and about 31% of deaths attributable to smoking are caused by lung cancer. A nuclear medicine physician's greatest impact on lung cancer may occur by encouraging smoking cessation in patients, in employees, and among friends.

HISTOLOGY

Lung cancer histology is complex. The most common types of lung cancer histologies are squamous cell cancer, adenocarcinoma, bronchioloalveolar cancer, large cell cancer, and small cell cancer. However, often a lung cancer will have histological features of more than one type. This is particularly true for bronchioloalveolar cancer, which is considered a subtype of adenocarcinoma. The portions of the cancer that have a more ground-glass appearance on CT are often classified as bronchioloalveolar cancer on histology, and the portions that appear more solid on CT are often classified adenocarcinoma on histology.

Squamous cell cancer tends to be more centrally located. It is well known in radiology because of its tendency to cavitate. Squamous cell cancer, which accounts for about one-third of lung cancer, appears to be decreasing in frequency in the United States, although not in Europe. Adenocarcinoma is often located more peripherally. It has a tendency to metastasize relatively early both to regional lymph nodes and to the brain.

The major distinction in terms of both staging and therapy is between **small cell lung cancer** (SCLC) and the other common histologies, which are grouped together as **non-small cell lung cancer** (NSCLC). It is common to use the abbreviations, SCLC and NSCLC; however, one needs to be careful about the single letter "N." That single letter in the acronym makes a big difference in therapy and prognosis.

Small cell lung cancer represents about 20–25% of lung cancer. It is different from the other types of lung cancer in staging and therapy. It metastasizes much more commonly. At the time of diagnosis, there are often metastases. Even when bulk metastases are not present, it is usually assumed that microscopic metastases are present. A pattern that is suggestive of small cell lung cancer is a small primary lung lesion with bulky mediastinal adenopathy.

The other reasonably common lung tumor is **pulmonary carcinoid**. Pulmonary carcinoid histology is divided into typical carcinoid and atypical carcinoid, with the atypical carcinoid being more aggressive.

Lung cancers often display **neuroendocrine differentiation**. Most commonly the tumors with neuroendocrine differentiation are small cell lung cancer or carcinoid tumors; however, non-small cell lung cancer can also show neuroendocrine differentiation.

CLINICAL PRESENTATION

There are many different clinical presentations of lung cancer. Patients may present with a cough, wheezing, hemoptysis, or chest pain, which may be pleuritic. They may have hoarseness or dysphagia due to involvement of the recurrent laryngeal nerve. Anorexia, weight loss, and weakness are relatively common at presentation. There are several well-known syndromes associated with lung cancer. Patients may present with superior vena cava syndrome or with Pancoast's syndrome (Horne's syndrome, shoulder pain, muscle wasting, and edema due to vascular compression). Several paraneoplastic syndromes may occur—syndrome of inappropriate antidiuretic hormone (SIADH), ectopic ACTH production, hypercalcemia, and ectopic human chorionic gonadotropin (hCG) production. There can be hypertrophic osteoarthropathy with bony changes and clubbing. Patients may be hypercoagulable and may present with pulmonary embolism. Patients may have nonbacterial endocarditis. The Eaton-Lambert syndrome, in which there is proximal muscle weakness on an autoimmune basis, may be seen with small cell lung cancer.

FDG UPTAKE IN LUNG CANCER

In general, lung cancer is very FDG-avid. There is relatively low uptake in the surrounding lung. This is especially true for aerated lung, where only about one-third of the volume is lung tissue, the rest being air with no FDG activity. Non-aerated lung should have about three times the activity of aerated lung. An area of atelectasis or a nodule that has uptake equal to lung tissue on a weight basis will have more uptake than surrounding lung on a volume basis. Thus, a nodule should not be compared to the surrounding aerated lung, but rather to other solid tissue. The typical comparison is with mediastinal soft tissues or blood pool.

Two lung tumors, pulmonary carcinoid and bronchioloaveolar cell cancer, are well known to be less FDG-avid and are frequently listed as causes of false negatives on FDG-PET. Although it is important to remember that these tumors may be a cause of false-negative scans, many of them are positive on FDG-PET. Bronchioloaveolar cell lung cancers with a prominent solid component on CT are more likely to be FDG-avid. Atypical carcinoid tumors are more likely to be FDG-avid than typical carcinoid tumors. Thus, FDG uptake should not be used to exclude either of these tumors. Necrotic lesions show little FDG activity in the region of necrosis, and this could potentially be a cause of a false-negative study; however, typically there is an FDG-avid rim, which can be easily detected.

The FDG-avidity of lung cancer is a valuable prognostic factor: the more FDG-avid the cancer; the worse the prognosis (see below). Buck et al. showed that FDG uptake correlated with tumor proliferation as measured by Ki-67 immunostaining in 18 lung cancers. They also compared the uptake of FDG with F-18-fluorothymidine (FLT). Although FDG had higher mean uptake as measured by SUV, the FLT had a better correlation with tumor proliferation. Studies of FLT as a prognostic indicator have not yet been done. These two PET tracers may provide different insight into cancer metabolism.

SINGLE PULMONARY NODULE (SPN)

FDG-PET scanning has an important role in diagnosis of lung cancer. A frequent referral to FDG-PET is a patient with a known lung nodule. Some of these lung nodules are detected incidentally, some by screening, and some by a symptom-directed workup. Regardless of exactly how the nodule was discovered, the patient has a known pulmonary nodule and the task is to determine if the nodule is malignant. Figure 1 shows two patients—one with FDG-avid non-small cell lung cancer and one with a benign nodule.

Using a single pulmonary nodule (SPN) to refer to lung cancer diagnosis is a bit of a misnomer, since patients present with a spectrum of disease.

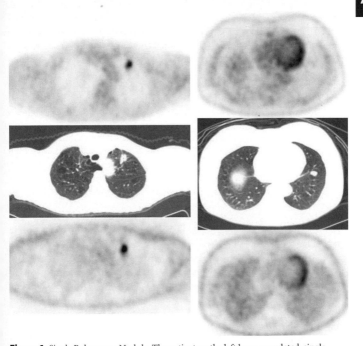

Figure 1: Single Pulmonary Nodule. The patient on the left has a speculated, single pulmonary nodule in the left upper lobe, which is FDG avid. Pathologically, this lesion was a poorly differentiated squamous cell cancer. The patient on the right has a lobular, single pulmonary nodule in the left lower lobe, which is not FDG avid. Six-month follow-up CT scan showed no change in the pulmonary nodule. On the top image is the attenuation corrected FDG-PET; in the middle image is the CT; and on the bottom image is the non-attenuation corrected FDG-PET.

Sometimes there is in fact only a single lung node. Sometimes there is a single dominant lung nodule with other small nodules (say, 2–6 mm). Sometimes there is more than one nodule in question. Sometimes there is other disease with a single suspicious nodule, e.g., a large, solid, speculated nodule. Pulmonary lesions, which are smaller than 3 cm and are surrounded by aerated lung, are called **pulmonary nodules**, while those that are greater than 3 cm are called **pulmonary masses**. However, the term *SPN* is sometimes also used to refer to these larger lesions. This section describes the evaluation of a lung lesion irrespective of whether there are other lung lesions and irrespective of size.

Resolution.   A key question is what size single pulmonary nodule can be reliably evaluated with FDG-PET. One answer is that FDG is hot spot imaging, so any size lesion can be seen so long as it is hot enough. However, the volume of a lesion goes as the cube of the dimension. A lesion that has one-half the diameter needs to have eight times the activity; a lesion that has one-quarter the diameter needs to have 64 times the activity. Thus, from a practical point of view, the size of the lesion is very important.

Miyaoka et al. performed a phantom study using a dual-head Anger camera PET. In that study, good sensitivity was obtained for lesions larger than about 15 mm. This size is compatible with a clinical study of dual-head Anger camera PET. For dedicated PET, lesions of about 8 mm can be detected with good sensitivity, although high-contrast lesions somewhat smaller in size can be detected in phantom studies. The ability to detect a small nodule will of course depend up the details of a particular situation. A lesion near the diaphragm where there is more motion will be more difficult to detect. A lesion adjacent to a hot myocardium will be more difficult to detect. Heavy patients are always harder to image than thin patients. A scan with a high noise equivalent count rate should out perform a scan with a low noise equivalent count rate. More avid lesions will be more readily detected. As a general rule of thumb, high sensitivity, say, 95%, can be achieved with dual-head Anger camera PET for a lesion of about 15 mm, and with dedicated PET for a lesion of about 8 mm. The potential trade-off between sensitivity and specificity is described below.

Criteria.   The standardized uptake value (SUV) has been used more extensively in lung cancer than in any other disease. The cut-off value between benign and malignant single pulmonary nodule in various studies has been in the range 2.0–2.5. Smaller lesions will have lower SUVs due to partial voluming. Most clinicians do not use the SUV directly, but rather compare the activity in the lesion to the mediastinal blood pool. A positive nodule has an uptake greater than the mediastinal blood pool. Using this internal control avoids errors in SUV calculations and the differences between normalizing for body weight, for lean body mass, or for surface area. Nonetheless, having an SUV value easily available during interpretation facilitates comparison with the mediastinal blood pool and provides a day-to-day normalization for the reader.

False-Positive Lesions.   Granulomatous disease is a common cause of false-positive single pulmonary nodule. Fungal granulomas due to coccidiomycosis, histoplasmosis, and aspergillosis are particularly common in patients who live or have lived in endemic areas. Coccidiomycosis is common in the San Joaquin Valley; in that region it is called valley fever. Histoplasmosis is common in the Ohio and Mississippi river basins. Granulomas due to tuberculosis are another cause of false positives. Sarcoidosis often has a characteristic pattern, but it can cause positive lung lesions.

Active infections are a cause of false positives when imaging for cancer. Often the pattern is not confused with a single pulmonary nodule on anatomic imaging, but occasionally post-infectious nodular findings can occur. Acute pulmonary infections can show marked FDG uptake. An endobronchial lesion can present as a chronic unresolved post-obstructive pneumonia. Typically, chronic post-obstructive pulmonary infections show relatively low level uptake. A very FDG-avid proximal lesion with an infiltrate with low-level FDG-avidity should make one think of this diagnosis. Figure 2 shows an example of a false-positive single pulmonary nodule.

Sensitivity and Specificity.   Gould et al. performed a meta-analysis to determine the accuracy of FDG-PET in the differentiation of benign and malignant pulmonary lesions. There is always a trade-off between sensitivity and specificity; so they used receiver operating characteristic methods to fit the data and pick an operating point. Using this methodology, they found that a sensitivity of 96.8% corresponded to specificity of 77.8%. Some very small, very FDG-avid lesions will be detected. However, in the 5–7 mm range, one should expect a decrease in sensitivity with the volume of the lesion. The specificity was more variable between the studies than the sensitivity. The variability in specificity may be due to different patient populations. In locations endemic for fungal granulomas, the specificity would be expected to be relatively low, whereas in locations with a low incidence of fungal granulomas, the specificity would be expected to be much higher.

The high sensitivity of FDG-PET is important clinically. A negative FDG-PET markedly reduces the chance that a lesion is malignant. This information may be adequate to obviate further clinical work-up. However, there are a few caveats to keep in mind. In the patient with a borderline-sized nodule or in whom there is a high suspicion of cancer, it may be wise to recommend further CT follow-up to assure two-year stability in size. If there are other smaller nodule(s), then it is important to follow-up these nodules. The FDG avidity of bronchioloaveolar cell cancer, especially pure bronchioloaveolar cell cancer, is reduced. In the case of a ground glass nodule, particularly a nodule with little

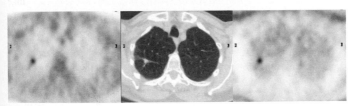

Figure 2: False-Positive Single Pulmonary Nodule. There was a persistent right upper lobe speculated nodule after resolution of pneumonia. The nodule was FDG avid. On pathology, the nodule was a necrotizing granuloma. On the left is the attenuation corrected FDG-PET; in the center is the CT; and on the right is the non-attenuation-corrected FDG-PET.

solid component, it may be wise to indicate the reduced sensitivity in the report and to recommend continued follow-up.

Competing Methods. There are several alternate methods of evaluating a single pulmonary nodule. A histological sample may be obtained from the nodule by transthoracic needle aspiration, by bronchoscopy with direct biopsy, transbronchial needle aspiration (TBNA) or bronchoalveolar lavage (BAL), or by surgical excision. Each of these methods has disadvantages. There is moderate morbidity from each procedure. Transthoracic needle aspiration is associated with pneumothorax, hemoptysis, and rarely air embolism. Methods using bronchoscopy are associated with hemoptysis, infection, and pneumothorax. Biopsy methods also suffer from sampling error. The complications associated with surgical excision depend on the method—video-assisted thoroscopic surgery (VATS) or thoracotomy. Depending up the exact location of the lesion, a biopsy may be more or less dangerous. However, the advantage of all of these methods is that they provide a histological sample.

A peripheral lesion, which is adherent to the chest wall, is ideal for transthoracic biopsy. An endobronchial lesion is ideal for bronchoscopy. A highly suspicious peripheral lesion, which is to be resected regardless of the findings on FDG, might be primarily resected. The details of a particular case often dictate the method that is most appropriate. However, in a large fraction of cases, FDG-PET will be the method of choice for characterizing a single pulmonary nodule.

STAGING

TNM Staging in Non-Small Cell Lung Cancer. Tumor (T), node (N), metastasis (M) staging is used for non-small cell lung cancer. The definition of the TNM descriptors is shown in Table 1. The size distinction between T1, a lesion ≤3 cm in size, and T2 corresponds to the distinction between a pulmonary nodule and a pulmonary mass. The distinction between T3 and T4 is basically whether the tumor is resectable or not; however, resectability will depend up surgeon and changes as technique improves.

The TNM evaluation is used to define cancer stage (see Table 2). Note that survival is very heavily dependent on tumor stage. Stages IA through IIIB are dependent on the T and N classification. Table 3 shows these stages using a tumor and node matrix. Stage IV disease is defined by metastatic disease. Staging is shown diagrammatically at the following web site, http://research. bidmc.harvard.edu/VPtutorials/pulmNodule/default.htm.

Therapy is also very dependent on stage. Stage IA and IB disease are usually treated with surgery alone, although adjuvant chemotherapy can be considered in stage IB. Stage II is treated with a combination of surgery and chemotherapy or radiotherapy. Stage IIIA patients typically have preoperative chemotherapy or radiotherapy. One effect of the neoadjuvant therapy is to shrink the tumor prior to resection. Stage IIIB and IV patients are generally considered incurable and they are treated with palliative therapy. A few, selected stage IIIB patients may be considered for an aggressive combined therapy approach. Stage IV patients with a single brain metastasis are a special case; a highly selected group of these patients are considered for curative resection. Therapy options are shown diagrammatically at the following web site, http:// research.bidmc.harvard.edu/VPtutorials/pulmNodule/images/Treatments.html.

Clinical PET and PET/CT

Table 1: TNM Descriptors for Non-Small Cell Lung Cancer

Primary tumor (T)

TX	Primary tumor cannot be assessed, or tumor proven by the presence of malignant cells in sputum or bronchial washings but not visualized by imaging or bronchoscopy
T0	No evidence of primary tumor
Tis	Carcinoma in situ
T1	Tumor ≤ 3 cm in greatest dimension, surrounded by lung or visceral pleura, without bronchoscopic evidence of invasion more proximal than the lobar bronchus (i.e., not in the main bronchus)
T2	Tumor with any of the following features of size or extent: • 3 cm in greatest dimension • Involves main bronchus, ≥ 2cm distal to the carina • Invades the visceral pleura • Associated with atelectasis or obstructive pneumonitis that extends to the hilar region but does not involve the entire lung.
T3	• Tumor of any size that directly invades any of the following: chest wall (including superior sulcus tumors), diaphragm, mediastinal pleura, parietal pericardium; or • tumor in the main bronchus < 2 cm distal to the carina, but without involvement of the carina; or • associated atelectasis or obstructive pneumonitis of the entire lung
T4	• Tumor of any size that invades any of the following: mediastinum, heart, great vessels, trachea, esophagus, vertebral body, carina; or • tumor with a malignant pleural or pericardial effusion, or with satellite tumor nodule(s) within the ipsilateral primary-tumor lobe of the lung

Regional lymph nodes (N)

NX	Regional lymph nodes cannot be assessed
N0	No regional lymph node metastasis
N1	Metastasis to ipsilateral peribronchial and/or ipsilateral hilar lymph nodes, and intrapulmonary nodes involved by direct extension of the primary tumor
N2	Metastasis to ipsilateral mediastinal and/or subcarinal lymph node(s)
N3	Metastasis to contralateral mediastinal, contralateral hilar, ipsilateral or contralateral scalene, or supraclavicular lymph node(s)

Distant metastasis (m)

MX	Presence of distant metastasis cannot be assessed
M0	No distant metastasis
M1	Distant metastasis present

After Mountain et al.[12]

Selection of therapy is well beyond the scope of this book. It depends on patient factors such as performance status and pulmonary function. It also depends on the details of the particular tumor. Anatomic imaging is often important in helping make important distinctions about issues such as invasion of structures, but FDG-PET also has an important role. Accurate staging is very important since it has such a major impact on both therapy and prognosis.

Table 2: TNM Staging

Stage	TNM	5-year Survival (%)
0	Carcinoma in situ	
IA	T1N0M0	61
IB	T2N0M0	38
IIA	T1N1M0	34
IIB	T2N1M0 T3N0M0	24
IIIA	T3N1M0 T1N2M0 T2-3N2M0	34
IIIB	T4N0-2 T1-4N3M0	5
IV	T1-4N0-3M1	1

After Mountain et al.[12]

Table 3: Staging—Tumor-Node Matrix

	N0	N1	N2	N3
T1	IA	IIA	IIIA	IIIB
T2	IB	IIB	IIIA	IIIB
T3	IIB	IIIA	IIIA	IIIB
T4	IIIB	IIIB	IIIB	IIIB

Lymph Node Stations.   Fairly precise lymph node localization is useful not only for staging, but also for communication with bronchoscopist or surgeon. Consequently there is a numbering system which is used to describe the various lymph node locations. Table 4 gives a brief description of each of the lymph node stations. The lymph node stations designated with a single digit, 1–9, are within the mediastinum. These lymph nodes are N2 nodes if ipsilateral to the tumor or N3 nodes if contralateral to the tumor in the TNM classification. Lymph node stations 10–14 correspond to N1 nodes, nodes that lie distal to the mediastinal pleural reflections. An "R" or an "L" can be appended to indicate if the lymph node is to the right or left of midline. An interactive depiction of the various lymph node stations is shown at http://research.bidmc.harvard.edu/VPtutorials/pulmNodule/images/Nodal%20Stations.html.

FDG-PET Staging in Non-Small Cell Lung Cancer.   FDG-PET has a major role to play in determining the nodal stage of the tumor. The typical CT criteria for a positive mediastinal node is based on a short axis size greater than 1 cm. However, this size-based criterion is known to be very inaccurate. FDG-PET can identify both positive nodes that are smaller in size and negative nodes that are large in size.

There is a relatively large distinction between N2 nodes, nodes in the ipsilateral mediastinum and N3 nodes, nodes in the contralateral mediastinum. Generally, that distinction separates resectable from non-repectable cancer. (There is considerable interest in aggressive protocols that use resection for

Table 4: Lymph Node Stations

N2 Nodes

N2 nodes stations are designated with a single digit
N2 nodes must lie within the mediastinal pleural envelope

1 Highest mediastinal nodes
Above the upper rim of the bracheocephalic (left innominate) vein where it ascends to the left, crossing in front of the trachea at its midline

2 Upper paratracheal nodes
Below #1 and above the upper margin of the aortic arch

3 Prevascular and retrotracheal nodes
3A: prevascular; 3P: retrotracheal. Midline nodes are ipsilateral for both sides

4 Lower paratracheal nodes
Below #2 and above the upper margin of the upper lobe bronchus and on the left, medial to the ligamentum arteriosum.

5 Subaortic (aorto-pulmonary window)
Lateral to the ligamentum arteriosum or the aorta or the left pulmonary artery, and proximal to the first branch of the left pulmonary artery

6 Para-aortic (ascending aorta or phrenic)
Anterior and lateral to the ascending aorta and the aortic arch or the innominate artery beneath a line tangential to the upper margin of the aortic arch

7 Subcarinal nodes
Caudal to the carina of the trachea, but not associated with the lower lobe bronchi or arteries within the lung

8 Paraesophageal nodes (below carina)
Adjacent to the wall of the esophagus, excluding subcarinal nodes

9 Pulmonary ligament nodes
Within the pulmonary ligament, including those in the posterior wall and lower part of the inferior pulmonary vein

N1 Nodes

N1 nodes are designated with two digits
N1 nodes must lie distal to the mediastinal pleural reflection

10 Hilar nodes
Distal to the mediastinal pleural reflection, adjacent to the proximal lobar bronchi and the bronchus intermedius

11 Interlobar nodes
Lying between lobar bronchi

12 Lobar nodes
Adjacent to the distal lobar bronchi

13 Segmental nodes
Adjacent to the segmental bronchi

14 Subsegmental nodes
Around the subsegmental bronchi

After Mountain et al.[13]

selected N3 disease.) PET imaging with anatomically fused images have a great advantage in being able to identify the exact location of mediastinal nodes.

One of the most important roles for FDG-PET is detection of distant metastases. It is common for non-small cell lung cancer to metastasize to the

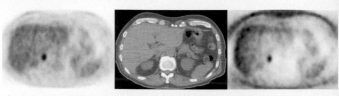

Figure 3: Adrenal Metastasis. The FDG-PET/CT shows a right renal metastasis. On the left is the attenuation corrected FDG-PET; in the center is the CT; and on the right is the non-corrected FDG-PET.

adrenal glands, the liver, and the bones. Figure 3 show a patient with an adrenal metastasis. Detection of a distant site of disease means the patient is stage IV and palliative chemotherapy is indicated. In general, it is most efficacious to biopsy the site that will confirm the highest stage of disease. If the FDG-PET scan identifies a distant site of disease, then that single site can be biopsied, often obviating biopsy of the primary lesion. Figure 4 shows a stage IV patient with a bone metastasis.

FDG-PET may also make the diagnostic work-up more effective. In complicated lesions, directing a biopsy to the most FDG-avid portion of the lesion may improve the yield. Figure 5 shows a patient with considerable chest disease and a single bone lesion in the ilium. Biopsy of the iliac lesion not only provides the diagnosis of cancer, but also provides pathologic confirmation of stage IV disease. A general rule is that biopsy of the lesion that confirms the highest stage will expedite the work-up.

Gould et al. performed a meta-analysis of studies comparing FDG-PET and CT evaluation of mediastinal lymph nodes. FDG-PET had a sensitivity of 85%

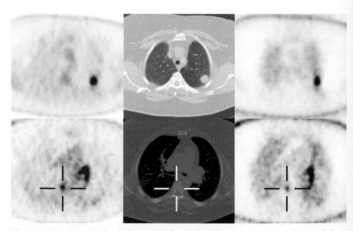

Figure 4: Stage IV: Vertebral Metastasis. The top line shows the primary left upper lobe lung cancer. The bottom line shows FDG uptake in a large hilar mass and uptake in a vertebra. Linked cursors show the relation of the uptake and the vertebra. The vertebral metastasis, which is not apparent on the CT scan, upstages this patient to stage IV. On the left are the attenuation-corrected FDG-PET images; in the center is the CT; and on the right is the non-attenuation-corrected FDG-PET.

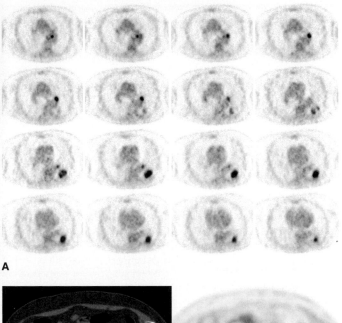

A

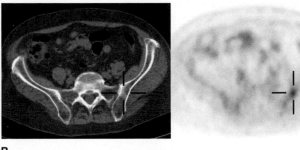

B

Figure 5: Biopsy Highest Stage Disease. Part **A** shows axial FDG-PET slices of the chest in a patient with left lower lobe lung cancer with ipsilateral hilar and mediastinal nodes. Part **B** shows a solitary iliac bone metastasis. Directing the biopsy to the iliac bone allows for diagnosis of cancer and for confirmation of stage IV disease.

and a specificity of 90%, whereas CT had a sensitivity of 61% and a specificity of 79%. FDG-PET was more sensitive but less specific in enlarged lymph nodes (sensitivity of 100%, specificity of 78%) than in normal-sized nodes (sensitivity of 82%, specificity of 93%). The receiver-operating-characteristic curves for these two cases were very similar; it appears that the size of the nodes changes the operating point, not the test accuracy. This type of behavior would be expected if a single cut-off for SUV were used without adjustment for partial volume effects.

Staging Small Cell Lung Cancer. Staging has a much smaller role in small cell lung cancer than in non-small cell lung cancer. Occasionally, localized small cell lung cancer (T1–2N0M0) can be cured with surgery followed by chemotherapy. Much more commonly, small cell lung cancer is metastatic at the time of presentation. Staging also has less prognostic importance in small cell lung cancer than in non-small cell lung cancer. The principle role of staging is to determine if radiotherapy will be used in addition to chemotherapy.

Small cell lung cancer is divided into two categories—limited disease and extensive disease. Limited disease is disease involving one hemithorax, including mediastinal and contralateral hilar lymph nodes. Ipsilateral, but not contralateral supraclavicular lymph nodes may also be involved. Patients with limited disease are considered for curative-intent combined chemotherapy and radiotherapy.

The role of FDG-PET scanning in small cell lung cancer is under investigation. A recent review noted the potential utility of FDG-PET but did not recommend it at the present time. Small cell lung cancer is very FDG-avid, and FDG-PET appears to upstage an important fraction of patients. However, exactly how to use FDG-PET in the context of a therapeutic regime has not been clearly established.

Radiation Treatment Planning.   FDG-PET may have an important role in radiation treatment planning in lung cancer. In addition to determining if radiation therapy is appropriate and whether therapy will be given with curative or palliative intent, FDG-PET is useful for determining therapy ports. It can be used both to limit ports to spare normal tissue and to include additional involved regions. Several studies have shown that PET has an impact on radiation treatment planning in an important fraction of patients. Hopefully, treatment plans that include all the FDG-avid lesions or the FDG-avid portions of a complex mass will result in more effective local control with less unnecessary tissue being treated.

Recurrent Laryngeal Nerve Palsy.   The recurrent laryngeal nerves, especially the left recurrent laryngeal nerve, may be involved with lung cancer causing recurrent laryngeal nerve palsy. In this case, the involved vocal chord does not function. The non-involved vocal chord must work harder than normal in order to make up for the loss in function of the involved vocal chord. Consequently, the ipsilateral vocal chord will not show any FDG uptake, and the contralateral vocal chord will show increase uptake, which can be quite intense. Unilateral FDG uptake in the vocal chord region especially with an appropriately placed mass can be used to suggest the diagnosis of recurrent laryngeal nerve palsy (see Figure 6). It should not be misinterpreted as spread of disease. http://www.med.harvard.edu/JPNM/TF03_04/Sept2/WriteUp.html.

MONITORING THERAPY

FDG-PET is playing an increasing role in monitoring therapy for lung cancer. A decrease in FDG uptake after therapy is very encouraging, although with lung cancer one often has to settle for stable findings. A new region of uptake indicates that therapy is not effective or no longer effective. The level of FDG uptake as measured by the SUV is a prognostic factor (see below) both before and during therapy. Remember that when comparing quantitative measures on sequential studies the details of the analysis become even more important. Quantitative measurement should be made at the same time after injection, and

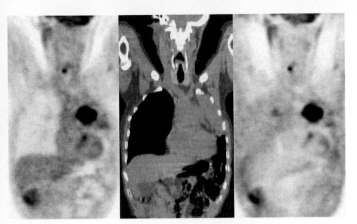

Figure 6: Recurrent Laryngeal Nerve Palsy. On the left is an attenuation-corrected coronal view of an FDG-PET study; in the center is the corresponding CT; and on the right is the corresponding uncorrected FDG-PET. There is a large FDG-avid mass abutting the aortic arch with secondary collapse of the left upper lobe. The recurrent laryngeal nerve separates from the vagus nerve and passes under the aortic arch passing behind the ligamentum arteriosum. The mass is in the region of the left recurrent laryngeal nerve. There is prominent FDG uptake in the right vocal chord, secondary to palsy of the left vocal chord.

the plasma glucose should be recorded for both studies. A simple way to normalize the SUV is to multiply by 100 and divide by the plasma glucose in mg/dL.

Some patients with bulky stage IIIA disease are borderline for surgical resection. Patients with stage IIIB disease are generally not considered for surgery; however, some of these patients may considered for more aggressive surgical protocols. These patients may be treated with neoadjuvant chemotherapy and radiotherapy and then reevaluated by FDG-PET. Marked improvement on FDG-PET imaging suggesting a good response to the neoadjuvant therapy may evolve as a method to decide if curative surgical therapy should be attempted. Figure 7 shows a patient with a good response to combined chemotherapy and radiotherapy. Figure 8 shows a different patient who shows progression of disease on neoadjuvant therapy.

Weber et al. studied 57 patients with stage IIIB or stage IV who were to undergo platinum-based chemotherapy. They used a decline in SUV of greater than 20% after one cycle of therapy to indicate a metabolic response response. There was a good correlation between a metabolic response after one cycle and the overall response to therapy. Metabolic response also correlated with mean time to progression and overall survival. A simple SUV measurement was as accurate as measuring the more complicated net influx constant.

When monitoring therapy with FDG-PET it is important to recognize the confounding effects of radiation therapy. In the area of radiation change there is typically low-level FDG uptake. Occasionally, there can be avid FDG uptake, especially when there is frank radiation pneumonitis. The FDG uptake often returns to normal after six months, but radiation change may persist for a longer period of time. There can be increased uptake in both the lung and the

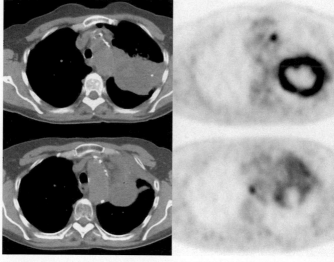

Figure 7: Response to Therapy. The top line shows the CT and FDG-PET at presentation. The left upper lobe mass shows peripheral FDG-avidity, but little activity in the center of the mass compatible with central necrosis. The para-aortic lymph node is also FDG-avid. The bottom line shows the CT and FDG-PET after chemotherapy and radiotherapy. There has been collapse of the left upper lobe, but marked decrease in uptake in the mass. Some low level uptake may be secondary to the collapsed lung tissue. The para-aortic lymph node is no longer FDG-avid. (Note increased uptake in the esophagus compatible with radiation esophagitis.) These findings represent a very good response to therapy. At operation, there were few viable tumor cells in the primary mass and no viable tumor in any lymph node.

chest wall after radiation therapy. A local region with the radiation port with more marked FDG uptake, or a region with increasing uptake, especially if it is associated with a mass on anatomic imaging, should be considered suspicious for recurrence. Mild to moderate uptake in a region corresponding to typical radiation changes does not suggest recurrence.

PROGNOSIS

The primary purpose of staging is to identify patients who may benefit from different therapies. In addition, staging is also a potent prognostic indicator. The five-year survival for patients with non-small cell lung cancer is 61% if they have stage I disease, and only 5% if they have stage IIIB disease (see Table 2). Since FDG imaging allows for more accurate staging, it should make TNM staging an even more accurate predictor of prognosis.

In addition to staging, the FDG avidity of the tumor is an independent prognostic factor. Duhaylongsod et al. showed that FDG uptake correlates with tumor growth rate. And, Buck et al. showed that FDG uptake correlated with Ki-67 immunostaining, a marker of tumor proliferation (see above). These studies provide a theoretical basis for why FDG avidity might identify more

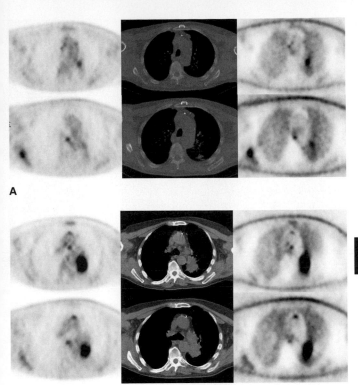

A

B

Figure 8: Disease Progression on Therapy. FDG-PET/CT scans were obtained on a patient before and after neoadjuvant. A. There is development of a right scapular metastasis. B. There is increase in the size and FDG-avidity of the mass and mediastinal lymph nodes.

aggressive tumors. Figure 9 show a patient with two lung lesions. The right upper lobe lesion showed relatively slow growth over a period of two years and three months, and the left lower lobe lesion showed a much faster rate of growth. The SUV for the FDG uptake in the right upper lobe lesion was 3.4 and the SUV of the left lower lobe lesion was 16.8.

In a retrospective study of 155 patients Ahuja et al. showed that the 118 patients with an SUV less than 10 had a median survival 24.6 months, while the 37 patients with an SUV greater than 10 had a median survival of 11.4 months. A multivariate analysis showed that SUV provided independent prognostic information when compared from the clinical stage and the lesion size. Vansteenkiste et al. found that performance status, stage, and SUV greater than 7 were prognostic factors. Tumor diameter and cell type were not independent predictors. Higashi et al. found that patients with an SUV less than or equal to 5 had a longer disease-free survival. SUV was an independent prognostic factor from the stage of disease of the tumor size. Of the patients with pathological stage I disease, those with an SUV less than or equal to 5 had a survival 88%,

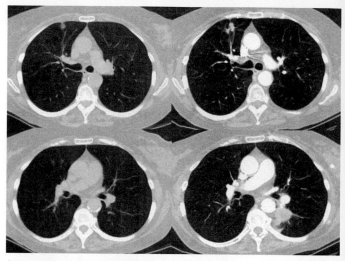

A

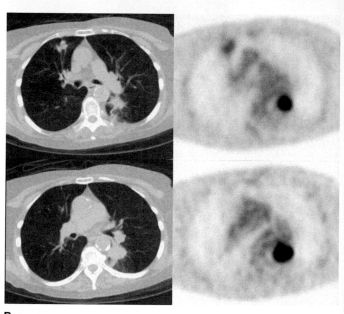

B

Figure 9: Growth Rate. **A.** The right side shows a CT scan obtained two years and three months after the CT scan on the left side. In the interval, there has been relatively slow growth of the nodule in the right upper lobe. By comparison, there has been rapid growth of the left lower lobe lesion. **B.** The top row shows a FDG-PET/CT centered over the right upper lobe lesion; the bottom row shows the same FDG-PET/CT centered over the left lower lobe lesion. The SUV of the right upper lobe lesion was 3.4, and the SUV of the left lower lobe lesion was 16.8.

while those with a SUV greater than 5 had a survival 17%. Jeong et al. found that patients with an SUV greater than or equal to 7 had 6.3 times the five-year mortality of those with an SUV less than 7.

Most of the information about prognosis has dealt with non-small cell lung cancer. But SUV may also provide prognostic information in small cell lung cancer.

Recurrent Lung Cancer/Second Primary.   There may be considerable post-operative and post-radiation therapy anatomic changes. These changes can make early detection of recurrent cancer a problem on anatomic imaging. In patients who have been successfully treated for lung cancer an important cause of mortality is the development of a second lung primary. In both recurrent and new primary lung cancer, FDG-PET imaging is valuable for detection of disease. Early detection is important, since new primaries are treated similarly to the initial primary and salvage therapies exist for localized recurrent lung cancer. Figure 10 shows detection of an FDG-avid lesion in a region with post treatment changes.

Patz et al. studied 113 patients a median of 8.1 months after primary therapy. The 100 patients with a positive scan had a mean survival of 12 months, while 11 of 13 patients with a negative scan were living after mean of 34 months. Hicks et al. studied patients with a suspected relapse greater than 6 after definitive therapy. Forty-one of 42 patients with recurrent disease were identified (sensitivity 98%). Fourteen of 17 patients who were disease free 12 months after scan had a negative scan (specificity 82%). The FDG-PET scan resulted in a major management change in 63% of patients. Both the presence and the extent of disease were important prognostic factors.

COST EFFECTIVENESS

The determination of cost effectiveness for most diagnostic studies uses a decision model where the clinical scenario is modeled mathematically, using assumptions about the accuracy of different tests and the utilities of different therapeutic regimes. Generally, more effective scenarios are associated with

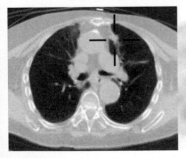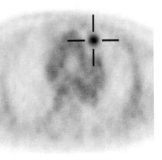

Figure 10: Post-Treatment Changes with FDG-avid Lesion. On the left is a CT scan and on the right is an FDG-PET scan. This patient had a right upper lobe lung cancer 13 years ago treated with combined chemotherapy and radiotherapy. Four years ago she had a left upper lobe lung cancer treated with a wedge resection. On the CT there post-treatment changes are seen with a somewhat nodular region medially in the left upper lobe. The FDG-PET clearly shows this region to be FDG-avid.

increased costs and then the cost per quality-adjusted life-year (QALY) is calculated. Gambhir et al. investigated use of FDG-PET in evaluation of single pulmonary nodule. Their results showed both increased survival and decreased cost using FDG-PET. The decreased costs were due to the decrease in the number of surgeries. Other investigators using different scenarios have come up with different degrees of cost effectiveness, but generally FDG-PET has a relatively low cost per QALY in the evaluation of single pulmonary nodule. The details of an individual case are often key in determining the utility of FDG-PET, but these decision analyses provide the background information for making individualized decisions.

Change in management based on a test result is a necessary condition for a study to be cost effective. Management efficacy is more easily studied than outcome efficacy. A test that results in a change in management in an important percentage of patients has the potential to have an important affect on outcome. It is common for diagnostic tests to result in a change in management in the 10–20% range. FDG-PET has been shown to result in changes in management in different non-small cell lung cancer groups in 27–67% of patients.

There is less data about small cell lung cancer. However, Kamel et al. found that management was changed in 12 of 42 patients (29%) with initial staging or restaging FDG-PET.

Screening.   Early stage lung cancer has a much better prognosis than more advanced lung cancer (see Table 2). Thus, it seems obvious that screening to find early-stage disease would improve patient survival. Although this strategy seems obvious, chest x-ray screening studies in the 1950s and 1960s did not demonstrate an improvement in survival. The many issues associated with efficaciousness of screening are complex, but given the improvement in imaging technology, it is hoped that more modern screening methods may prove to be effective. Particularly interesting is the potential for low-dose CT screening of high-risk patients. The American College of Radiology Imaging Network (ACRIN) is currently conducting a multicenter National Cancer Institute (NCI) sponsored trial, National Lung Screening Trial (NLST), to compare low-dose CT and chest x-ray in screening for lung cancer (http://www.acrin-nlst.org/).

Some investigators have advocated FDG-PET for screening. There is as of yet no compelling data to suggest that FDG-PET should be used for screening.

SUMMARY

Diagnosis, staging, and restaging of lung cancer are among the most extensively studied applications of FDG-PET. With the exception of bronchioloaveolar cell cancer and carcinoid, lung cancer is very FDG-avid. Lung cancer is one of the most common indications for FDG-PET, and FDG-PET has a large impact on lung cancer management.

BIBLIOGRAPHY

1. Ahuja V, Coleman RE, Herndon J, Patz EF, Jr. The prognostic significance of fluorodeoxyglucose positron emission tomography imaging for patients with non-small cell lung carcinoma. *Cancer* 1998; 83(5):918–24.
2. Belhocine T, Foidart J, Rigo P, et al. Fluorodeoxyglucose positron emission tomography and somatostatin receptor scintigraphy for diagnosing and staging carcinoid

tumours: correlations with the pathological indexes p53 and Ki-67. *Nucl Med Commun* 2002; 23(8):727–34.

3. Boiselle PM, Ernst A, Karp DD. Lung cancer detection in the 21st century: potential contributions and challenges of emerging technologies. *AJR Am J Roentgenol* 2000; 175(5):1215–21.
4. Buck AK, Halter G, Schirrmeister H, et al. Imaging Proliferation in Lung Tumors with PET: (18)F-FLT Versus (18)F-FDG. *J Nucl Med* 2003; 44(9):1426–31.
5. Coleman RE, Laymon CM, Turkington TG. FDG imaging of lung nodules: a phantom study comparing SPECT, camera-based PET, and dedicated PET. *Radiology* 1999; 210(3):823–8.
6. Dizendorf EV, Baumert BG, von Schulthess GK, et al. Impact of whole-body 18F-FDG PET on staging and managing patients for radiation therapy. *J Nucl Med* 2003; 44(1):24–9.
7. Duhaylongsod FG, Lowe VJ, Patz EF, Jr., et al. Lung tumor growth correlates with glucose metabolism measured by fluoride-18 fluorodeoxyglucose positron emission tomography. *Ann Thorac Surg* 1995; 60(5):1348–52.
8. Gambhir SS, Hoh CK, Phelps ME, et al. Decision tree sensitivity analysis for cost-effectiveness of FDG-PET in the staging and management of non-small-cell lung carcinoma. *J Nucl Med* 1996; 37(9):1428–36.
9. Gould MK, Maclean CC, Kuschner WG, et al. Accuracy of positron emission tomography for diagnosis of pulmonary nodules and mass lesions: a meta-analysis. *Jama* 2001; 285(7):914–24.
10. Gould MK, Sanders GD, Barnett PG, et al. Cost-effectiveness of alternative management strategies for patients with solitary pulmonary nodules. *Ann Intern Med* 2003; 138(9):724–35.
11. Hauber HP, Bohuslavizki KH, Lund CH, et al. Positron emission tomography in the staging of small-cell lung cancer: a preliminary study. *Chest* 2001; 119(3):950–4.
12. Heyneman LE, Patz EF. PET imaging in patients with bronchioloalveolar cell carcinoma. *Lung Cancer* 2002; 38(3):261–6.
13. Hicks RJ, Kalff V, MacManus MP, et al. The utility of (18)F-FDG PET for suspected recurrent non-small cell lung cancer after potentially curative therapy: impact on management and prognostic stratification. *J Nucl Med* 2001; 42(11):1605–13.
14. Higashi K, Ueda Y, Arisaka Y, et al. 18F-FDG uptake as a biologic prognostic factor for recurrence in patients with surgically resected non-small cell lung cancer. *J Nucl Med* 2002; 43(1):39–45.
15. Hoekstra CJ, Hoekstra OS, Stroobants SG, et al. Methods to monitor response to chemotherapy in non-small cell lung cancer with 18F-FDG PET. *J Nucl Med* 2002; 43(10):1304–9.
16. Jadvar H, Segall GM. False-negative fluorine-18-FDG PET in metastatic carcinoid. *J Nucl Med* 1997; 38(9):1382–3.
17. Jemal A, Murray T, Samuels A, et al. Cancer statistics, 2003. *CA Cancer J Clin* 2003; 53(1):5–26.
18. Jeong HJ, Min JJ, Park JM, et al. Determination of the prognostic value of [(18)F]fluorodeoxyglucose uptake by using positron emission tomography in patients with non-small cell lung cancer. *Nucl Med Commun* 2002; 23(9):865–70.
19. Kalff V, Hicks RJ, MacManus MP, et al. Clinical impact of (18)F fluorodeoxyglucose positron emission tomography in patients with non-small-cell lung cancer: a prospective study. *J Clin Oncol* 2001; 19(1):111–8.
20. Kamel EM, Zwahlen D, Wyss MT, et al. Whole-Body (18)F-FDG PET Improves the Management of Patients with Small Cell Lung Cancer. *J Nucl Med* 2003; 44(12):1911–7.
21. Lardinois D, Weder W, Hany TF, et al. Staging of non-small cell lung cancer with integrated positron-emission tomography and computed tomography. *New Engl J Med* 2003; 348:2500–7.
22. Miyaoka RS, Kohlmyer SG, Lewellen TK. Hot sphere detection limits for a dual head coincidence imaging system. *IEEE Trans Nucl Sci* 1999; 46(6):2185–2191.

7

23. Mountain CF, Dresler CM. Regional lymph node classification for lung cancer staging. *Chest* 1997; 111(6):1718–23.

24. Mountain CF. Revisions in the International System for Staging Lung Cancer. *Chest* 1997; 111(6):1710–7.

25. Nestle U, Hellwig D, Fleckenstein J, et al. Comparison of early pulmonary changes in 18FDG-PET and CT after combined radiochemotherapy for advanced non-small-cell lung cancer: a study in 15 patients. *Front Radiat Ther Oncol* 2002; 37:26–33.

26. Nestle U, Hellwig D, Schmidt S, et al. 2-Deoxy-2-[18F]fluoro-D-glucose positron emission tomography in target volume definition for radiotherapy of patients with non-small-cell lung cancer. *Mol Imaging Biol* 2002; 4(3):257–63.

27. Pandit N, Gonen M, Krug L, Larson SM. Prognostic value of [18F]FDG-PET imaging in small cell lung cancer. *Eur J Nucl Med Mol Imaging* 2003; 30(1):78–84.

28. Patz EF, Jr., Connolly J, Herndon J. Prognostic value of thoracic FDG PET imaging after treatment for non-small cell lung cancer. *AJR Am J Roentgenol* 2000; 174(3):769–74.

29. Seltzer MA, Yap CS, Silverman DH, et al. The impact of PET on the management of lung cancer: the referring physician's perspective. *J Nucl Med* 2002; 43(6):752–6.

30. Simon GR, Wagner H. Small cell lung cancer. *Chest* 2003; 123(1 Suppl):259S–271S.

31. Vansteenkiste JF, Stroobants SG, Dupont PJ, et al. Prognostic importance of the standardized uptake value on (18)F-fluoro-2-deoxy-glucose-positron emission tomography scan in non-small-cell lung cancer: An analysis of 125 cases. Leuven Lung Cancer Group. *J Clin Oncol* 1999; 17(10):3201–6.

32. Weber W, Young C, Abdel-Dayem HM, et al. Assessment of pulmonary lesions with 18F-fluorodeoxyglucose positron imaging using coincidence mode gamma cameras. *J Nucl Med* 1999; 40(4):574–8.

33. Weber WA, Petersen V, Schmidt B, et al. Positron emission tomography in non-small-cell lung cancer: prediction of response to chemotherapy by quantitative assessment of glucose use. *J Clin Oncol* 2003; 21(14):2651–7.

34. Weir HK, Thun MJ, Hankey BF, et al. Annual report to the nation on the status of cancer, 1975–2000, featuring the uses of surveillance data for cancer prevention and control. *J Natl Cancer Inst* 2003; 95(17):1276–99.

35. Yap CS, Schiepers C, Fishbein MC, et al. FDG-PET imaging in lung cancer: how sensitive is it for bronchioloalveolar carcinoma? *Eur J Nucl Med Mol Imaging* 2002; 29(9):1166–73.

Oncology—Digestive Tract

I. ESOPHAGEAL CANCER

Esophageal cancer accounts for about 4% of all digestive tract cancers. In many patients, the tumor has metastasized before the initial diagnosis. The distal esophagus is most often involved and the overall prognosis is generally poor. The presenting symptoms may include dysphagia, odynophagia, and hematemesis. The diagnostic procedures include esophagoscopy with biopsy. Squamous cell carcinoma accounts for two-thirds of esophageal carcinomas. Adenocarcinoma is the second most common histology and usually arises from Barrett esophagus. Other, less common, malignancies include sarcoma, primary melanoma, and oat cell carcinoma (apudoma). Currently, CT and endoscopic ultrasound (EUS) are the mainstays in the clinical staging of esophageal carcinoma. However, imaging evaluation with CT is not a reliable index of resectability. Surgical resection and radiation therapy remain the standard treatment for patients with esophageal carcinoma. Aggressive surgical intervention provides for a chance of cure while radiation therapy offers palliation for obstructive symptoms. Chemotherapy may also be considered for metastatic disease.

FDG PET is currently approved by the Center for Medicare and Medicaid Services for staging, restaging, and assessing treatment response in esophageal cancer. Primary esophageal carcinoma is highly FDG-avid (mean SUV of 11), which is correlated to increased Glut-1 expression in the tumor (Fig. 1). Despite this, however, small cancers may be missed, especially in the gastroesophageal junction, where there may be mild physiologic FDG accumulation. FDG PET has proved more valuable than CT in determining tumor resectability. The ability of FDG PET in detecting locoregional lymph node metastases depends on many factors, including the tumor volume in the lymph node, the node size, and the background activity. PET has relatively low sensitivity (about 50%) but relatively high specificity (about 90%) in detecting local invasion and loco-regional lymph node metastases. Despite this, combination of PET and EUS with fine-needle aspiration biopsy (PET+EUS-FNA) is suggested as the most cost-effective staging procedure for patients with esophageal cancer, unless resources are scarce or PET is unavailable.

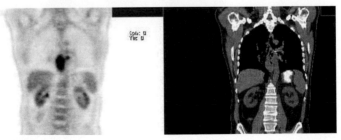

Figure 1: Intensely hypermetabolic distal esophageal adenocarcinoma without evidence of distant metastatic disease.

FDG PET appears to be most useful in assessing for recurrent and distant metastatic disease (Figs. 2–4). For the detection of recurrent disease, PET is very sensitive, although the combination of conventional methods and PET is most helpful in characterizing anastomotic recurrences. PET is more sensitive than and as specific as CT for the detection of systemic metastatic disease. However, in this clinical setting, PET may provide additional diagnostic information, which may lead to management changes in nearly 20% of patients. False-positive results may

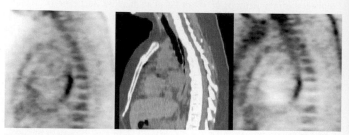

Figure 2: Esophageal Cancer. A sagittal slice from an FDG-PET/CT is shown from a patient with esophageal cancer. On the left is the attenuation corrected PET; in the center is the CT; on the right is the non-corrected PET.

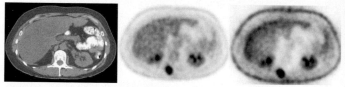

Figure 3: Esophageal Adenocarcinoma Muscle Metastasis. FDG-PET/CT showing intense uptake in a muscle metastasis from adenocarcinoma of the esophagus. On the left is the CT; in the center is the attenuation-corrected PET; and on the right is the non-attenuation-corrected PET.

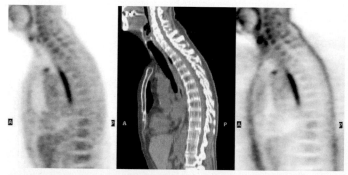

Figure 4: Esophageal Uptake After Radiation Therapy. Sagittal slices from an FDG-PET/CT in a patient with small cell lung cancer shows uptake in the esophagus in the area of the radiation port. Note that there is also decreased uptake in the bone marrow in this same region. Post-radiation therapy changes should not be confused with esophageal cancer.

occur in patients with benign strictures after dilation and with esophagitis. The diagnostic utility of FDG PET in monitoring histopathologic tumor response to therapy, such as neoadjuvant radiotherapy and chemotherapy, has also been reported. Responders show a decline in lesion FDG accumulation, while non-responders show minimal decline or no significant change in FDG uptake. The PET evidence of response is associated with longer disease-free period and better overall survival in comparison to nonresponders who have worse prognosis.

In summary, FDG PET scanning improves the clinical staging and restaging of patients with esophageal cancer by providing additional and complementary information to conventional imaging and allows for an objective assessment of tumor response to treatment, while offering important prognostic information. Therefore, the management of most patients with esophageal cancer is enhanced with use of FDG PET.

II. GASTRIC CANCER

Gastric cancer is common worldwide, most notably in East Asia, Chile, and Ireland. Adenocarcinoma accounts for the great majority of cases, while lymphoma and leiomyosarcoma are less common. Traditional diagnostic studies include upper gastrointestinal contrast radiologic examination and gastroscopy. After diagnosis, treatment usually involves gastrectomy followed by chemoradiation. Prognosis for patients with gastric carcinoma depends on a variety of factors, including tumor histology and grade, stage of disease, presence and extent of lymph node metastasis, and extent of lymph node dissection. Despite overall poor prognosis and relatively limited treatment options, studies have shown that the five-year survival after radical gastrectomy may be 37% and the mean time to recurrence may be close to two years.

Patterns of gastric cancer recurrence, in decreasing frequency, are distant sites only, peritoneal seeding only, combined peritoneal and locoregional disease, locoregional sites only, and combined distant and locoregional disease. The diagnosis of presence and extent of recurrent gastric cancer is difficult. Changes in serum tumor marker levels such as carcinoembryonic antigen (CEA) and carbohydrate antigen 19-9 (CA 19-9) may be useful as a predictor of treatment effect in patients with gastric cancer and serve as good prognostic factors. However, tumor markers cannot localize the sites and extent of residual or recurrent disease, and therefore imaging evaluation is often employed.

The experience with the utility of FDG PET in gastric carcinoma is limited. FDG PET has been shown to have higher sensitivity for detecting hepatic and distant metastases and higher accuracy for determining resectability of the primary tumor in comparison to CT (Fig. 5). However, PET appears to be limited in locoregional nodal staging and in assessing peritoneal spread. Peritoneal recurrence in gastric cancer is common and may occur in nearly half of the patients following curative tumor resection. FDG PET has low sensitivity for detection of the intra-peritoneal spread of disease. Differentiation between normal bowel FDG uptake and uptake related to carcinomatosis peritonei can be difficult. However, the sensitivity may be improved in close association with the clinical information (e.g., malignant ascites), direct careful visual correlation with potential clues on CT such as peritoneal caking, nodularity, and beaded thickening and with the expected preferential sites of seeding in the lower small bowel mesentery near the ileocecal junction and the sigmoid mesocolon.

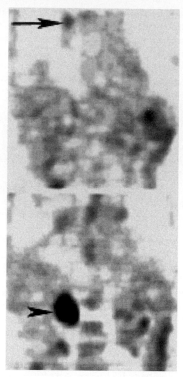

Figure 5: A 77-year-old male with a history of gastric adenocarcinoma treated with partial gastrectomy and chemotherapy. FDG PET was performed for evaluation for recurrent and metastatic disease eight months after the end of treatment. Whole-body PET scan shows intensely hypermetabolic lesions involving the right adrenal gland (arrowhead), right hilum (arrow) and the peritoneal surfaces concordant with subsequent CT studies. The patient underwent additional chemotherapy based on PET localization of extensive metastatic disease.

In patients with gastric non-Hodgkin's lymphoma, PET can detect high-grade and some of the low-grade tumors but may miss mucosa-associated lymphoid tissue (MALT) type tumors and tumors with large mucinous component. PET may also have a role in the assessment of response to chemotherapy in patients with gastric cancer.

PET has limitations in specific clinical situations. FDG PET may be falsely positive in patients with gastritis, which can also demonstrate high FDG uptake similar to neoplasm. Gastritis usually displays diffuse increased gastric FDG localization, while cancer often presents as a focal hypermetabolic lesion. This difference in tracer distribution pattern, however, may not necessarily hold as inflammation can be occasionally focal and cancer may be disseminated to involve nearly the entire stomach. However, clinical, laboratory, and the findings of the other imaging studies may be helpful in differentiating cancer from inflammation. Normal stomach may also demonstrate FDG uptake, but the uptake level is low and conforms to gastric configuration. The physiological gastric FDG uptake is significantly higher at the oral end. A stronger gastric FDG uptake at the anal end may be suggestive of a pathological uptake. Nevertheless, a normal contracted stomach can also appear as a focal lesion. In general, however, anatomic imaging correlation would be needed to localize the finding since abnormalities in adjacent structures such as a regional lymph node, or a lesion in the left hepatic lobe, the pancreatic tail or the adrenal gland may be indistinguishable from a focal gastric abnormality.

III. COLORECTAL CANCER

Colorectal cancer is the third most common malignancy in the United States. Most cancers occur after age 50 unless there are predisposing conditions such as familial polyposis or ulcerative colitis. Digital rectal exam, fecal occult blood test, and endoscopy are used for screening. Barium enema or and the recently developed CT colonography may also employed for the imaging evaluation of patients with suspected colorectal cancer. The vast majority of colon cancers are adenocarcinomas. The tumor spread sequentially from the primary site to adjacent lymph nodes and then up to the mesenteric lymph node chain. Low rectal and anal cancers tend to spread laterally to perineal nodes and may appear in inguinal nodes rather than in retroperitoneal nodes. Primary tumor is removed even in the presence of distant metastases since local symptoms are relieved and the quality of life is enhanced. Post-operative adjuvant radiation therapy may also be beneficial. Palliative radiation therapy is used in unresectable tumors that cause pain or excessive bleeding. Chemotherapy has been employed for palliation and a radiation sensitizer. In post-operative patients, an elevated serum carcinoembryonic antigen (CEA) level suggests recurrent and/or metastatic disease. The most common sites of metastases include the liver, lung and brain. Resection of isolated metastases is associated with improve survival while multifocal metastatic lesions are associated with less favorable prognosis.

The utility of FDG PET in colorectal carcinoma has been studied relatively extensively. For preoperative diagnosis, both CT and FDG PET may miss the involvement of the local lymph nodes. However, FDG PET is superior to CT for detecting liver metastases. The detection of the primary tumor depends on the size of the tumor and the background activity. Colon may occasionally

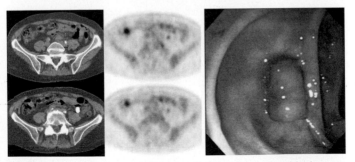

Figure 6: Colonic Polyp. A patient with non-small cell lung cancer showed focal increased uptake in the colon shown on a PET/CT scan (top left). A four-month follow-up scan showed the same finding (bottom left). A 3-cm adenomatous polyp was removed at colonoscopy (right).

demonstrate high FDG localization. However, focal intense hypermetabolism is highly suspicious for neoplasm that may include carcinoma, although focal inflammation and infection can have similar appearance (Figs. 6–8). False negatives may also result in subcentimeter and mucinous tumors.

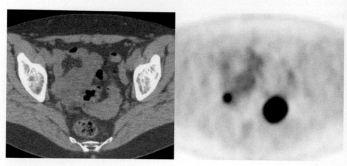

Figure 7: Colon Cancer. FDG-PET/CT in a patient with papillary thyroid cancer showed a previously unknown adenocarcinoma of the colon. The smaller bright focus on the patients right is due to urine in a ureter.

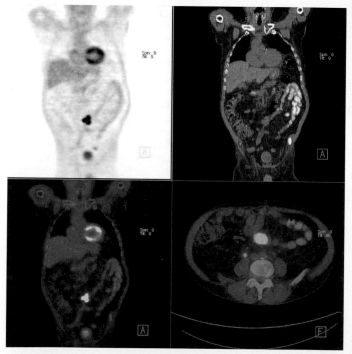

Figure 8: Midline distal left primary colon carcinoma at an unusual location related to anatomical variation. The hypermeatbolic activity in midline pelvis is related to the urinary bladder.

Clinical PET and PET/CT

FDG PET is particularly useful in the restaging of colorectal cancer for detection of recurrence and metastatic disease. Cancer tends to recur in up to one-third of patients within two years after the primary curative therapy. In patients with elevated or increasing serum CEA level, imaging is used to localize the site of recurrence. CT is often used in this clinical setting. However, CT may miss both hepatic and extrahepatic metastases in a significant number of patients and cannot differentiate postsurgical anatomic alterations from tumor recurrence. In general, however, combined functional and anatomic imaging provides valuable complementary information on localization and characterization of lesions (Figs. 9, 10). For example, in a recent case report, a curative abdominosacral resection of recurrent rectal cancer was performed based on the diagnostic information of PET-CT fusion images. FDG PET has also been shown to be more accurate than CT portography for detection of hepatic metastases (92% vs. 80%, respectively).

FDG PET has been shown to be particularly advantageous in the clinical setting of suspected recurrent and metastatic disease. A recent meta-analysis synthesizing the findings of 11 peer-reviewed articles in 281 patients reported an overall sensitivity of 97% (95% confidence level, 95–99%) and a specificity of 76% (95% confidence level, 64–88%) for FDG PET in detecting recurrent colorectal cancer throughout the whole body. An overall FDG PET-directed

8

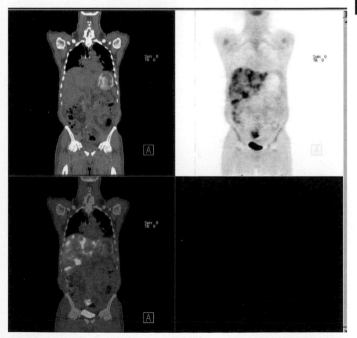

Figure 9: A 54-year-old man with recent diagnosis of colon carcinoma and liver metastases. There is a large focus of increased tracer activity in the known primary sigmoid tumor with panlobar hepatic metastases and possibly peritoneal deposits in the right paracolic gutter.

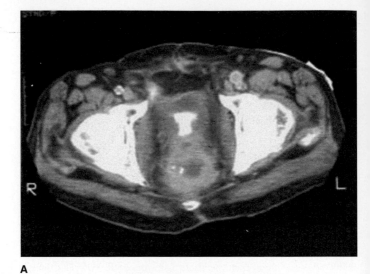

A

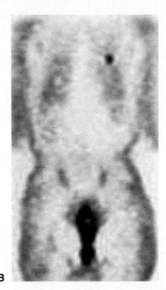

B

Figure 10: A 75-year-old male with a history of rectal cancer s/p low anterior resection and chemotherapy and an elevated serum CEA level of 22. **A.** CT shows a presacral pelvic mass with obscuration of fat planes. **B.** PET shows intense hypermetabolism in the pelvic mass compatible with locally recurrent disease and an unsuspected right upper lung metastatic lesion. Perineal and right lung lesion biopsies confirmed the PET findings.

change in management of 29% (95% confidence level, 25–34%) was also reported. In another study, a survey of referring physicians indicated that FDG PET had a major impact on the management of their patients with a change in clinical stage in 42% and a change in clinical management in more than 60% of patients with colorectal cancer. FDG PET is also cost-effective when included in the evaluation of patients with colorectal cancer. In one study of patients undergoing preoperative restaging, FDG PET resulted in substantial potential savings primarily as a result of detecting nonresectable disease thereby avoiding unnecessary surgery. FDG PET also resulted in cost savings with the use of a decision-tree model and sensitivity analysis. In a blinded prospective comparative study of FDG PET and CEA scan (Tc 99m-labeled arcitumomab) with surgical exploration as "gold standard," FDG-PET scans predicted unresectable disease in 90% of patients, while CEA scans failed to predict unresectable disease in any patient. In patients found to have resectable disease or disease that could be treated with regional therapy, FDG-PET scan prediction rate was 81% and that of CEA scan was only 13%.

FDG PET has been shown to be useful in monitoring tumor response to treatment that may include radiation therapy, chemotherapy, and hepatic chemoembolization or radiofrequency ablation (Figs. 11, 12). Lesions that show decline in FDG uptake after therapy demonstrate favorable response, while presence of residual FDG uptake can lead to additional treatment. Radiation therapy is often associated with intense inflammatory reaction which hinders detection of residual cancer with FDG PET performed early after completion of therapy. The exact time course of the FDG uptake in relation to the post-radiation inflammatory reaction remains undefined. However, use of semi-quantitative measures such as the retention index (RI), defined as RI = (SUV on delayed image − SUV on early image)/SUV on early image, soon after irradiation may be able to distinguish between patients with residual tumor and those without residual tumor. Presence of hypermetabolism several months (arbitrarily ≥ 6 months) after the completion of the radiation therapy raises the suspicion for residual cancer.

FDG PET is approved by the Center for Medicare and Medicaid Services for the imaging evaluation of patients with colorectal cancer. PET is complementary to CT for preoperative staging at the time of initial diagnosis. PET is

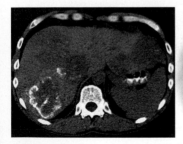
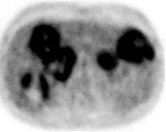

Figure 11: Colon Cancer Post-Chemoembolization. Colonic adenocarcinoma was previously treated with chemoembolization. There is relatively less FDG avidity in the region of prior chemoemoliztion, which is shown by the high density due to Lipiodol. The FDG-avid metastases show central necrosis with decreased density and decreased FDG uptake.

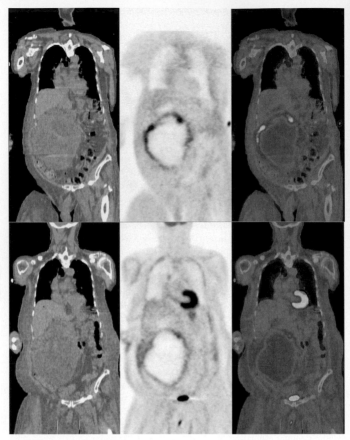

Figure 12: GIST Pre- and Post-Therapy. FDG-PET/CT studies in a patient with a gastrointestinal stromal tumor (GIST) before and after 10 days of therapy with Gleevec. The pre-therapy study shows a very large lesion with very prominent central necrosis. The post-therapy study shows a prompt decrease in FDG avidity in the viable portions of the tumor. GIST was formerly called leiomyosarcoma.

particularly indicated for restaging in patients with suspected recurrent and metastatic disease based on elevated or rising serum CEA level. PET is also useful for differentiating post-treatment changes from residual/recurrent cancer and in monitoring tumor response to therapy. The inclusion of FDG PET in the imaging evaluation of patients with recurrent colorectal cancer can have significant impact on the clinical management of these patients in a cost-effective manner.

BIBLIOGRAPHY

Gastroesophageal Cancer

1. Arslan N, Miller TR, Dehdashti F, et al. Evaluation of response to neoadjuvant therapy by quantitative 2-deoxy-2-[18F]fluoro-D-glucose with positron emission tomography in patients with esophageal cancer. Mol Imaging Biol 2002; 4:301–10.

2. Bakheet SM, Amin T, Alia AG, et al. F-18 FDG uptake in benign esophageal disease. Clin Nucl Med 1999; 24:995–7.

3. Berger KL, Nicholson SA, Dehdashti F, Siegel BA. FDG PET evaluation of mucinous neoplasms: correlation of FDG uptake with histopathologic features. AJR Am J Roentgenol 2000; 74:1005–1008.

4. Block MI, Patterson GA, Sundaresan RS, et al. Improvement in staging of esophageal cancer with the addition of positron emission tomography. Ann Thorac Surg 1997; 64:770–6.

5. Brucher BL, Weber W, Bauer M, et al. Neoadjuvant therapy of esophageal squamous cell carcinoma: response evaluation by positron emission tomography. Ann Surg 2001; 233:300–9.

6. Chin BB, Wahl RL. 18F-Fluoro-2-deoxyglucose positron emission tomography in the evaluation of gastrointestinal malignancies. Gut 2003; 52 Suppl 4:iv23–9.

7. Choi JY, Lee KH, Shim YM, et al. Improved detection of individual nodal involvement in squamous cell carcinoma of the esophagus by FDG PET. J Nucl Med 2000; 41:808–15.

8. Couper GW, McAteer D, Wallis F, et al. Detection of response to chemotherapy using positron emission tomography in patients with esophageal and gastric cancer. Br J Surg 1998; 85:1403–1406.

9. De Potter T, Flamen P, Van Cutsem E, et al. Whole-body PET with FDG for the diagnosis of recurrent gastric cancer. Eur J Nucl Med Mol Imaging 2002; 29:525–9.

10. DeYoung CM, Suntharalingam M, Line BR, et al. The ability of whole body FDG18 PET imaging to predict pathologic response to induction chemoradiotherapy in locally advanced esophageal cancer. A prospective phase II trial. Int J Radiat Oncol Biol Phys 2003; 57(2 Suppl):S165–6.

11. Downey RJ, Akhurst T, Ilson D, et al. Whole body 18FDG-PET and the response of esophageal cancer to induction therapy: results of a prospective trial. J Clin Oncol 2003; 21:428–32.

12. Flamen P, Lerut A, Van Cutsem E, et al. The utility of positron emission tomography for the diagnosis and staging of recurrent esophageal cancer. J Thorac Cardiovasc Surg 2000; 120:1085–92.

13. Flamen P, Lerut A, Van Cutsem E, et al. Utility of positron emission tomography for the staging of patients with potentially operable esophageal carcinoma. J Clin Oncol 2000; 18:3202–10.

14. Flamen P, Van Cutsem E, Lerut A, et al. Positron emission tomography for assessment of the response to induction radiochemotherapy in locally advanced esophageal cancer. Ann Oncol 2002; 13:361–8.

15. Flanagan FL, Dehdashti F, Siegel BA, et al. Staging of esophageal cancer with 18F-fluorodeoxyglucose positron emission tomography. AJR Am J Roentgenol. 1997; 168:417–24.

16. Fukunaga T, Okazumi S, Koide Y, et al. Evaluation of esophageal cancers using fluorine-18-fluorodeoxyglucose PET. J Nucl Med 1998; 39:1002–7.

17. Hoffmann M, Kletter K, Diemling M, et al. Positron emission tomography with fluorine-18-2-fluoro-2-deoxy-D-glucose (F18-FDG) dose not visualize extranodal B-cell lymphoma of the mucosa-associated lymphoid tissue (MALT)-type. Ann Oncol 1999; 10:1185–1189.

18. Ichiya Y, Kuwabara Y, Otsuka M, et al. Assessment of response to cancer therapy using fluorine-18-fluorodeoxyglucose and positron emission tomography. J Nucl Med 1991; 32:1655–60.

8

19. Jadvar H, Cham DK, Conti PS. Diagnostic evaluation of esophageal carcinoma with [F-18]-FDG PET/CT. Mol Imaging Biol 2003; 5:188.

20. Jadvar H, Tatlidil R, Garcia AA, Conti PS. Evaluation of recurrent gastric malignancy with [F-18]-FDG positron emission tomography. Clin Radiol 2003; 58:215–21.

21. Kato H, Kuwano H, Nakajima M, et al. Usefulness of positron emission tomography for assessing the response of neoadjuvant chemoradiotherapy in patients with esophageal cancer. Am J Surg 2002; 184:279–83.

22. Kato H, Kuwano H, Nakajima M, et al. Comparison between positron emission tomography and computed tomography in the use of the assessment of esophageal carcinoma. Cancer 2002; 94:921–8.

23. Kato H, Takita J, Miyazaki T, et al. Correlation of 18-F-fluorodeoxyglucose (FDG) accumulation with glucose transporter (Glut-1) expression in esophageal squamous cell carcinoma. Anticancer Res 2003; 23:3263–72.

24. Kawamura T, Kusakabe T, Sugino T, et al. Expression of glucose transporter-1 in human gastric carcinoma: association with tumor aggressiveness, metastasis, and patient survival. Cancer 2001; 92:634–641.

25. Kim K, Park SJ, Kim BT, et al. Evaluation of lymph node metastases in squamous cell carcinoma of the esophagus with positron emission tomography. Ann Thorac Surg 2001; 71:290–4.

26. Kneist W, Schreckenberger M, Bartenstein P, et al. Positron emission tomography for staging esophageal cancer: does it lead to a different therapeutic approach? World J Surg 2003; 27:1105–12.

27. Koga H, Sasaki M, Kuwabara Y, et al. An analysis of the physiological FDG uptake pattern in the stomach. Ann Nucl Med 2003; 17:733–8.

28. Kole AC, Plukker JT, Nieweg OE, Vaalburg W. Positron emission tomography for staging of esophageal and gastroesophageal malignancy. Br J Cancer 1998; 78:521–527.

29. Lerut T, Flamen P, Ectors N, et al. Histopathologic validation of lymph node staging with FDG-PET scan in cancer of the esophagus and gastroesophageal junction: A prospective study based on primary surgery with extensive lymphadenectomy. Ann Surg 2000; 232:743–52.

30. Lin EC, Lear J, Quaife RA. Metastatic peritoneal seeding patterns demonstrated by FDG positron emission tomographic imaging. Clin Nucl Med 2001; 29:249–250

31. Luketich JD, Friedman DM, Weigel TL, et al. Evaluation of distant metastases in esophageal cancer: 100 consecutive positron emission tomography scans. Ann Thorac Surg 1999; 68:1133–6.

32. Luketich JD, Schauer PR, Meltzer CC, et al. Role of positron emission tomography in staging esophageal cancer. Ann Thorac Surg 1997; 64:765–9.

33. McAteer D, Wallis F, Couper G, et al. Evaluation of 18F-FDG positron emission tomography in gastric and esophageal carcinoma. Br J Radiol 1999; 72:525–529.

34. Meltzer CC, Luketich JD, Friedman D, et al. Whole-body FDG positron emission tomographic imaging for staging esophageal cancer comparison with computed tomography. Clin Nucl Med 2000; 25:882–7.

35. Noguchi Y, Marat D, Saito A, et al. Expression of facilitative glucose transporters in gastric tumors. Hepatogastroenterology 1999; 46:2683–89.

36. Nunez RF, Yeung HW, Macapinlac H. Increased F-18 FDG uptake in the stomach. Clin Nucl Med 1999; 24:281–282.

37. Ott K, Fink U, Becker K, et al. Prediction of response to preoperative chemotherapy in gastric carcinoma by metabolic imaging: results of a prospective trial. J Clin Oncol 2003; 21:4604–10.

38. Pectasides D, Mylonakis A, Kostopoulou M, et al. CEA, CA 19-9, and CA-50 in monitoring gastric carcinoma. Am J Clin Oncol 1997; 20:348–353.

39. Rankin SC, Taylor H, Cook GJ, Mason R. Computed tomography and positron emission tomography in the pre-operative staging of esophageal carcinoma. Clin Radiol 1998; 53:659–65.

40. Rasanen JV, Sihvo EI, Knuuti MJ, et al. Prospective analysis of accuracy of positron emission tomography, computed tomography, and endoscopic ultrasonography in

staging of adenocarcinoma of the esophagus and the esophagogastric junction. Ann Surg Oncol 2003; 10:954–60.

41. Rice TW. Clinical staging of esophageal carcinoma. CT, EUS, and PET. Chest Surg Clin N Am 2000; 10:471–85.

42. Rodriguez M, Ahlstrom H, Sundin A, et al. [18F] FDG PET in gastric non-Hodgkin's lymphoma. Acta Oncol 1997; 36:577–584.

43. Schwarz RE, Zagala-Nevarez K. Recurrence patterns after radical gastrectomy for gastric cancer: prognostic factors and implications for postoperative adjuvant therapy. Ann Surg Oncol 2002; 9:394–400.

44. Shiraishi N, Inomata M, Osawa N, Yasuda K, Adachi Y, Kitano S. Early and late recurrence after gastrectomy for gastric carcinoma. Univariate and multivariate analyses. Cancer 2000; 89:255–261.

45. Skehan SJ, Brown AL, Thompson M, et al. Imaging features of primary and recurrent esophageal cancer at FDG PET. Radiographics 2000; 20:713–23.

46. Stahl A, Ott K, Weber WA, et al. FDG PET imaging of locally advanced gastric carcinomas: correlation with endoscopic and histopathological findings. Eur J Nucl Med Mol Imaging 2003; 30:288–95.

47. van Westreenen HL, Heeren PA, Jager PL, et al. Pitfalls of positive findings in staging esophageal cancer with F-18-fluorodeoxyglucose positron emission tomography. Ann Surg Oncol 2003; 10:1100–5.

48. Wallace MB, Nietert PJ, Earle C, et al. An analysis of multiple staging management strategies for carcinoma of the esophagus: computed tomography, endoscopic ultrasound, positron emission tomography, and thoracoscopy/laparoscopy. Ann Thorac Surg 2002; 74:1026–32.

49. Weber WA, Ott K, Becker K, et al. Prediction of response to preoperative chemotherapy in adenocarcinomas of the esophagogastric junction by metabolic imaging. J Clin Oncol 2001; 19:3058–65.

50. Wren SM, Stijns P, Srinivas S. Positron emission tomography in the initial staging of esophageal cancer. Arch Surg 2002; 137:1001–6.

51. Yeung HW, Macapinlac H, Karpeh M, et al. Accuracy of FDG-PET in gastric cancer. preliminary experience. Clin Positron Imaging 1998; 1:213–221.

52. Yeung HW, Macapinlac HA, Mazumdar M, et al. FDG-PET in esophageal cancer. incremental value over computed tomography. Clin Positron Imaging 1999; 2:255–260.

53. Yoo CH, Noh SH, Shin DW, Choi SH, Min JS. Recurrence following curative resection for gastric carcinoma. Br J Surg 2000; 87:236–242.

54. Yoon YC, Lee KS, Shim YM, et al. Metastasis to regional lymph nodes in patients with esophageal squamous cell carcinoma: CT versus FDG PET for presurgical detection prospective study. Radiology 2003; 227:764–70.

55. Yoshioka T, Yamaguchi K, Kubota K, et al. Evaluation of 18F-FDG PET in patients with metastatic or recurrent gastric cancer. J Nucl Med 2003; 44:690–9.

Colorectal Cancer

1. Abdel-Nabi H, Doerr RJ, Lamonica DM, et al. Staging of primary colorectal carcinoma with fluorine-18 fluorodeoxyglucose whole-body PET: correlation with histopathologic and CT findings. Radiology 1998; 206:755–60.

2. Akhurst T, Larson SM. Positron emission tomography imaging of colorectal cancer. Semin Oncol 1999; 26:577–83.

3. Beets G, Penninckx F, Schiepers C, et al. Clinical value of whole-body positron emission tomography with [18F]fluorodeoxyglucose in recurrent colorectal cancer. Br J Surg 1994; 81:1666–70.

4. Delbeke D, Vitola J, Sandler MP, et al. Staging recurrent metastatic colorectal carcinoma with PET. J Nucl Med 1997; 38:1196–1201.

5. Donckier V, Van Laethem JL, Goldman S, et al. [F-18] fluorodeoxyglucose positron emission tomography as a tool for early recognition of incomplete tumor destruction after radiofrequency ablation for liver metastases. J Surg Oncol 2003; 84:215–23.

6. Drenth JP, Nagengast FM, Oyen WJ. Evaluation of (pre-)malignant colonic abnormalities: endoscopic validation of FDG-PET findings. Eur J Nucl Med 2001; 28:1766–9.

7. Falk PM, Gupta NC, Thorson AG, et al. Positron emission tomography for preoperative staging of colorectal carcinoma. Dis Colon Rectum 1994; 37:153–6.

8. Findlay M, Young H, Cunningham D, et al. Noninvasive monitoring of tumor metabolism using fluorodeoxyglucose and positron emission tomography in colorectal cancer liver metastases: correlation with tumor response to fluorouracil. J Clin Oncol 1996; 14:700–8.

9. Flamen P, Stroobants S, Van Cutsem E, et al. Additional value of whole-body positron emission tomography with fluorine-18-2-fluoro-2-deoxy-D-glucose in recurrent colorectal cancer. J Clin Oncol 1999; 17:894–901.

10. Flanagan FL, Dehdashti F, Qgunbiyi OA, et al. Utility of FDG PET for investigating unexplained plasma CEA elevation in patients with colorectal cancer. Ann Surg 1998; 227:319–23.

11. Gambhir SS, Valk P, Shepherd J, et al. Cost effective analysis modeling of the role of FDG PET in the management of patients with recurrent colorectal cancer. J Nucl Med 1997; 38:90P.

12. Guillem J, Calle J, Akhurst T, et al. Preoperative assessment of primary rectal cancer response to preoperative radiation and chemotherapy using 18-fluorodeoxyglucose positron emission tomography. Dis Colon Rectum 2000; 43:18–24.

13. Huebner RH, Park KC, Shepherd JE, et al. A meta-analysis of the literature for whole-body FDG PET detection of recurrent colorectal cancer. J Nucl Med. 2000; 41:1177–89.

14. Imdahl A, Reinhardt MJ, Nitzsche EU, et al. Impact of 18F-FDG positron emission tomography for decision making in colorectal cancer recurrences. Arch Surg 2000; 385:129–134.

15. Ito K, Kato T, Tadokoro M, et al. Recurrent rectal cancer and scar: differentiation with PET and MR imaging. Radiology 1992; 182:549–52.

16. Jadvar H, Johnson DL, Abella-Columna E, et al. Staging colorectal carcinoma with FDG PET at the time of initial diagnosis. Radiology 1997; 205(P):399.

17. Kim EE, Chung SK, Haynie TP, et al. Differentiation of residual or recurrent tumors from post-treatment changes with F-18 FDG PET. Radiographics 1992; 12:269–79.

18. Koike I, Ohmura M, Hata M, et al. FDG-PET scanning after radiation can predict tumor regrowth three months later. Int J Radiat Oncol Biol Phys 2003; 57:1231–8.

19. Libutti SK, Alexander HR Jr, Choyke P, et al. A prospective study of 2-[18F] fluoro-2-deoxy-D-glucose/positron emission tomography scan, 99mTc-labeled arcitumomab (CEA-scan), and blind second-look laparotomy for detecting colon cancer recurrence in patients with increasing carcinoembryonic antigen levels. Ann Surg Oncol 2001; 8:779–86.

20. Meta J, Seltzer M, Schiepers C, et al. Impact of 18F-FDG PET on managing patients with colorectal cancer: the referring physician's perspective. J Nucl Med 2001; 42:586–90.

21. Ohue M, Sekimoto M, Fukunaga H, et al. A case of curative resection of local recurrence after abdominosacral resection of recurrent rectal cancer based on the diagnosis of PET/CT fusion images. Gan To Kagaku Ryoho 2003; 30:1829–32.

22. Schiepers C, Penninckx F, De Vadder N, et al. Contribution of PET in the diagnosis of recurrent colorectal cancer: comparison with conventional imaging. Eur J Surg Oncol 1995; 21:517–22.

23. Staib L, Schirrmeister H, Reske SN, et al. Is (18F)F-fluorodeoxyglucose positron emission tomography in recurrent colorectal cancer a contribution to surgical decision making? Am J Surg 2000; 180:1–5.

24. Strauss LG, Clorius JH, Schlag P, et al. Recurrence of colorectal tumors: PET evaluation. Radiology 1989; 170:329–32.

25. Tatlidil R, Jadvar H, Bading JR, Conti PS. Incidental colonic [F-18]fluorodeoxyglucose uptake: correlation with colonoscopy and histopathology. Radiology 2002; 224:783–7.

26. Valk PE, Abella-Columna E, Haseman MK, et al. Whole-body PET imaging with F-18-fluorodeoxyglucose in management of recurrent colorectal cancer. Arch Surg 1999; 134:503–11.

27. Vitola JV, Delbeke D, Meranze SG, et al. Positron emission tomography with F-18-fluorodeoxyglucose to evaluate the results of hepatic chemoembolization. Cancer 1996; 78:2216–22.

28. Vitola JV, Delbeke D, Sandler MP, et al. Positron emission tomography to stage metastatic colorectal carcinoma to the liver. Am J Surg 1996; 171:21–6.

29. Whiteford MH, Whiteford HM, Yee LF, et al. Usefulness of FDG-PET scan in the assessment of suspected metastatic or recurrent adenocarcinoma of the colon and rectum. Dis Colon Rectum 2000; 43:759–67.

30. Zhuang H, Hickeson M, Chacko TK, et al. Incidental detection of colon cancer by FDG positron emission tomography in patients examined for pulmonary nodules. Clin Nucl Med 2002; 27:628–32.

8

9
Oncology—Pancreas and Hepatobiliary System

I. PANCREATIC CANCER

Pancreatic ductal adenocarcinoma is a dreadful disease with a poor prognosis. Diagnosis at an early stage when the tumor is small and localized is therefore very important for potential cure with surgery. Unfortunately the disease commonly presents in the late stages, primarily due to nonspecific clinical signs and symptoms. Carbohydrate antigen 19-9 (CA 19-9) has been identified as a useful serologic marker for predicting prognosis and relapse in patients with known or suspected recurrent pancreatic carcinoma. A level greater than 1,000 U/ml (normal level <37 U/ml) suggests unresectability, while normalization after therapy predicts relatively longer survival. However, CA19-9 is nonspecific and can be elevated in a variety of benign (e.g., pancreatitis, cholangitis, cirrhosis) and malignant (e.g., gastrointestinal cancers, cholangiocarcinoma, hepatocellular cancer) conditions. CA19-9 is also not suitable for screening, as the level is frequently normal in the early stages of pancreatic carcinoma. Furthermore, about 5% of the population cannot synthesize the CA 19-9 antigen. Despite these limitations, CA 19-9 is a reliable biological marker for monitoring of patients with known or suspected pancreatic cancer, which can prompt imaging evaluation.

Abdominal US, CT, and endoscopic retrograde cholangiopancreatography (ERCP) are the most frequent diagnostic methods used for evaluation of patients with clinical suspicion for pancreatic cancer. However, these methods have difficulty in distinguishing pancreatic cancer from chronic mass-forming pancreatitis, and in differentiating viable tumor from post-therapy changes. Percutaneous biopsy or fine-needle aspiration with CT or US guidance may also be inconclusive. as inflammation and fibrosis around the tumor may impede accurate sampling. The exact role of MRI remains unclear, although recent reports have indicated an advantage over CT.

Pancreatic ductal adenocarcinoma is FDG-avid. The high FDG uptake is due to overexpression of Glut-1 in the pancreatic tumor. FDG PET has been used in preoperative diagnosis of pancreatic carcinoma in differentiating benign from malignant lesions. In this clinical setting, various studies have reported a sensitivity of 85–100% and a specificity of 67–99%, and is a valuable companion to CT for lesion characterization. Once the diagnosis of pancreatic cancer is established, FDG PET is useful for staging by detecting unsuspected distant metastases, which may lead to significant changes in treatment planning. FDG PET, however, may not be superior to anatomic imaging, although it can be a useful adjunct, in assessing local tumor extension and resectability, in detecting metastatic involvement of the adjacent regional lymph nodes and peritoneal carcinomatosis.

FDG PET is particularly useful in the imaging evaluation of patients with suspected recurrent and distant metastatic pancreatic carcinoma based on rising serum tumor marker levels (e.g., CA19-9) and negative or equivocal CT

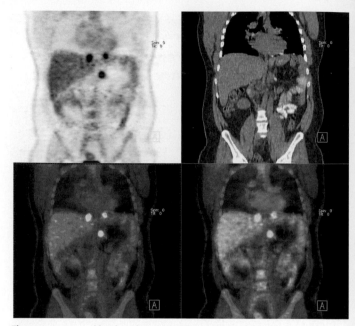

Figure 1: A 50-year-old male with metastatic pancreatic cancer treated one month earlier with wedge liver resection of metastases, partial pancreatectomy, and splenectomy. PET-CT shows hypermetabolic residual hepatic and peripancreatic metastases.

(Figs. 1, 2). Post-treatment anatomic alterations often result in equivocal CT for detection of recurrent disease. Functional imaging with PET, however, can distinguish recurrent tumor from fibrosis and scar based on the high level of FDG localization in the tumor in comparison to low FDG accumulation in treatment-related scar. The complementary diagnostic information provided by FDG PET also impacts the management of patients with pancreatic carcinoma. The impact is particularly important in the form of avoiding unnecessary surgery in unresectable disease or detecting previously unsuspected metastatic disease. FDG PET can also document tumor response to treatment by demonstrating decline in FDG accumulation in responding lesions and stable or increase in FDG uptake in nonresponding lesions. The treatment-related metabolic changes occur earlier than anatomic alterations and therefore can provide an earlier indication of the treatment efficacy, which is especially important in clinical situations where therapeutic options are limited, such as in pancreatic cancer; and the rapid selection of the most effective treatment is pivotal for improving overall survival. In fact the intensity of FDG accumulation as measured by SUV has prognostic value. Patients who have lesions with lower SUV have longer mean survival (SUV < 3, 14 months) in comparison to those with lesions that display higher SUV (SUV >3, 5 months).

In summary, FDG PET has been demonstrated to be useful in the evaluation of indeterminate pancreatic masses, staging of pancreatic cancer, detection of metastatic disease, differentiation of viable tumor from post-therapy

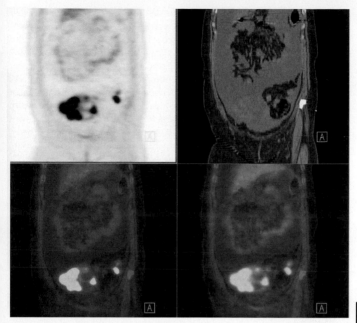

Figure 2: A 41-year-old female with pancreatic cancer treated with tumor resection followed by radiotherapy and one year later by chemotherapy. PET-CT two months after the end of last treatment shows large ascites with extensive hypermetabolism in the right and left lower abdomen corresponding to metastatic disease involving the peritoneum and the mesentery.

changes, and in monitoring response to therapy. However, false negatives may occur with small lesions and in the presence of hyperglycemia, while false-positive results may be seen with chronic and acute pancreatitis.

II. HEPATOBILIARY TUMORS

Hepatocellular carcinoma (HCC) occurs more commonly in the tropics and is associated with exposure to carcinogens and chronic liver disease, such as cirrhosis and viral hepatitis. HCC occurs in two gross patterns, a diffuse form and a nodular form. The fibrolamellar variant is of particular interest, since this variety is more amenable to surgical resection. HCC metastasizes to the regional lymph nodes, lung, and the skeleton. The most common presenting symptoms are abdominal pain, anorexia, weight loss, right-upper-quadrant mass, and ascites. However, one-third of patients may be asymptomatic. Tumor markers associated with HCC include alpha-fetoprotein (AFP) and alpha-1-globulin. Traditional diagnostic imaging evaluation may include US, CT, MRI, and scintigraphy with Tl-201 or Ga-67 citrate.

The exact role of FDG PET in HCC has not been established. Differentiated HCC has relatively high glucose-6-phosphatase activity, which leads to diminished FDG retention in the tumor. FDG PET has a relatively low sensitivity for HCC but may detect up to 70% of HCC lesions (false-negative rate of 30%). FDG PET may, however, be particularly useful in detecting poorly differentiated tumors in view of elevated serum AFP levels. If FDG accumulates in the primary HCC, then PET may be helpful for staging by detecting sites of metastatic disease. PET positivity appears to be correlated with higher histopathologic grade and intratumoral fibrosis but not necrosis or cirrhosis. FDG PET may also be useful in the differential diagnosis with focal nodular hyperplasia (FNH) lesions since FNH frequently demonstrates normal or even decreased accumulation of 18F-FDG (mean SUV 2.12 ± 0.38). FDG PET may, however, be limited in differentiating HCC from benign liver diseases in hepatitis B virus carriers and in patients with chronic hepatitis C virus infection. False positives may also occur with hepatic adenoma.

FDG-PET imaging may have a clinically significant impact in up to 30% of patients with HCC. In FDG-avid HCC, PET has an advantage over CT for monitoring response to treatments (e.g., chemotherapy, surgical cryoablation, radiofrequency ablation, hepatic arterial chemoembolization, etc.) such that the detection of residual or recurrent tumor may prompt appropriate alterations in treatment strategy. The intensity of FDG accumulation in HCC may have prognostic value in predicting the clinical outcome in these patients. C-11 acetate has also been studied in HCC and appears to offer high sensitivity and specificity in this clinical setting. Histopathologic correlation suggests that the well-differentiated HCC tumors are best detected by C-11 acetate and the poorly differentiated types are more FDG-avid.

Cholangiocarcinoma has a poor prognosis. The tumor may develop within the liver or be extrahepatic. There may be predisposing conditions such as sclerosing cholangitis and ulcerative colitis. Lungs are most affected with metastases. Gallbladder carcinoma has a relatively strong association with cholelithiais. Treatment depends on the stage of disease at presentation. Early-stage disease that is confined to the gallbladder is treated with cholecystectomy, which may be extended to the resection of a section of adjacent liver and regional lymph nodes. Palliative therapy is offered to patients with advanced disease which is not infrequently seen when there is clinical suspicion for gallbladder carcinoma. The prognosis is dismal with 5-year survival less than 5%.

FDG accumulates in both gallbladder cancer and in cholangiocarcinoma (Fig. 3). A recent study in 36 patients with suspected cholangiocarcinoma and 14 patients with suspected gallbladder carcinoma demonstrated a sensitivity of 85% for nodular cholangiocarcinoma, 18% for infiltrating cholangiocarcinoma, and 78% for gallbladder cancer. PET led to a change in surgical management in 30% of patients with cholangiocarcinoma because of detection of unsuspected metastases. PET was also helpful for detecting residual gallbladder carcinoma following cholecystectomy but was not helpful in patients with carcinomatosis. False positives occurred with primary sclerosing cholangitis, inflammatory changes related to biliary stents, and granulomatous disease. In another study, PET was performed for preoperative diagnosis of gallbladder malignancy. The sensitivity and specificity of FDG-PET were 75% and 87.5%, respectively. Xanthogranulomatous cholecystitis resulted in the only false-positive case. Therefore, FDG PET may be used for the differential diagnostic imaging evaluation of polypoid lesions of gallbladder.

FDG PET has also been found to be useful in detecting the primary lesion in both hilar and peripheral intrahepatic cholangiocarcinoma and distant metas-

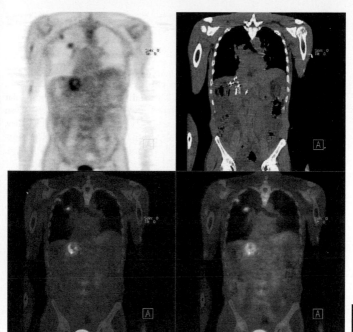

Figure 3: A 57-year-old male with cholangiocarcinoma treated with t3 months earlier with trisegmentectomy and percutaneous biliary stenting. PET-CT shows metastatic deposits in the right lung and a combination of chronic inflammation and probable residual tumor in the surgical hepatic bed.

tases in patients with peripheral cholangiocarcinoma. FDG PET may be false-positively indicate Klatskin tumor-mimicking lesions and falsely negative in mucinous cholangiocarcinoma and in detecting regional lymph node metastases.

REFERENCES

Pancreatic Cancer

1. Bares R, Dohman BM, Klever P, et al. FDG-PET for preoperative assessment of pancreatic masses: results of a prospective study. J Nucl Med 1995; 36:224P.

2. Bares R, Klever P, Hambuechen U, et al. Positron emission tomography (PET) with fluorine-18-labeled deoxyglucose (FDG) for detection of pancreatic cancer (PC): comparison with CT, ultrasonography (US), and ERCP. J Nucl Med 1993; 34:98P.

3. Bares R, Klever P, Hauptmann S, et al. F-18 fluorodeoxyglucose PET in vivo evaluation of pancreatic glucose metabolism for detection of pancreatic cancer. Radiology 1994; 192:79–86.

4. Bares R, Klever P, Hellwig D, et al. Pancreatic cancer detected by positron emission tomography with 18F-labelled deoxyglucose: methods and first results. Nucl Med Commun 1993; 14:596–601.

5. Delbeke D, Rose DM, Chapman WC, et al. Optimal interpretation of FDG PET in the diagnosis, staging and management of pancreatic carcinoma. J Nucl Med 1999; 40:1784–91.

6. Diederichs CG, Staib L, Glatting G, Beger HG, Reske SN. FDG PET: elevated plasma glucose reduces both uptake and detection rate of pancreatic malignancies. J Nucl Med 1998; 39:1030–3.

7. Friess H, Langhans J, Ebert M, et al. Diagnosis of pancreatic cancer by 2[18F]-fluoro-2-deoxy-D-glucose positron emission tomography. Gut 1995; 36:771–7.

8. Higashi T, Sakahara H, Torizuka T, et al. Evaluation of intraoperative radiation therapy for unresectable pancreatic cancer with FDG PET. J Nucl Med 1999; 40:1424–3.

9. Higashi T, Tamaki N, Torizuka Tet al. Differentiation of malignant from benign pancreatic tumors by FDG-PET: comparison with CT, US, and endoscopic ultrasonogrpahy. J Nucl Med 1995; 36:224P.

10. Ho CL, Dehdashti F, Griffeth LK, et al. FDG-PET evaluation of indeterminate pancreatic masses. J Comput Assist Tomogr 1996; 20:363–369.

11. Inokuma T, Tamaki N, Torizuka T, et al. Evaluation of pancreatic tumors with positron emission tomogrpahy and F-18 fluorodeoxyglucose: comparison with CT and US. Radiology 1995; 195:345–352.

12. Jadvar H, Fischman AJ. Evaluation of pancreatic carcinoma with FDG PET. Abdom Imaging 2001; 26:254–9.

13. Keogan MT, Tyler D, Clark L, et al. Diagnosis of pancreatic carcinoma: role of FDG PET. AJR Am J Roentgenol 1998; 171:1565–1570.

14. Klever P, Bares R, Fass J, et al. PET with fluorine-18 deoxyglucose for pancreatic disease. Lancet 1992; 340:1158–1159.

15. Reske SN, Grillenberger KG, Glatting G, et al. Overexpression of glucose transporter 1 and increased FDG uptake in pancreatic carcinoma. J Nucl Med 1997; 38:1344–1348.

16. Shreve PD. Focal fluorine-18 fluorodeoxyglucose accumulation in inflammatory pancreatic disease. Eur J Nucl Med 1998; 25:259–264.

17. Stollfuss JC, Glatting G, Friess H, et al. 2-(fluorine-18)-fluoro-2-deoxy-D-glucose PET in detection of pancreatic cancer: value of quantitative image interpretation. Radiology 1995; 195:339–344.

18. Stollfuss JC, Kocher F, Glatting G, Reske SN. Pancreatic cancer vs. chronic pancreatitis: diagnosis with [18F]-FDG PET, CT and ERCP. J Nucl Med 1995; 36: 223–224.

19. Stollfuss JC, Schonberger JA, Fries H, et al. Improved diagnosis of pancreatic carcinoma with FDG-PET compared to CT in non-invasive imaging modalities. Eur J Nucl Med 1994; 22: 759P.

20. Zimny M, Buell U. 18FDG-positron emission tomography in pancreatic cancer. Ann Oncol 1999; 10(Suppl. 4): 28–32.

21. Safi F, Roscher R, Beger HG. The clinical relevance of tumor marker CA 19-9 in the diagnosing and monitoring of pancreatic carcinoma. Bull Cancer 1990; 77: 83–91.

22. Steinberg W. The clinical utility of the CA 19-9 tumor-associated antigen. Am J Gastroenterology 1990; 85: 350–5.

Hepatobiliary Cancer

1. Anderson CD, Rice MH, Pinson CW, et al. Fluorodeoxyglucose PET imaging in the evaluation of gallbladder carcinoma and cholangiocarcinoma. J Gastroint Surg 2004; 8:90–7.

2. Anderson GS, Brinkmann F, Soulen MC, et al. FDG positron emission tomography in the surveillance of hepatic tumors treated with radiofrequency ablation. Clin Nucl Med. 2003; 28:192–7.

3. Braga FJ, Flamen P, Mortelmans L, et al. Ga-67-positive and F-18 FDG-negative imaging in well-differentiated hepatocellular carcinoma. Clin Nucl Med 2001; 26:642.

4. Delbeke D, Martin WH, Sandler MP, et al. Evaluation of benign vs malignant hepatic lesions with positron emission tomography. Arch Surg 1998; 133:510–5.

5. Donckier V, Van Laethem JL, Goldman S, et al. F-18] fluorodeoxyglucose positron emission tomography as a tool for early recognition of incomplete tumor destruction after radiofrequency ablation for liver metastases. J Surg Oncol 2003; 84:215–23.

6. Fritscher-Ravens A, Bohuslavizki KH, Broering DC, et al. FDG PET in the diagnosis of hilar cholangiocarcinoma. Nucl Med Commun 2001; 22:1277–85.

7. Ho CL, Yu SC, Yeung DW. 11C-acetate PET imaging in hepatocellular carcinoma and other liver masses. J Nucl Med 2003; 44:213–21.

8. Iwata Y, Shiomi S, Sasaki N, et al. Clinical usefulness of positron emission tomography with fluorine-18-fluorodeoxyglucose in the diagnosis of liver tumors. Ann Nucl Med 2000; 14:121–6.

9. Jeng LB, Changlai SP, Shen YY, et al. Limited value of 18F-2-deoxyglucose positron emission tomography to detect hepatocellular carcinoma in hepatitis B virus carriers. Hepatogastroenterology 2003; 50:2154–6.

10. Keiding S, Hansen SB, Rasmussen HH, et al. Detection of cholangiocarcinoma in primary sclerosing cholangitis by positron emission tomography. Hepatology 1998; 28:700–6.

11. Khan MA, Combs CS, Brunt EM, et al. Positron emission tomography scanning in the evaluation of hepatocellular carcinoma. J Hepatol 2000; 32:792–7.

12. Kim YJ, Yun M, Lee WJ, et al. Usefulness of 18F-FDG PET in intrahepatic cholangio-carcinoma. Eur J Nucl Med Mol Imaging 2003; 30:1467–72.

13. Kluge R, Schmidt F, Caca K, et al. Positron emission tomography with [(18)F]fluoro-2-deoxy-D-glucose for diagnosis and staging of bile duct cancer. Hepatology 2001; 33(5):1029–35.

14. Koh T, Taniguchi H, Yamaguchi A, et al. Differential diagnosis of gallbladder cancer using positron emission tomography with fluorine-18-labeled fluoro-deoxyglucose (FDG-PET). J Surg Oncol 2003; 84:74–81.

15. Krug B, Martinet JP, Lacrosse M, et al. A well-differentiated hepatocellular carcinoma detected only by F-18 FDG positron emission tomography. Clin Nucl Med 2003; 28:606–7.

16. Kurtaran A, Becherer A, Pfeffel F, et al. 18F-fluorodeoxyglucose (FDG)-PET features of focal nodular hyperplasia (FNH) of the liver. Liver 2000; 20:487–90.

17. Lomis KD, Vitola JV, Delbeke D, et al. Recurrent gallbladder carcinoma at laparoscopy port sites diagnosed by PET scan: implications for primary and radical second operations. Ann Surg 1997; 63:341–5.

18. Patel PM, Alibazoglu H, Ali A, et al. 'False-positive' uptake of FDG in a hepatic adenoma. Clin Nucl Med 1997; 22:490–1.

19. Schroder O, Trojan J, Zeuzem S, et al. Limited value of fluorine-18-fluorodeoxyglucose PET for the differential diagnosis of focal liver lesions in patients with chronic hepatitis C virus infection. Nuklearmedizin 1998; 37:279–85.

20. Shiomi S, Nishiguchi S, Ishizu H, et al. Usefulness of positron emission tomography with fluorine-18-fluorodeoxyglucose for predicting outcome in patients with hepatocellular carcinoma. Am J Gastroenterol 2001; 96:1877–80.

21. Torizuka T, Tamaki N, Inokuma T, et al. In vivo assessment of glucose metabolism in hepatocellular carcinoma with FDG-PET. J Nucl Med 1995; 36:1811–7.

22. Torizuka T, Tamaki N, Inokuma T, et al. Value of fluorine-18-FDG-PET to monitor hepatocellular carcinoma after interventional therapy. J Nucl Med 1994; 35:1965–9.

23. Trojan J, Schroeder O, Raedle J, et al. Fluorine-18 FDG positron emission tomography for imaging of hepatocellular carcinoma. Am J Gastroenterol 1999; 94:3314–9.

24. Widjaja A, Mix H, Wagner S, et al. Positron emission tomography and cholangiocarcinoma in primary sclerosing cholangitis. Z Gastroenterol 1999; 37:731–3.

25. Wudel LJ Jr, Delbeke D, Morris D, et al. The role of [18F]fluorodeoxyglucose positron emission tomography imaging in the evaluation of hepatocellular carcinoma. Am Surg 2003; 69:117–24.

Oncology—Breast and Female Reproductive System

I. BREAST CANCER

Breast cancer is the most common cancer in women in the United States. The lifetime risk of breast cancer is about one in eight in the American women. The histopathologic types of breast cancer include ductal adenocarcinoma, lobular carcinoma, lymphoma, sarcoma, and the Paget's disease of the nipple. Mammography and ultrasound are currently the principal imaging modalities for screening. Mammography has low specificity, and although it is relatively sensitive for detecting suspicious lesions in fatty breasts, it has lower sensitivity in detecting lesions in dense and augmented breasts. Breast MRI has also been employed for characterization of breast lesions and for determination of tumor relationship to the axillary and supraclavicular neurovascular structures. Scintimammography with Tc-99m sestamibi may be helpful in the evaluation of radiographically dense breasts. Bone scintigraphy is useful for the detection of osseous metastatic disease. There has also been a fast-growing utilization of preoperative mapping of the sentinel lymph node(s) with scintigraphy in order to stage the axilla in order to avoid complete axillary nodal dissection with its associated potential morbidity (chronic pain, numbness, lymphedema, etc.).

FDG PET has been evaluated for diagnosis, staging, restaging, and monitoring therapy response in patients with breast cancer (Figs. 1–5). Although the current data suggest that FDG PET may have limited diagnostic utility in the detection of small primary tumors, in staging the axilla, and in detecting blastic osseous metastatic lesions, but PET has superiority over conventional imaging in detecting distant metastases and recurrent disease, and in monitoring therapy response The Centers for Medicare and Medicaid Services has recently provided coverage for the procedure.

Although few studies have demonstrated overexpression of Glut-1 in untreated primary breast cancer, others have reported no clear relationship between tumor FDG uptake and Glut-1 overexpression. FDG localization is significantly higher in ductal carcinoma than in lobular (median SUV 5.6 for infiltrating ductal carcinomas vs. 3.8 for lobular carcinomas). Breast density and hormonal status affect the FDG uptake in the breast tissue. Dense breasts demonstrate higher FDG uptake than nondense breasts. However, the highest SUV observed in dense breasts is relatively low at about 1.4.

Lactating breast shows high FDG localization that appears to be related to suckling. The high FDG uptake in the breast, however, may impede tumor detection in this subset of patients. Similarly acute or chronic infectious mastitis and post-surgical hemorrhagic mastitis may lead to breast hypermetabolism.

Mammography and ultrasound remain the main diagnostic imaging tools for the diagnosis of primary breast cancer. However, the metabolic information provided by FDG PET may be useful in the noninvasive characterization of the indeterminate lesions. The development of the new combined PET and

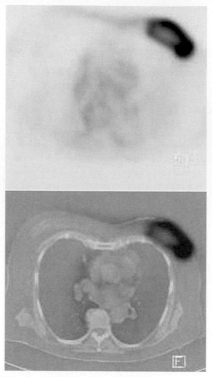

Figure 1: Marked hypermetabolism in a large left breast mass. Surgical specimen demonstrated infiltrating ductal adenocarcinoma.

radiographic imaging systems (a positron emission mammography device mounted on a sterotactic X-ray mammography system) and the positron-sensitive probe may help in discriminating between benign and malignant breast masses, in guiding biopsy, and in reducing costly surgical procedures. PET is also useful in the evaluation of patients with augmented breasts in whom the other traditional diagnostic imaging techniques may be inconclusive. For the diagnosis of breast cancer, lesion detectabilility appears to increase with the more delayed scan time of 3 h than the usual scan time of 1–1.5 h (93% vs. 83%, respectively) after the intravenous administration of FDG. It is also of note that false-positive PET may occur in specific conditions such as fibroadenoma, but this is similar to the case with Tc-99m sestamibi imaging. However, in general it appears that SUV of benign lesion is lower than that of the malignant lesion, although there is significant overlap.

FDG PET has limited sensitivity in staging the axilla in patients with early breast cancer, with a false-negative rate that may approach over 20%. A recent prospective multi-center study of axillary nodal staging with FDG PET demonstrated mean sensitivity, specificity, positive, and negative predictive values of 61%, 80%, 62%, and 79%, respectively. FDG PET appears to be a specific method for staging the axilla such that sentinel lymph node biopsy may be

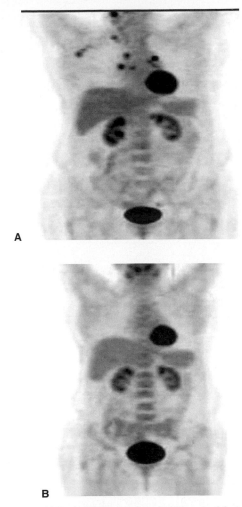

A

B

Figure 2: A 53-year-old female with history of poorly differentiated ductal right breast cancer initially treated with right mastectomy who now presents with palpable right axillary nodes. **A.** Pre-therapy FDG PET demonstrates extensive metastatic nodal disease in the right neck, right axilla, and the mediastinum. **B.** Post-therapy FDG PET shows no evident disease compatible with good therapy response.

avoided in patients with positive axilla on the PET study. The overall sensitivity and specificity for the detection of the axillary metastases on FDG PET does not appear to be related to the SUV of the primary carcinoma. The differences among studies in the reported diagnostic performance of PET in relation to axillary nodal staging are likely because of several factors, including differences in the tumor type, the prevalence of disease in the study population, the

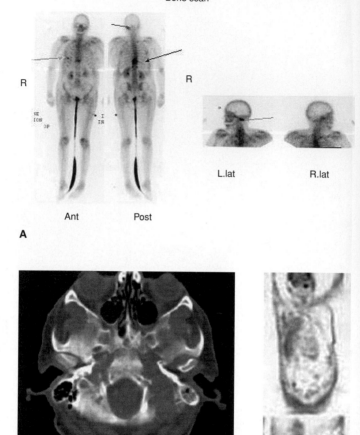

Bone scan

R   R

Ant   Post   L.lat   R.lat

A

B

C

Figure 3: A 59-year-old female with a history of breast cancer s/p spinal decompression for metastatic disease. **A.** Bone scan shows active lesions in the left temporal skull, thoracolumbar spine, and the fifth right anterolateral rib. **B.** Head CT at bone window level shows a large lytic lesion in the left mastoid area. **C.** PET scan demonstrates the corresponding hypermetabolic lesions (rib lesion not shown).

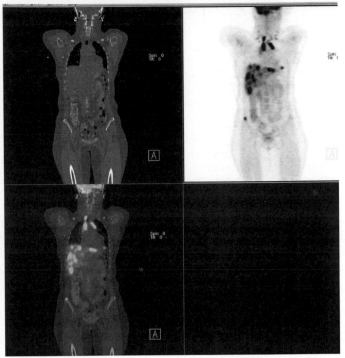

Figure 4: A 43-year-old female with a history of right breast carcinoma treated with mastectomy and reconstruction followed by chemotherapy. PET-CT images show extensive upper mediastinal, hepatic, and several skeletal metastases.

10

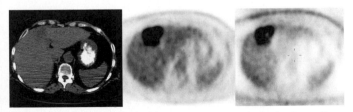

Figure 5: Solitary Liver Metastasis from Breast Cancer. FDG-PET/CT showing a solitary liver metastasis in the medial segment of the left lobe in a patient with a history of breast cancer eight years prior to presentation. Biopsy showed adenocarcinoma which was estrogen receptor positive. The solitary metastasis was resected.

imaging methodology, and the image interpretation criteria. However, detection of micrometastases and small tumor-infiltrated lymph nodes is limited by the spatial resolution of the current PET imaging systems.

FDG PET has also been reported to be a useful tool in the evaluation of patients with suspected metastatic plexopathy, particularly if the other imaging studies are unremarkable. PET can also differentiate between radiation-induced plexopathy and metastatic plexopathy. FDG PET has been found to be helpful in the evaluation of patients with inflammatory breast cancer. Mammography usually demonstrates parenchymal distortion, diffuse increased density, and skin thickening. On FDG PET, the diffuse pattern of breast FDG uptake reflects the dermal lymphatic spread of the malignancy. In another uncommon malignancy, cystic infiltrating ductal carcinoma, PET shows intense focal FDG localization in the solid component and a ring-like increased uptake, corresponding to the wall of the cystic component of the tumor.

FDG PET has been demonstrated to be accurate in the diagnosis of recurrent and metastatic disease not recognized by conventional imaging methods. In a study comparing FDG PET and MRI for detecting recurrent disease, the sensitivity and specificity were 79% and 100% for MRI and 94% and 72% for PET. Additional unknown metastases were detected by whole-body PET in a few patients that influenced the clinical management. A comparative study of FDG PET and conventional imaging in patients with clinical suspicion of local recurrence or distant metastatic disease demonstrated sensitivity, specificity, positive and negative predictive values of 97%, 82%, 87%, 96% for FDG PET in comparison to 84%, 60%, 73%, and 75% for conventional imaging. FDG PET up-staged the disease in 10% and down-staged the disease in 13% of patients and lead to a change in therapeutic management in 21% of patients. PET is also more sensitive than serum tumor markers (CA 15-3 and CEA) in detecting relapsed breast cancer. FDG PET has been compared with bone scan in the detection of osseous metastases. PET and bone scan appear to offer similar sensitivity in this regard, but PET provides a specificity advantage over bone scan. Bone metastases of the osteolytic or mixed type are usually better visualized on PET than the sclerotic bony lesions. In general, FDG PET may impact the clinical stage and management of about 30% of patients with suspected recurrent and metastatic breast cancer.

FDG PET has been shown to be useful in the assessment of therapy response in patients with breast cancer by demonstrating decline in the tumor glucose metabolism with successful chemotherapy in correlation with decline in serum tumor markers. In one study, in patients who responded to chemotherapy the median SUV of the lesions decreased from 7.7 at baseline to 5.7 after the first chemotherapy course to 1.2 at the end of the chemotherapy regimen. In patients with stable disease as the best response, no significant decrease in tumor glucose SUV was noted in comparison to the baseline level. A complete response was predicted after the first course of chemotherapy with a sensitivity of 90% and a specificity of 74%. Moreover, FDG PET has been demonstrated to be useful in evaluating response to the new therapies such as stereotactic interstitial laser therapy, which is emerging as a promising alternative to surgery for treating early-stage breast cancer.

PET can also stratify the clinical outcome more accurately than conventional imaging, such that a negative PET predicts longer disease-free survival in comparison to a positive PET. FDG PET can provide quantitative metabolic information that may be used to predict overall and relapse-free survival in patients with breast cancer. Patients with lesions that demonstrate high FDG uptake have significantly poorer prognoses than those with lesions that have low FDG uptake.

II. CERVICAL CANCER

Papanicolaou (Pap) smear screening has resulted in a sharp decline in the mortality from cervical cancer. However, cervical cancer still remains a leading cause of death in relatively young women in the developing countries where screening is less prevalent. Most cervical cancers are squamous cell carcinomas, but some are adnocarcinomas. Staging provides important information about the choice of treatment protocol and prognosis. The staging of disease is based on the International Federation of Gynecology and Obstetrics (FIGO) classification. The cure rate is nearly 100% in early-stage disease, while it is less than 5% in the late stages. Choice of therapy, including surgery, radiation therapy, and chemotherapy depends primarily on the disease stage. The disease-free interval after treatment depends on the initial stage of the tumor and the adequacy of the initial treatment. Recurrent disease is associated with a poor prognosis and the tumor tends to relapse in the pelvis, retroperitoneum, and distant sites.

The utility of FDG PET in staging of cervical carcinoma has been studied by several investigators (Fig. 6). Early studies showed high accumulation of

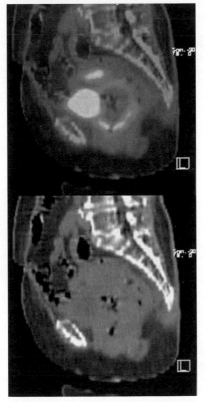

10

Figure 6: A 69-year-old female with recurrent cervical cancer. PET-CT shows a pelvic soft tissue mass with a hypermetabolic rim posterior to the urinary bladder compatible with tumor recurrence surrounding necrotic tumor.

FDG in both the primary tumor and the metastatic lesions. The high FDG uptake is related to the overexpression of Glut-1 in the tumor and does not correlate with the initial grade of histologic differentiation and FIGO staging. Lesion visualization in the pelvis is improved by obtaining postvoid FDG PET images, which substantially reduce the bladder urinary activity. PET has been demonstrated to have a competitive advantage over CT in the diagnostic imaging evaluation of cervical cancer, although CT provides important information on the anatomic localization of the lesions. In one study of patients with advanced cervical cancer confined to the pelvis and negative abdominal CT studies for nodal disease, FDG PET demonstrated a sensitivity of 86% and a specificity of 94% in detecting para-aortic lymph nodal disease with retroperitoneal surgical exploration as the diagnostic "gold" standard. In a similar study of patients with advanced cervical cancer and negative abdominal MRI studies for nodal disease, FDG PET showed a sensitivity of 83% and specificity of 97% for assessment of para-aortic lymph node metastases. MRI appears to have insufficient accuracy for nodal staging, while high positive predictive value of PET can obviate the need for nodal sampling with the caveat that microscopic disease may be missed by either imaging modality. FDG PET has been shown to be not only more accurate than CT for lymph node staging but also a better predictor of survival in patients with cervical cancer.

Several studies have shown the utility of FDG PET in the diagnosis of recurrent and metastatic disease. In a recent investigation, feasibility of FDG PET in the early detection of recurrent disease was evaluated retrospectively in patients without evidence of cervical cancer after therapy. The sensitivity and specificity of PET for detection of early recurrence were 90% and 76%, respectively. The sensitivity was higher in the spine, liver, and the mediastinal, hilar, and scalene lymph node basins and relatively lower in the lung and retrovesical and para-aortic lymph node chains. In another retrospective study comparing CT and PET in the detection of recurrent disease, the sensitivity and specificity were 78% and 83% for CT and 100% and 94% for PET, respectively. The diagnostic performance of PET in relation to specific sites of disease has also been investigated. The sensitivity and specificity of FDG PET were 90% and 100% for detecting local recurrence, 100% and 94% for pelvic lymph node metastases, 100% and 100% for para-aortic lymph node metastases, and 100% and 100% for distal metastases, respectively. In other studies, dual phase FDG PET scanning at 40 min and at 3 h after tracer administration followed by calculation of a lesion retention index (defined as subtraction of the 40-min lesion SUV from that at 3 h) was shown to be not only highly accurate but also significantly superior to MRI and CT in detecting metastases. The performance of PET may also be improved with PET-CT in view of precise localization of hypermetabolic lesions.

Staging based on PET may significantly influence the choice of treatment. FDG PET can also provide important information for radiation treatment planning, which improves isodose tumor coverage and spares the nearby critical structures. Similar findings have also been reported with the use of semi-quantitative measures such as SUV in detecting active cervical cancer after radiation and in monitoring therapy response in metastatic disease. PET may measure tumor volume accurately in patients with advanced disease and provide important information about prognosis including the progression-free survival and the overall survival.

FDG PET has been shown to be valuable in predicting the outcomes of patients with cervical cancer. In one study, based on the PET detection of the extent of lymph node metastatic involvement, the three-year cause-specific survival was 73% for those patients without lymph node metastases, 58% for those with only pelvic lymphadenopathy, 29% for those with pelvic and para-aortic lymph node metastases, and 0% for those with pelvic, para-aortic, and supra-clavicular metastatic nodal disease. Post-treatment surveillance monitoring of cervical cancer by FDG PET has also been studied. The two-year progression-free survival rate was 86% for patients with unremarkable FDG PET scans, 40% for those with persistent abnormal FDG uptake, and 0% for those with new sites of hypermetablic disease

III. UTERINE CANCER

Endometrial tumor is not only the most common type of uterine cancer but also the most common type of female genital cancer in the United States. Endometrial adenocarcinoma is the predominant malignant neoplasm of the uterus. The tumor tends to spread along the surface of the uterine cavity before penetrating the uterine corpus. Metastases may spread via the blood vessels, through the lymphatic system, or may seed the peritoneum via the fallopian tube. The cure rate for endometrial cancer is high. Hysterectomy is the primary treatment. However, radiation therapy, hormonal therapy, and chemotherapy may also be employed in infrequent inoperable cases.

Several single case studies and case-series studies have reported on the usefulness of PET in endometrial cancer (Figs. 7, 8). In one study, FDG PET

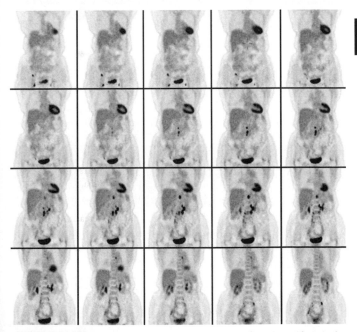

Figure 7: Uterine Cancer Staging. Coronal FDG-PET images of a patient with a mixed Mullerian tumor of the uterus shows widespread abdominal nodal metastases as well as a paraesophageal node in the mediastinum.

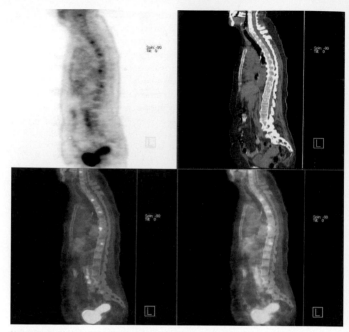

Figure 8: A patient with hypermetabolic endometrial cancer (posterior to urinary bladder) and evidence for multiple osseous metastases in the thoracic spine.

detected unsuspected asymptomatic recurrences in 12% of cases but missed microscopic lung metastases. PET demonstrated a sensitivity of 96%, a specificity of 78%, a positive predictive value of 89%, a negative predictive value of 91%. PET findings also altered the treatment choice by detecting unsuspected distant metastases. Although FDG PET appears to be very useful for the imaging evaluation of endometrial carcinoma, benign uterine conditions, such as uterine leiomyoma, may also result in relatively high FDG accumulation and be cause for false-positive finding. The physiologic endometrial FDG uptake may also change cyclically, increasing during the ovulatory and menstrual phases (Figs. 9–10).

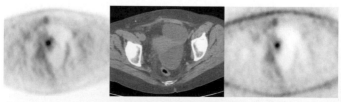

Figure 9: Endometrial Uptake. FDG-PET/CT shows endometrial activity at the time of menses. Also note the absence of uptake in two adnexal cysts.

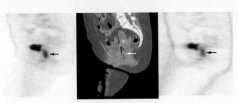

Figure 10: Activity in Tampon. Sagittal slice from an FDG-PET/CT in a patient who was menstruating at the time of scan. There is increased activity in a tampon (shown by an arrow). Although there is little blood activity at the time of scan, shortly after injection the blood activity is high. Furthermore, there is endometrial uptake of FDG at the time of menses. On the left is an attenuation-corrected FDG image; in the center is a CT image; on the right is a non-corrected FDG image.

FDG PET may also be useful in the evaluation of the less common uterine sarcomas by demonstrating relatively high FDG accumulation in the tumor. FDG PET appears to have a competitive diagnostic advantage over MRI and US in the imaging assessment of uterine sarcoma.

IV. OVARIAN CANCER

Ovarian carcinoma is one of the deadliest and the most difficult of all gynecologic cancers to control because it often presents in the late stages of disease. Clinical symptoms such as abdominal distension and discomfort develop when the disease is advanced. Serum tumor markers such as CA-125 are useful in patients with epithelial ovarian cancer. Staging is according to the FIGO classification scheme. Definitive staging usually includes abdominal surgery accompanied by biopsy of suspicious areas and cytologic evaluation of the ascetic fluid, and the washings of the cul-de-sac, the lateral and paracolic gutters, and the subdiaphragmatic areas, as well as scrapings of the visceral and the parietal surfaces. Cytoreductive surgery is employed with the goal of removing as much of the tumor as possible. Post-operative treatment includes chemotherapy and/or radiotherapy. Second-look surgical exploration has been used to determine the need for further therapy in patients who appear to be free of clinically evident disease. The choice of post-operative therapy is dependent on the properties of the tumor, the age and reproductive status of the patient, and the co-morbid conditions. Intra-peritoneal administration of chemotherapeutic agents, whole abdomen external radiotherapy, and hormonal therapy are other therapeutic alternatives. Survival depends on the initial stage of disease, the lesion grade, and the amount of residual disease following therapy. The five-year survival is about 70% in patients with stage I disease and about 4% in patients with stage IV disease.

The diagnostic utility of PET in ovarian carcinoma has been investigated relatively extensively (Figs. 11, 12). Most reported studies with FDG use post-void pelvis images to reduce bladder urine activity and do not incorporate bladder irrigation. In premenopausal women, normal ovaries may demonstrate relatively high FDG uptake that appears to be related to the menstrual cycle. A group of investigators compared the diagnostic performances of US, MRI, and FDG PET with histopathology, as the standard of reference for the detection of malignancy, in patients with asymptomatic adnexal masses. The overall

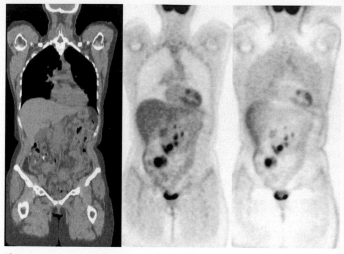

Figure 11: Ovarian Cancer Staging. Coronal FDG-PET/CT in a patient with ovarian cancer shows multiple sites of interabdominal spread of disease.

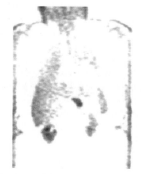

Figure 12: A 54-year-old patient with history of ovarian cancer s/p BSO and chemotherapy. Recurrence was suspected based on elevated serum CA-125 level (71 U/ml). PET scan demonstrated abnormal focal hypermetabolic activity in the epigastric region. Second-look surgery revealed metastatic disease involving the gastrocolic ligament and omentum.

sensitivities and specificities were 58% and 76% for PET, 92% and 60% for US, 83% and 84% for MRI, and 92% and 85% for the combined imaging modalities, respectively. The combination of all three modalities was considered the method of choice for the imaging assessment of asymptomatic adnexal masses for malignancy. Similarly, the addition of FDG PET to CT increases accuracy in staging ovarian cancer. In one study, the lesion-based sensitivity, specificity, and negative predictive value were 70%, 83%, and 59%, respectively, for CT alone and 83%, 92%, and 73%, respectively, for combined PET and CT. Although PET imaging may be useful for identifying macroscopic disease when other imaging modalities are negative or equivocal, both PET and the other imaging modalities are limited in detecting the peritoneal micrometastases as well as the low-grade malignancies and cannot currently substitute for a second-look operation. Imaging detection of peritoneal carcinomatosis can be difficult on both CT and PET. However, attention to certain characteristic scintigraphic patterns, including the presence of either nodular or diffuse peritoneal activity, can be helpful for recognition of peritoneal pathology. Overall, the encouraging results of the diagnostic performance of FDG PET have rendered significant impact on the clinical staging (18–57%) and the clinical management (17–67%) of patients with ovarian cancer.

The utility of the new hybrid PET-CT imaging system has also been assessed in the detection of recurrent ovarian carcinoma in a recent retrospective study. Recurrent disease was correctly identified in 62% of patients who had negative CT and positive PET-CT studies, which suggested such patients might directly proceed to salvage treatment and avoid the morbidity and expense of surgical evaluation. Other studies have also documented the incremental diagnostic utility of PET-CT in comparison to PET alone. In one study, PET-CT identified additional lesions compared to CT in 80% and changed management in 73% of the patients.

PET has been found to be more sensitive than CT in the evaluation of patients with suspected recurrent disease based on elevated serum tumor marker CA-125 (>35 U/ml). In a study of patients with asymptomatic elevated serum tumor marker and equivocal or negative other imaging studies, FDG PET detected sites of recurrent disease with a sensitivity of 95% and specificity of 88%. In a similar study, FDG PET was found to be accurate in detecting ovarian cancer recurrence with a sensitivity of 80% and a specificity of 100% in comparison to sensitivities and specificities of 55% and 100%, respectively, for conventional imaging (CT and MRI), and 75% and 100%, respectively, for CA-125 serum tumor marker. In patients with rising CA-125 levels within the normal range, FDG PET may also be useful in detecting an early small region of relapse even when the other imaging studies and the physical examination are unremarkable. Other reports suggest that combined conventional imaging and PET results in the highest diagnostic yield for detecting the sites of recurrent disease. There are also recent encouraging reports on the utility of combined PET-CT imaging systems for localizing and differentiating pathologic activity from physiologic activity in women with recurrent ovarian carcinoma. Specifically, PET-CT imaging has a high predictive value of 94% in detecting recurrent disease equal to or larger than 1 cm among patients with biochemical evidence of recurrence and negative or equivocal conventional CT findings. The PET-CT detection of macroscopic recurrent lesions may thus facilitate complete surgical cytoreduction.

The prognostic utility of FDG PET has also been studied. A negative PET scan during the follow-up period after the primary treatment predicts longer relapse-free interval than a positive PET scan does.

BIBLIOGRAPHY

Breast Cancer

1. Adler LP, Faulhaber PF, Schnur KC, et al. Axillary lymph node metastases: screening with [F-18]2-deoxy-2-fluoro-D-glucose (FDG) PET. Radiology 1997; 203:323–7.

2. Adler LP, Weinberg IN, Bradbury MS, et al. Method for combined FDG-PET and radiographic imaging of primary breast cancers. Breast J 2003; 9:163–6.

3. Ahmad A, Barrington S, Maisey M, et al. Use of positron emission tomography in evaluation of brachial plexopathy in breast cancer patients. Br J Cancer 1999; 478–82.

4. Avril N, Dose J, Janicke F, et al. Assessment of axillary lymph node involvement in breast cancer patients with positron emission tomography using radiolabeled 2-(fluorine-18)-fluoro-2-deoxy-D-glucose. J Natl Cancer Inst 1996; 88:1204–9.

5. Avril N, Menzel M, Dose J, et al. Glucose metabolism of breast cancer assessed by 18F-FDG PET: histologic and immunohistochemical tissue analysis. J Nucl Med 2001; 42:9–16.

6. Avril N, Rose CA, Schelling M, et al. Breast imaging with positron emission tomography and fluorine-18 fluorodeoxyglucose: use and limitations. J Clin Oncol 2000; 18:3495–502.

7. Barranger E, Grahek D, Antoine M, et al. Evaluation of fluorodeoxyglucose positron emission tomography in the detection of axillary lymph node metastases in patients with early-stage breast cancer. Ann Surg Oncol 2003; 10:622–7.

8. Bassa P, Kim EE, Inoue T, et al. Evaluation of preoperative chemotherapy using PET with fluorine-18-deoxyglucose in breast cancer. J Nucl Med 1996; 37:931–8.

9. Bender H, Kirst J, Palmedo H, et al. Value of 18-fluoro-deoxyglucose positron emission tomography in the staging of recurrent breast carcinoma. Anticancer Res 1997; 17:1687–92.

10. Bombardieri E, Crippa F. PET imaging in breast cancer. Q J Nucl Med 2001; 45:245–56.

11. Brix G, Henze M, Knopp MV, et al. Comparison of pharmacokinetic MRI and [18F]fluorodeoxyglucose PET in the diagnosis of breast cancer: initial experience. Eur Radiol 2001; 11:2058–70.

12. Brown RS, Goodman TM, Zasadny KR, et al. Expression of hexokinase II and Glut-1 in untreated human breast cancer. Nucl Med Biol 2002; 29:443–53.

13. Buck A, Schirrmeister H, Kuhn T, et al. FDG uptake in breast cancer: correlation with biological and clinical prognostic parameters. Eur J Nucl Med Mol Imaging 2002; 29:1317–23.

14. Burcombe RJ, Makris A, Pittam M, et al. Evaluation of good clinical response to neoadjuvant chemotherapy in primary breast cancer using [18F]-fluorodeoxyglucose positron emission tomography. Eur J Cancer 2002; 38:375–9.

15. Crippa F, Agresti R, Seregni E, et al. Prospective evaluation of fluorine-18-FDG PET in presurgical staging of the axilla in breast cancer. J Nucl Med 1998; 39:4–8.

16. Crowe JP Jr, Adler LP, Shenk RR, et al. Positron emission tomography and breast masses: comparison with clinical, mammographic and pathological findings. Ann Surg Oncol 1994; 1:132–40.

17. Dose J, Bleckmann C, Bachmann S, et al. Comparison of fluorodeoxyglucose positron emission tomography and "conventional diagnostic procedures" for the detection of distant metastases in breast cancer patients. Nul Med Commun 2002; 23:857–64.

18. Eubank WB, Mankoff DA, Vesselle HJ, et al. Detection of locoregional and distant recurrences in breast cancer patients by using FDG PET. Radiographics 2002; 22:5–17.

19. Flanagan FL, Dehdashti F, Siegel BA. PET in breast cancer. Semin Nucl Med 1998; 28:290–302.

20. Gennari A, Donati S, Salvadori B, et al. Role of 2-[18F]-fluorodeoxyglucose (FDG) positron emission tomography (PET) in the early assessment of response to chemotherapy in metastatic breast cancer patients. Clin Breast Cancer 2000; 1:156–61.

21. Goerres GW, Miche SC, Fehr MK, et al. Follow-up of women with breast cancer: comparison between MRI and FDG PET. Eur Radiol 2003; 13:1633–44.

22. Greco M, Crippa M, Agresti R, et al. Axillary lymph node staging in breast cancer by 2-fluoro-2-deoxy-D-glucose positron emission tomography: clinical evaluation and alternative management. J Natl Cancer Inst 2001; 93:630–5.

23. Hoh CK, Schipers C. 18-FDG imaging in breast cancer. Semin Nucl Med 1999; 29:49–56.

24. Hubner KF, Smith GT, Thie JA, et al. The potential of F-18-FDG PET in breast cancer. Detection of primary lesions, axillary lymph node metastases, or distant metastases. Clin Positron Imaging 2000; 3:197–205.

25. Jadvar H, Epstein A, Conti PS. Evaluation of suspected recurrent and metastatic breast carcinoma with ^{18}F-FDG PET. J Nucl Med 2003; 44 (5 Suppl):170P.

26. Kamel EM, Wyss MT, Fehr MK, et al. [18F]-Fluorodeoxyglucose positron emission tomography in patients with suspected recurrence of breast cancer. J Cancer Res Clin Oncol 2003; 129:147–53.

27. Minn H, Soini I. [18F]fluorodeoxyglucose scintigraphy in diagnosis and follow-up of treatment in advanced breast cancer. Eur J Nucl Med 1989; 15:61–6.

28. Moon DH, Maddahi J, Silverman DH, et al. Accuracy of whole-body fluorine-18-FDG PET for the detection of recurrent or metastatic breast carcinoma. J Nucl Med 1998; 39:431–5.

29. Nair N, Ali A, Dowlatshahi K, et al. Positron emission tomography with fluorine-18 fluorodeoxyglucose to evaluate response of early breast carcinoma treated with stereotactic interstitial laser therapy. Clin Nucl Med 2000; 25:505–7.

30. Nieweg OE, Kim EE, Wong WH, et al. Positron emission tomography with fluorine-18-deoxyglucose in the detection and staging of breast cancer. Cancer 1993; 71:3920–5.

31. Oshida M, Uno K, Suzuki M, et al. Predicting the prognoses of breast carcinoma patients with positron emission tomography using 2-deoxy-2-fluoro[18F]-D-glucose. Cancer 1998; 82:2227–34.

32. Raylman RR, Majewski S, Weisenberger AG, et al. Positron emission mammography-guided breast biopsy. J Nucl Med 2001; 42:960–6.

33. Rose C, Dose J, Avril N. Positron emission tomography for the diagnosis of breast cancer. Nucl Med Commun 2002; 23:613–8.

34. Schelling M, Avril N, Nahrig J, et al. Positron emission tomography using [(18)F]fluorodeoxyglucose for monitoring primary chemotherapy in breast cancer. J Clin Oncol 2000; 18:1689–95.

35. Scirrmeister H, Kuhn T, Guhlmann A, et al. Fluorine-18 2-deoxy-2-fluoro-D-glucose PET in the preoperative staging of breast cancer: comparison with the standard staging procedures. Eur J Nucl Med 2001; 28:351–8.

36. Siggelkow W, Zimmy M, Faridi A, et al. The value of positron emission tomography in the follow-up for breast cancer. Anticancer Res 2003; 23:1859–67.

37. Smith IC, Ogston KN, Whitford P, et al. Staging of the axilla in breast cancer: accurate in vivo assessment using positron emission tomography with 2-(fluorine-18)-fluoro-2-deoxy-D-glucose. Ann Surg 1998; 228:220–7.

38. Smith IC, Welch AE, Hutcheon AW, et al. Positron emission tomography using [(18)F]-fluorodeoxy-D-glucose to predict the pathologic response of breast cancer to primary chemotherapy. J Clin Oncol 2000; 18:1676–88.

39. Suarez M, Perez-Castejon MJ, Jimenez A, et al. Early diagnosis of recurrent breast cancer with FDG-PET in patients with progressive elevation of serum tumor markers. Q J Nucl Med 2002; 46:113–21.

40. Tse NY, Hoh CK, Hawkins RA, et al. The application of positron emission tomographic imaging with fluorodeoxyglucose to the evaluation of breast disease. Ann Surg 1992; 216:27–34.

41. van der Hoeven JJ, Hoekstra OS, Comans EF, et al. Determinants of diagnostic performance of [F-18]fluorodeoxyglucose positron emission tomography for axillary staging in breast cancer. Ann Surg 2002; 236:619–24.

42. Vranjesevic D, Filmont JE, Meta J, et al. Whole-body (18)F-FDG PET and conventional imaging for predicting outcome in previously treated breast cancer patients. J Nucl Med 2002; 43:325–9.

43. Vranjesevic D, Schiepers C, Silverman DH, et al. Relationship between 18F-FDG uptake and breast density in women with normal breast tissue. J Nucl Med 2003; 44:1238–42.

10

44. Wahl RL, Cody RL, Hutchins GD, et al. Primary and metastatic breast carcinoma: initial clinical evaluation with PET with the radiolabeled glucose analog 2-[F-18]-fluoro-2-deoxy-D-glucose. Radiology 1991; 179:765–70.

45. Wahl RL, Helvie MA, Chang AE, et al. Detection of breast cancer in women after augmentation mammoplasty using fluorine-18-fluorodeoxyglucose PET. J Nucl Med 1994; 35:872–5.

46. Wahl RL, Siegel BA, Coleman RE, et al. Prospective multi-center study of axillary nodal staging with FDG positron emission tomography in breast cancer. J Nucl Med 2003; 44(5 Suppl):77P.

47. Wahl RL, Zasadny K, Helvie M, et al. Metabolic monitoring of breast cancer chemo-hormonotherapy using positron emission tomography: initial evaluation. J Clin Oncol 1993; 11:2101–11.

48. Wahl RL. Current status of PET in breast cancer imaging, staging, and therapy. Semin Roentgenol 2001; 36:250–60.

49. Wu D, Gambhir SS. Positron emission tomography in diagnosis and management of invasive breast cancer: current status and future perspectives. Clin Breast Cancer 2003; 4(Suppl 1):S55–63.

50. Yap CS, Seltzer MA, Schiepers C, et al. Impact of whole-body 18F-FDG PET on staging and managing patients with breast cancer: the referring physician's perspective. J Nucl Med 2001; 42:1334–7.

Ovarian Cancer

1. Blodgett TM, Meltzer CC, Townsend DW, et al. PET/CT in re-staging patients with ovarian carcinoma. J Nucl Med 2002; 5(suppl):310P.

2. Bristow RE, del Carmen MG, Pannu HK, et al. Clinically occult recurrent ovarian cancer: patient selection for secondary cytoreductive surgery using combined PET/CT. Gynecol Oncol 2003; 90:519–28.

3. Bristow RE, Simpkins F, Pannu HK, et al. Positron emission tomography for detecting clinically occult surgically respectable metastatic ovarian cancer. Gynecol Oncol 2002; 85:196–200.

4. Casey MJ, Gupta NC, Muths CK: Experience with positron emission tomography (PET) scans in patients with ovarian cancer. Gynecol Oncol 1994; 53:331–8.

5. Chang WC, Hung YC, Kao CH, et al. Usefulness of whole body positron emission tomography (PET) with 18F-fluoro-2-deoxyglucose (FDG) to detect recurrent ovarian cancer based on asymptomatically elevated serum levels of tumor marker. Neoplasm 2002; 49:329–33.

6. Cho SM, Ha HK, Byaun JY, et al. Usefulness of FDG PET for assessment of early recurrent epithelial ovarian cancer. AJR 2002; 179:391–5.

7. Cohade C, Mourtziks KA, Pannu HK, et al. Direct comparison of PET and PET/CT in the detection of recurrent ovarian cancer. J Nucl Med 2003; 5(suppl):129P.

8. Dadparvar S, Chotipanich C, Guan L, et al. 18FDG-PET imaging in detection of recurrent ovarian carcinoma. J Nucl Med 2003; 5(suppl):131P.

9. Drieskens O, Stroobants S, Gysen M, et al. Positron emission tomography with FDG in the detection of peritoneal and retroperitoneal metastases of ovarian cancer. Gynecol Obstet Invest 2003; 55:130–4.

10. Fenchel S, Grab D, Nuessle K, et al. Asymptomatic adnexal masses: correlation of FDG PET and histopathologic findings. Radiology 2002; 223:780–8.

11. Fenchel S, Kotzerke J, Stohr I, et al. Preoperative assessment of asymptomatic adnexal tumors by positron emission tomography and F-18 fluorodeoxyglucose. Nukleramedizin 1999; 38:101–7.

12. Garcia Velloso MJ, Boan Garcia JF, Villar Luque LM, et al. F-18-FDG positron emission tomography in the diagnosis of ovarian recurrence. Comparison with CT scan and CA-125. Rev Esp Med Nucl 2003; 22:217–23.

13. Holschneider CH, Manuel M, Williams CM, et al. FDG-PET in ovarian cancer: use of the standardized uptake value (SUV) to differentiate physiological bowel cavity from intraperitoneal metastatic tumor. J Nucl Med 2002; 5(suppl):29P.

14. Hubner KF, McDonald TW, Niethammer JG, et al. Assessment of primary and metastatic ovarian cancer by positron emission tomography (PET) using 2-[18F]deoxyglucose (2-[18F]FDG). Gynecol Oncol 1993; 51:197–204.

15. Hubner KF, McDonald TW, Smith GT, Thie JA. Detection of recurrent ovarian cancer by PET using FDG. Clin Positron Imaging 1999; 2:346.

16. Ishiko O, Honda K, Hirai K, et al. Diagnosis of metastasis of ovarian clear cell carcinoma to the peritoneum of the abdominal wall by positron emission tomography with (fluorine-18)-2-deoxyglucose. Oncol Rep 2001; 8:67–9.

17. Israel O, Keidar Z, Bar-Shalom R, et al. Hybrid PET/CT imaging with FDG in management of patients with gynecologic malignancies. J Nucl Med 2003; 5(suppl):129P.

18. Jadvar H, Tatlidil R, Conti PS: FDG-PET in the evaluation of recurrent ovarian cancer. J Nucl Med 2001; 42(5 Suppl): 286P.

19. Karlan BY, Hawkins R, Hoh C, et al. Whole-body positron emission tomography with 2-[18F]-fluoro-2-deoxy-D-glucose can detect recurrent ovarian carcinoma. Gynecol Oncol 1993; 51:175–81.

20. Kubik-Huch RA, Dorffler W, von Schulthess GK, et al. Value of (18F)-FDG positron emission tomography, computed tomography, and magnetic resonance imaging in diagnosing primary and recurrent ovarian carcinoma. Eur Radiol 2000; 10:761–7.

21. Kurokawa T, Yoshida Y, Kawahara K, et al. Whole-body PET with FDG is useful for following up an ovarian cancer patient with only rising CA-125 levels within the normal range. Ann Nucl Med 2002; 16:491–3.

22. Lerman H, Metser U, Grisaru D, et al. Normal and abnormal 18F-FDG endometrial and ovarian uptake in pre- and postmenopausal patients: assessment by PET/CT. J Nucl Med 2004; 45:266–71.

23. Mahy N, Mathieu I, Willemart B, et al. The place of PET-FDG in the diagnosis of recurrent ovarian cancer. J Nucl Med 2003; 5(suppl):130P.

24. Makhija S, Howden N, Edwards R, et al. Positron emission tomography/computed tomography imaging for the detection of recurrent ovarian and fallopian tube carcinoma: a retrospective review. Gynecol Oncol 2002; 85:53–8.

25. Manuel M, Holschneider CH, Williams CM, et al. Correlation of FDG-PET scans with surgicopathologic findings in ovarian cancers. J Nucl Med 2002; 5(suppl):29P.

26. Nakamoto Y, Saga T, Ishimori T, et al. Clinical value of positron emission tomography with FDG for recurrent ovarian cancer. AJR 176:1449–54.

27. Pannu HK, Bristow RE, Cohade C, et al. PET-CT in recurrent ovarian cancer: initial observations. Radiographics 2004; 24:209–23.

28. Picchio M, Sironi S, Messa C, et al. Advanced ovarian carcinoma: usefulness of ([[(180F]FDG-PET in combination with CT for lesion detection after primary treatment. Q J Nucl Med 2000; 47:77–84.

29. Rieber A, Nussie K, Stohr I, et al. Preoperative diagnosis of ovarian tumors with MR imaging: comparison with transvaginal sonography, positron emission tomography, and histologic findings. AJR 2001; 177:123–9.

30. Rose PG, Faulhaber P, Miraldi F, et al. Positive emission tomography for evaluating a complete clinical response in patients with ovarian or peritoneal carcinoma: correlation with second-look laparotomy. Gynecol Oncol 2001; 82:17–21.

31. Ryu S, Kim J, Kim Bg, et al. FDG-PET scan cannot substitute for second look operation in patients with ovarian cancer showing clinical complete response with chemotherapy. J Nucl Med 2001; 5(suppl): 286P.

32. Safaei A, Meta J, Gambhir SS, et al. Impact of whole body PET imaging with FDG on staging and managing patients with ovarian cancer: the referring physician's point of view. J Nucl Med 2001; 5(suppl):285P.

33. Schroder W, Zimmy M, Rudlowski C, et al. The role of 18F-fluoro-deoxyglucose positron emission tomography (18F-FDG PET) in diagnosis of ovarian cancer. Int J Gynecol Cancer 1999; 9:117–122.

34. Smith GT, Hubner KF, McDonald T, Thie JA. Avoiding second-look surgery and reducing costs in managing patients with ovarian cancer by applying F-18-FDG PET. Clin Positron Imaging 1998; 1:263.

10

35. Smith GT, Hubner KF, McDonald T, Thie JA. Cost analysis of FDG PET for managing patients with ovarian cancer. Clin Positron Imaging 1999; 2:63–70.

36. Torizuka T, Nobezawa S, Kanno T, et al. Ovarian cancer recurrence: role of whole–body positron emission tomography using 2-[fluoro-18]-fluoro-2-deoxy-D-glucose. Eur J Nucl Med Mol Imaging 2002; 29:797-803.

37. Yen RF, Sun SS, Shen YY, et al. Whole body positron emission tomography with 18F-fluoro-2-deoxyglucose for the detection recurrent ovarian cancer. Anticancer Res 2001; 21:3691–4.

38. Yoshida Y, Kurokawa T, Kawahara K, et al. Incremental benefits of FDG positron emission tomography over CT alone for the preoperative staging of ovarian cancer. AJR 2004; 182:227–33.

39. Yuan CC, Liu RS, Wang PH, et al. Whole-body PET with (fluorine-18)-2-deoxyglucose for detecting recurrent ovarian carcinoma. Initial Report. J Reprod Med 1999; 44:775–8.

40. Zimmy M, Siggelkow W, Schroder W, et al. 2-[Fluorine-18]-fluoro-2-deoxy-d-glucose positron emission tomography in the diagnosis of recurrent ovarian cancer. Gynecol Oncol 2001; 83:310–5.

Uterine Cancer

1. Belhocine T. An appraisal of 18F-FDG PET imaging in post-therapy surveillance of uterine cancers: clinical evidence and a research proposal. Int J Gynecol Cancer 2003; 13:228–33.

2. Belhocine T, De Barsy C, Hustinx R, et al. Usefulness of (18)F-FDG PET in the post-therapy surveillance of endometrial carcinoma. Eur J Nucl Med Mol Imaging 2002; 29:1132–9.

3. Cher S, Lay Ergun E. Positron emission tomographic-computed tomographic imaging of a uterine sarcoma. Clin Nucl Med 2003; 28:443–4.

4. Kao CH. FDG uptake in a huge uterine myoma. Clin Nucl Med 2003; 28:249.

5. Lapela M, Leskinen-Kallio S, Varpula M, et al. Imaging of uterine carcinoma by carbon-11-methionine and PET. J Nucl Med 1994; 35:1618–23.

6. Lentz SS. Endometrial carcinoma diagnosed by positron emission tomography: a case report. Gynecol Oncol 2002; 86:223–4.

7. Nakahara T, Fujii H, Ide M, et al. F-18 FDG uptake in endometrial cancer. Clin Nucl Med 2001; 26:82–3.

8. Saga T, Higashi T, Ishimori T, et al. Clinical value of FDG-PET in the follow-up of post-operative patients with endometrial cancer. J Nucl Med 2003; 5(suppl):385P.

9. Umesaki N, Tanaka T, Miyama M, et al. Positron emission tomography using 2-[(18)F]fluoro-2-deoxy-D-glucose in the diagnosis of uterine leiomyosarcoma : a case report. Clin Imaging 2001; 25:203–5.

10. Umesaki N, Tanaka T, Miyama M, et al. Positron emission tomography with (18)F-fluorodeoxyglucose of uterine sarcoma: a comparison with magnetic resonance imaging and power Doppler imaging. Gynecol Oncol 2001; 80:372–7.

Cervical Cancer

1. Aizer-Dannon A, Bar-Am A, Ron IG, et al. Fused functional-anatomic images of metastatic cancer of cervix obtained by a combined gamma camera and X-ray tube hybrid system with an illustrative case and review of the (18)F-fluorodeoxyglucose literature. Gynecol Oncol 2003; 90:453–7.

2. Belhocine T, Thille A, Fridman V, et al. Contribution of whole-body 18FDG PET imaging in the management of cervical cancer. Gynecol Oncol 2002; 87:90–7.

3. Dose J, Hemminger GE, Bohuslavizki KH: Therapy monitoring using FDG-PET in metastatic cervical cancer. Lancet Oncol 2000; 1:106.

4. Follen M, Levenback CF, Iyer RB, et al. Imaging in cervical cancer. Cancer 2003; 98:2028–38.

5. Grigsby PW, Siegel BA, Dehdashti F, et al. Posttherapy surveillance monitoring of cervical cancer by FDG-PET. Int J Radiat Oncol Biol Phys 2003; 55:907–13.

6. Grigsby PW, Siegel BA, Dehdashti F. Lymph node staging by positron emission tomography in patients with carcinoma of the cervix. J Clin Oncol 2001; 19:3745–9.

7. Havrilesky LJ, Wong TZ, Secord AA, et al. The role of PET scanning in the detection of recurrent cervical cancer. Gynecol Oncol 2003; 90:186–90.

8. Jadvar H, Conti PS. FDG PET in the evaluation of women with cervical carcinoma. Radiology 2001; 221(P):386.

9. Karlan BY, Hoh C, Tse N, et al. Whole-body positron emission tomography with (fluorine-18)-2-deoxyglucose can detect metastatic carcinoma of the fallopian tube. Gynecol Oncol 1993; 49:383–8.

10. Kerr IG, Manji MF, Powe J, et al. Positron emission tomography for the evaluation of metastases in patients with carcinoma of the cervix: a retrospective review. Gynecol Oncol 2001; 81:477–80.

11. Kuhnel G, Horn LC, Fischer U, et al. 18F-FDG positron emission tomography in cervical carcinoma: preliminary findings. Zentralbl Gynakol 2001; 123:229–35.

12. Lin WC, Hung YC, Yeh LS, et al. Usefulness of (18)F-fluorodeoxyglucose positron emission tomography to detect para-aortic lymph nodal metastasis in advanced cervical cancer with negative computed tomography findings. Gynecol Oncol 2003; 89:73–6.

13. Ma SY, See LC, Lai CH, et al. Delayed (18)F-FDG PET for detection of paraaortic lymph node metastases in cervical cancer patients. J Nucl Med 2003; 44:1775–83.

14. Miller TR, Grisby PW. Measurement of tumor volume by PET to evaluate prognosis in patients with advanced cervical cancer treated by radiation therapy. Int J Radiat Oncol Biol Phys 2002; 53:353–9.

15. Miller TR, Pinkus E, Dehdashti F, et al. Improved prognostic value of 18F-FDG PET using a simple visual analysis of tumor characteristics in patients with cervical cancer. J Nucl Med 2003; 44:192–7.

16. Nakamoto Y, Eisbruch A, Achtyes ED, et al. Prognostic value of positron emission tomography using F-18-fluorodeoxyglucose in patients with cervical cancer undergoing radiotherapy. Gynecol Oncol 2002; 84:289–95.

17. Narayan K, Hicks RJ, Jobling T, et al. A comparison of MRI and PET scanning in surgically staged loco-regionally advanced cervical cancer: potential impact on treatment. Int J Gynecol cancer 2001; 11:263–71.

18. Reinhardt MJ, Ehritt-Braun C, Vogelgesang D, et al. Metastatic lymph nodes in patients with cervical cancer: detection with MR imaging and FDG PET. Radiology 2001; 218:776–82.

19. Rose PG, Adler LP, Rodriguez M, et al. Positron emission tomography for evaluating para-aortic nodal metastasis in locally advanced cervical cancer before surgical staging: a surgicopathologic study. J Clin Oncol 1999; 17:41–5.

20. Ryu SY, Kim MH, Choi SC, et al. Detection of early recurrence with 18F-FDG PET in patients with cervical cancer. J Nucl Med 2003; 44:347–52.

21. Singh AK, Grigsby PW, Dehdashti F, et al. FDG-PET lymph node staging and survival of patients with FIGO stage IIIb cervical carcinoma. Int J Radiat Oncol Biol Phys 2003; 56:489–93.

22. Sugawara Y, Eisbruch A, Kosuda S, et al. Evaluation of FDG PET in patients with cervical cancer. J Nucl Med 1999; 40:1125–31.

23. Sun SS, Chen TC, Yen RF, et al. Value of whole body 18F-fluoro-deoxyglucose positron emission tomography in the evaluation of recurrent cervical cancer. Anticancer Res 2001; 21(4B):2957–61.

24. Tatsumi M, Cohade C, Zellars R, et al. Initial experience in imaging uterine cervical cancer with FDG PET-CT: direct comparison with PET. J Nucl Med 2003; 5(suppl):394P.

25. Tran BN, Grigsby PW, Dehdashti F, et al. Occult supraclavicular lymph node metastasis identified by FDG-PET in patients with carcinoma of the uterine cervix. Gynecol Oncol 2003; 90:572–6.

26. Umesaki N, Tanaka T, Miyama M, et al. Early and evaluation of therapy in postoperative recurrent cervical cancers by positron emission tomography. Oncol Rep 2000; 7:53–6.
27. Umesaki N, Tanaka T, Miyama M, et al. The role of 18F-fluoro-2-deoxy-D-glucose positron emission tomography (18F-FDG-PET) in the diagnosis of recurrence and lymph node metastasis of cervical cancer. Oncol Rep 2000; 7:1261–4.
28. Yeh LS, Hung YC, Shen YY, et al. Detecting para-aortic lymph nodal metastasis by positron emission tomography of 18F-fluorodeoxyglucose in advanced cervical cancer with negative magnetic resonance imaging findings. Oncol Rep 2002; 9:1289–92.
29. Yen TC, Ng KK, Ma SY, et al. Value of dual-phase 2-fluoro-2-deoxy-d-glucose positron emission tomography in cervical cancer. J Clin Oncol 2003; 21:3651–8.
30. Yen TC, See LC, Lai CH, et al. 18F-FDG uptake in squamous cell carcinoma of the cervix is correlated with glucose transporter 1 expression. J Nucl Med 2004; 45:22–9.

Oncology—Male Reproductive System

I. TESTICULAR CANCER

Testicular cancer represents about 1% of all cancers in males, but it is one of the most frequent cancers in young adult men and is more common in whites than in blacks. With the current treatment strategies overall cure rates of approximately 95% may be achieved. Typical disease presentation is an asymptomatic testicular mass. Diagnostic procedures include physical examination, serum tumor marker (alpha-fetoprotein, human chorionic gonadotropin) assays, and imaging. Scrotal US can delineate the intrascrotal mass. CT is usually employed for staging. Treatment and prognosis depends on the stage of disease and the histopathology of the cancer. Surgery with bilateral retroperitoneal lymph node dissection is usually carried out in seminoma preceded occasionally by chemotherapy-induced debulking of lymphadenopathy. In nonseminomas, cytoreductive surgery and chemotherapy has replaced radiation therapy in the low-stage disease, although irradiation of the nonresectable localized metastatic disease may be helpful. Complete remission can be obtained in up to 70% of patients with metastatic disease by chemotherapy alone. Another 15% of patients may become disease-free by surgical excision of the residual tumor.

The normal testis demonstrates variable FDG uptake. The range of SUV varies from a minimum of 0.9 to a maximum of 5.7 with a mean of 2.2. There may be a moderate correlation between decreasing testicular FDG uptake and increasing age, probably as a result of age-related decline in androgen production. The diagnostic utility of PET in testicular cancer has been evaluated. In general it appears that seminomas accumulate more FDG than nonseminomas. However, tumors may display very heterogeneous FDG uptake with an SUV ranging from as low as 1.8 to as high as 17.3. For staging, the typical reported sensitivities and specificities are 87% and 94% for PET, 73% and 94% for CT, and 67% and 100% for serum tumor markers.

FDG PET not only detects retroperitoneal relapse earlier than CT but has an advantage over CT in restaging with a high negative predictive value in predicting treatment-related fibrosis (Fig. 1). FDG PET may be false-positive early after chemotherapy due to reactive inflammatory processes. Despite this potential pitfall, PET appears to be more advantageous than CT and serum tumor markers in assessing early response to chemotherapy and in identifying those patients who may benefit from high-dose salvage chemotherapy (Fig. 2). It has been suggested that FDG PET must be performed at least two weeks after completion of chemotherapy to reduce the false-positive findings. PET is also useful for the detection of malignant nodes that do not meet the size criteria at CT or when the lack of retroperitoneal fat makes it difficult to identify retroperitoneal nodes with CT. In a difficult case when there is urgency in treatment decision-making, FDG PET may be useful in directing CT-guided needle biopsy of the residual lesions for distinguishing viable tumor or teratoma from residual fibrosis and necrosis. Similarly, in patients with bulky seminoma who have been treated with chemotherapy, FDG PET performs well in detecting residual viable tumor, especially those greater than 3 cm. In a subset of patients

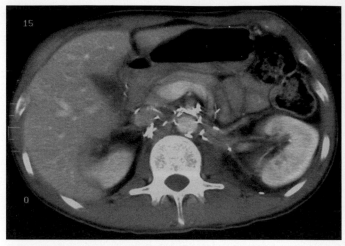

A

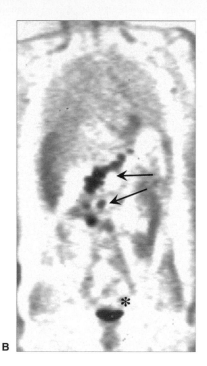

B

Figure 1: A 36-year-old male with nonseminomatous testicular cancer treated with orchiectomy and retroperitoneal lymph node dissection followed by chemotherapy; βhcG = 34. **A.** CT shows post-operative changes. **B.** PET shows extensive hypermetabolic recurrent disease confirmed by biopsy.

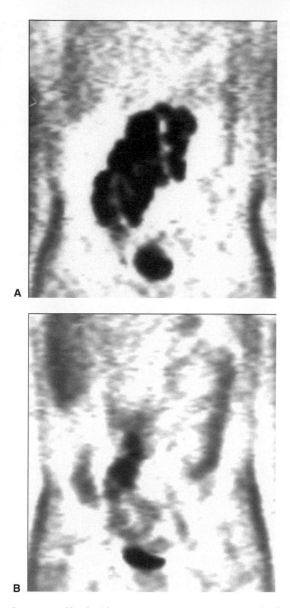

Figure 2: A 44-year-old male with seminomatous testicular cancer treated with orchiectomy followed by chemotherapy. **A.** Prechemotherapy PET shows extensive hypermetabolic nodal metastatic disease. **B.** Post-chemotherapy PET shows decline in the extent of disease compatible with partial treatment response.

with raised serum tumor markers alone, a positive predictive value of 92% and a negative predictive value of 50% have been reported. Although the exact role of FDG PET in the imaging evaluation of testicular cancer is not yet established, strong evidence is accumulating for its relevant clinical utility.

II. PROSTATE CANCER

Prostate cancer is the most common cancer affecting men in the United States. As life expectancy increases, so will the incidence of this disease, creating what will become an epidemic male health problem. The common histology is adenocarcinoma. Digital rectal examination is considered the standard of reference for detection of prostate cancer. About 50% of all palpable nodules are carcinomas. Neither prostatic acid phosphatase (PAP) nor prostate specific antigen (PSA) are useful for screening prostate cancer, although elevated serum levels of these substances are usually suggestive of locally advanced or metastatic disease. The commonly used Gleason Score, which ranges from a minimum of 2 to a maximum of 10, is based on both the tumor's glandular differentiation as well as its growth pattern and has been shown to be associated with the clinical stage of disease. Current imaging tests, including ultrasound, CT, MRI, and In-111 capromab pendetide (Prostascint) are not sufficiently accurate to detect local recurrence or metastatic disease. Although bone scintigraphy can be useful in detecting osseous metastases, the false-positive rate is high. Bone scintigraphy also cannot detect soft tissue or lymph nodal involvement, quite prevalent with metastatic spread of this disease.

Early studies of FDG PET in prostate cancer have shown that FDG accumulation in the primary prostate cancer is generally low, and may overlap with the uptake in benign prostatic hyperplasia (BPH), in the normal gland and in the postoperative scar or local recurrence. However, animal and preliminary clinical studies have demonstrated that FDG PET may be useful in the evaluation of advanced androgen-independent disease and in patients with high Gleason scores and serum PSA level, in the detection of active osseous and soft tissue metastases, and in the assessment of response after androgen ablation and treatment with novel chemotherapies. For metastatic disease, FDG localization in the lesions may display a standardized uptake value (SUV) of up to 5.7 at a positive predictive value of 98%. Moreover, FDG PET may be more useful than In-111 Prostascint in the detection of metastatic disease in patients with high PSA or PSA velocity. FDG PET appears to be more useful in the detection of soft tissue metastases than osseous metastases, although it has been suggested that FDG PET may discriminate active osseous disease from the scintigraphically quiescent lesions. Other clinical situations that FDG PET may be appropriate are patients who have had incomplete response to therapy or who have a rising PSA level despite treatment. In particular, animal and pilot human clinical studies have demonstrated that FDG accumulation in both the primary tumor and the metastatic sites decreases in as early as one to five months after androgen ablation, which is concordant with decline in lesion size on CT and the serum PSA level. Additionally, it has been suggested that FDG PET has a better specificity but lower sensitivity for detecting osseous metastases in comparison to bone scintigraphy and is useful in differential diagnosis of flare reaction after endocrine therapy. FDG PET has been shown to have prognostic value in patients undergoing radical prostatectomy. Patients with lesions that demonstrated high FDG accumulation (i.e., high SUV) had poorer prognosis in comparison to those with low SUV.

There has also been a growing interest in the utility of other PET radio-tracers for imaging of prostate cancer. Acetate participates in cytoplasmic lipid synthesis, which is believed to be increased in tumors. Cellular retention of radiolabeled acetate in prostate cancer cell lines is primarily due to incorporation of the radiocarbon into phosphatidylcholine and neutral lipids of the cells. The lack of accumulation of acetate in urine is also advantageous to imaging prostate cancer in particular, because the prostate bed remains unobstructed by the adjacent high levels of radioactivity in the urinary bladder, commonly a problem with FDG. Although there can be a considerable overlap between the uptake level in primary cancer and in the normal prostate gland, generally, the uptake appears to be greater in the tumor than in the normal tissue. C-11 acetate may also be useful in detection of tumor recurrence in patients who had been treated previously with prostatectomy or radiation therapy.

Choline PET may also be useful in imaging prostate cancer. The biological basis for radiolabeled choline uptake in tumors is the malignancy-induced up-regulation of choline kinase, which leads to the incorporation and trapping of choline in the form of phosphatidylcholine (lecithin) in the tumor cell membrane in proportion to the rate of tumor duplication. The tracer uptake has been noted to decrease in both the primary tumor and in the metastases after hormonal therapy and increase after relapse as measured by the increase in the serum PSA level.

Although both acetate and choline appear to be more or less equally useful in imaging prostate cancer in individual patients and are more advantageous than FDG in some clinical circumstances, such as detection of the locally recurrent disease, large clinical studies in well-defined clinical situations will be needed to determine their exact diagnostic role before other important practical issues such as easy accessibility to these tracers are addressed. The diagnostic potential of other tracers such as radiolabeled androgen analog F-18 fluoro-5a-dihydrotestosterone (FDHT) for imaging androgen receptors will also need to be established.

11

BIBLIOGRAPHY

Testicular Cancer

1. Albers P, Bender H, Yilmaz H, et al. Positron emission tomography in the clinical staging of patients with stage I and II testicular germ cell tumors. Urology 1999; 53:808–11.
2. Becherer A, De Santis M, Bokemeyer C, et al. FDG-PET as prognostic indicator for seminoma residuals: an update from the SEMPET trial. J Nucl Med 2003; 5(suppl):174P.
3. Bokemeyer C, Kollmannsberger C, Oechsle K, et al. Early prediction of treatment response to high-dose salvage chemotherapy in patients with relapsed germ cell cancer using [(18)F]FDG PET. Br J Cancer 2002; 86:506–11.
4. Cremerius U, Effert PJ, Adam G, et al. FDG PET for detection and therapy control of metastatic germ cell tumor. J Nucl Med 1998; 39:815–22.
5. Cremerius U, Wildberger JE, Borchers H, et al. Dose positron emission tomography using 18-fluoro-2-deoxyglucose improve clinical staging of testicular cancer? Results of a study in 50 patients. Urology 1999; 54:900–4.
6. de Geus-Oei LF, Spermon JR, Kiemeney LA, et al. Chemotherapy response monitoring with 18FDG-PET in patients with high stage testicular germ cell cancer. J Nucl Med 2003; 5(Suppl):131P.

7. De Santis M, Bokemeyer C, Becherer A, et al. Predictive impact of 2-18fluoro-2-deoxy-D-glucose positron emission tomography for residual postchemotherapy masses in patients with bulky seminoma. J Clin Oncol 2001; 19:3740–4.

8. Frank IN, Graham Jr SD, Nabors WL: Urologic and Male Genital Cancers, in Holleb AI, Fink DJ, Murphy GP (eds): Clinical Oncology. Atlanta, American Cancer Society, 1991.

9. Ganjoo KN, Chan RJ, Sharma M, et al. Positron emission tomography scans in the evaluation of postchemotherapy residual masses in patients with seminoma. J Clin Oncol 1999; 17:3457–60.

10. Hain SF, O'Doherty MJ, Timothy AR, et al. Fluorodeoxyglucose PET in the initial staging of germ cell tumors. Eur J Nucl Med 2000; 27:590–4.

11. Hain SF, O'Doherty MJ, Timothy AR, et al. Fluorodeoxyglucose positron emission tomography in the evaluation of germ cell tumors at relapse. Br J Cancer 2000; 83:863–9.

12. Huddart RA. Use of FDG-PET in testicular tumors. Clin Oncol (R Coll Radiol) 2003; 15:123–7.

13. Karapetis CS, Strickland AH, Yip D, et al. Use of fluorodeoxyglucose positron emission tomography scans in patients with advanced germ cell tumor following chemotherapy: single-center experience with long-term follow up. Intern Med J 2003; 33:427–35.

14. Lassen U, Daugaard G, Eigtved A, et al. Whole-body FDG-PET in patients with stage I non-seminomatous germ cell tumors. Eur J Nucl Med Mol Imaging 2003; 396–402.

15. Muller-Mattheis V, Reinhardt M, Gerharz CD, et al. Positron emission tomography with [18F]-2-fluoro-2-deoxy-D-glucose (18FDG-PET) in diagnosis of retroperitoneal lymph node metastases of testicular tumors. Urologe A 1998; 37:609–20.

16. Nuutinen JM, Leskinen S, Elomaa I, et al. Detection of residual tumors in postchemotherapy testicular cancer by FDG-PET. Eur J Cancer 1997; 33:1234–41.

17. Pandit-Taskar N, Sinha A, Gonen M, et al. Testicular uptake in 18FDG PET scan. J Nucl Med 2003; 5(Suppl): 143P.

18. Reinhardt MJ, Matthies A, Biersack HJ: PET-imaging in tumors of the reproductive tract. Q J Nucl Med 2002; 46:105–12.

19. Reinhardt MJ, Muller-Mattheis VG, Gerharz CD, et al. FDG-PET evaluation of retroperitoneal metastases of testicular cancer before and after chemotherapy. J Nucl Med 1997; 38:99–101.

20. Sanchez D, Zudaire JJ, Fernandez JM, et al. 18F-fluoro-2-deoxyglucose-positron emission tomography in the evaluation of nonseminomatous germ cell tumors at relapse. BJU Int 2002; 89:912–6.

21. Spermon JR, De Geus-Oei LF, Kiemeney LA, et al. The role of (18)fluoro-2-deoxyglucose positron emission tomography in initial staging and re-staging after chemotherapy for testicular germ cell tumors. BJU Int 2002; 89(6):549–56.

22. Tatlidil R, Jadvar H, Conti PS. Utility of FDG-PET in the evaluation of residual or recurrent testicular carcinoma: comparison to CT and serum tumor markers. Radiology 2000; 217(P):220.

23. Tsatalpas P, Beuthien-Baumann B, Kropp J, et al. Diagnostic value of 18F-FDG positron emission tomography for detection and treatment control of malignant germ cell tumors. Urol Int 2002; 68:157–63.

24. Wilson CB, Young HE, Ott RJ, et al. Imaging metastatic testicular germ cell tumors with 18FDG positron emission tomography: prospects for detection and management. Eur J Nucl Med 1995; 22:508–13.

25. Yun M, Jang S, Kim W, et al. Pattern of testicular uptake with age and the effect of chemotherapy on testicular uptake determined by FDG PET. J Nucl Med 2001; 5(Suppl): 287P.

Prostate Cancer

1. Chang CH, Wu HC, Tsai JJ, et al. Detecting metastatic pelvic lymph nodes by (18)f-2-deoxyglucose positron emission tomography in patients with prostate-specific antigen relapse after treatment for localized prostate cancer. Urol Int 2003; 70(4):311–315.

2. de Jong IJ, Pruim J, Elsinga PH, et al. Preoperative staging of pelvic lymph nodes in prostate cancer by 11C-choline PET. J Nucl Med 2003; 44:331–335.

3. Dimitrakopoulou-Strauss A, Strauss LG. PET imaging of prostate cancer with 11C-acetate. J Nucl Med 2003; 44:556–558.

4. Fricke E, Machtens S, Hofmann M, et al. Positron emission tomography with (11)C-acetate and (18)F-FDG in prostate cancer patients. Eur J Nucl Med Mol Imaging 2003; 30:607–611.

5. Hara T, Kosaka N, Kishi H. PET imaging of prostate cancer using carbon-11-choline. J Nucl Med 1998; 39(6):990–995.

6. Hofer C, Laubenbacher C, Block T, et al. Fluorine-18-fluorodeoxyglucose positron emission tomography is useless for the detection of local recurrence after radical prostatectomy. Eur Urol 1999; 36:31–35.

7. Jadvar H, Pinski JK, Conti PS. FDG PET in suspected recurrent and metastatic prostate cancer. Oncol Rep 2003; 10:1485–8.

8. Kato T, Tsukamoto E, Kuge Y, et al. Accumulation of [(11)C]acetate in normal prostate and benign prostatic hyperplasia: comparison with prostate cancer. Eur J Nucl Med Mol Imaging 2002; 29(11):1492–1495.

9. Kotzerke J, Volkmer BG, Glatting G, et al. Intra-individual comparison of [11C]acetate and [11C]choline PET for detection of metastases of prostate cancer. Nuklearmedizin 2003; 42:25–30.

10. Larson SM, Morris M, Gunther I, et al. Tumor localization of 16beta-(18)F-Fluoro-5alpha-Dihydrotestosterone versus (18)F-FDG in patients with progressive, metastatic prostate cancer. J Nucl Med 2004; 45:366–373.

11. Liu IJ, Zafar MB, Lai YH, et al. Fluorodeoxyglucose positron emission tomography studies in diagnosis and staging of clinically organ-confined prostate cancer. Urology 2001; 57:108–111.

12. Morris MJ, Akhurst T, Osman I, et al. Fluorinated deoxyglucose positron emission tomography imaging in progressive metastatic prostate cancer. Urology 2002; 59:913–18.

13. Oyama N, Akino H, Suzuki Y, et al. FDG PET for evaluating the change of glucose metabolism in prostate cancer after androgen ablation. Nucl Med Commun 2001; 22:963–969.

14. Oyama N, Akino H, Suzuki Y, et al. Prognostic value of 2-deoxy-2-[F-18]fluoro-D-glucose positron emission tomography imaging for patients with prostate cancer. Mol Imaging Biol 2002; 4:99–104.

15. Patel P, Cohade C, DeWeese T, et al. Evaluation of metabolic activity of prostate gland with PET-CT. J Nucl Med 2002; 43(5 Suppl):119P.

16. Picchio M, Messa C, Landoni C, et al. Value of [11C]choline-positron emission tomography for re-staging prostate cancer: a comparison with [18F]fluorodeoxyglucose-positron emission tomography. J Urol 2003; 169(4):1337–1340.

17. Price DT, Coleman RE, Liao RP, et al. Comparison of [18 F]fluorocholine and [18 F]fluorodeoxyglucose for positron emission tomography of androgen dependent and androgen independent prostate cancer. J Urol 2002; 168:273–280.

18. Salminen E, Hogg A, Binns D, et al. Investigations with FDG-PET scanning in prostate cancer show limited value for clinical practice. Acta Oncol 2002; 41(5):425–429.

19. Sanz G, Robles JE, Gimenez M, et al. Positron emission tomography with 18fluorine-labelled deoxyglucose: utility in localized and advanced prostate cancer. BJU Int 1999; 84:1028–1031.

20. Seltzer MA, Barbaric Z, Belldegrun A, et al. Comparison of helical computerized tomography, positron emission tomography and monoclonal antibody scans for evaluation of lymph node metastases in patients with prostate specific antigen relapse after treatment for localized prostate cancer. J Urol 1999; 162:1322–1328.

21. Shimizu N, Masuda H, Yamanaka H, et al. Fluorodeoxyglucose positron emission tomography scan of prostate cancer bone metastases with flare reaction after endocrine therapy. J Urol 1999; 161:608–609.

11

22. Shreve PD, Grossman HB, Gross MD, Wahl RL. Metastatic prostate cancer: initial findings of PET with FDG. Radiology 1996; 199:751–756.
23. Shreve PD, Iannone P, Weinhold P. Cellular metabolism of [1-C14]-acetate in prostate cancer cells in vitro. J Nucl Med 2002; 43(5 Suppl):272P.
24. Sung J, Espiritu JI, Segall GM, Terris MK. Fluorodeoxyglucose positron emission tomography studies in the diagnosis and staging of clinically advanced prostate cancer. BJU Int 2003; 92:24–7.
25. Yeh SD, Imbriaco M, Larson SM, et al. Detection of bony metastases of androgen-independent prostate cancer by PET-FDG. Nucl Med Biol 1996; 23:693–697.

Oncology—Urology

I. KIDNEY CANCER

Renal cell carcinoma (RCC) arises from the renal tubular epithelium and accounts for the majority of the adult kidney tumors. The tumor is highly angioinvasive and results in widespread hematogenous and lymphatic metastases especially to the lung, liver, lymph nodes, bone, and brain. Metastases are present in about 50% of patients at initial presentation. Radical nephrectomy is the main treatment for the early stages of disease, although palliative nephrectomy may also be performed in advanced disease with intractable bleeding. Solitary metastasis may also be resected. RCC responds poorly to chemotherapy. Radiation therapy for RCC is used for palliation of metastatic sites, specifically, bone and brain. Immunotherapy with biologic response modifiers such as interleukin-2 and interferon alpha has the most impact on the treatment of metastatic disease. The five-year survival may be as high as 80–90% for early stages of disease, while advanced disease carries a poor prognosis.

Current imaging tests, including CT, MRI, and skeletal scintigraphy, are not sufficiently accurate to detect recurrent and metastatic disease. Preliminary studies of PET imaging of RCC have revealed a promising role in the evaluation of indeterminate renal masses, in pre-operative staging and assessment of tumor burden, in detection of osseous and non-osseous metastases, in restaging after therapy, and in the determination of effect of imaging findings on clinical management. However, few other PET studies have demonstrated less enthusiastic results and no advantage over standard imaging methods.

A relatively high false-negative rate of 23% has been reported with FDG PET in the preoperative staging of RCC when compared to histological analysis of surgical specimens. Other studies have reported high accuracy in characterizing indeterminate renal masses with a mean tumor-to-kidney uptake ratio of 3.0 for malignancy. The superiority of FDG PET in evaluating skeletal metastases as compared to bone scintigraphy has also been shown. These mixed observations are probably related to the heterogeneous expression of GLUT-1 in RCC, which may not correlate with the tumor grade or extent.

FDG PET can also alter clinical management in up to 40% of patients with suspicious locally recurrent and metastatic renal cancer (Fig. 1). In a recent study of the utility of FDG PET in re-staging RCC, a sensitivity of 87% was reported at a specificity of 100%. In another report, the diagnostic performance of FDG revealed a sensitivity of 71%, specificity of 75%, accuracy of 72%, negative predictive value of 33%, and positive predictive value of 94%. Therefore, FDG PET appears to offer modest diagnostic accuracy in re-staging RCC. A negative study may not exclude disease, while a positive study is highly suspicious for malignancy. The diagnostic accuracy of FDG PET appears not to be improved by semi-quantitative analysis, which is probably due to the fundamental variability of glucometabolism in RCC. Since FDG is excreted in the urine, the intense urine activity may confound lesion detection in and near the renal bed. Intravenous administration of furosemide (lasix) has been proposed to improve urine clearance from the renal collecting system, although the exact

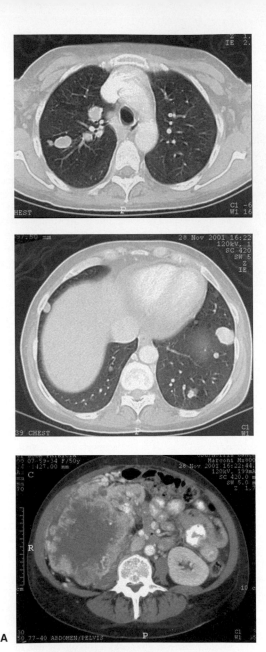

Figure 1: A 49-year-old male with metastatic right renal cell carcinoma. A: Chest and abdomen CT studies demonstrate multiple bilateral pulmonary lesions and a large necrotic right renal mass.

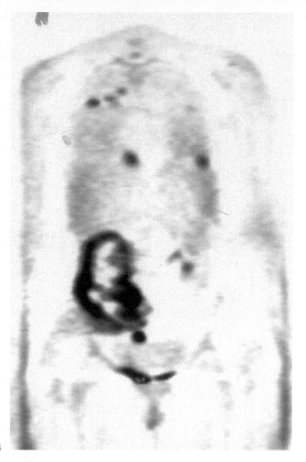

B

Figure 1: (Continued) B. Coronal PET shows intense hypermetabolism at the rim of the renal mass and in the pulmonary lesions.

benefit of such intervention in improving lesion detection remains undefined. Other PET tracers (e.g., C-11 acetate) may also suitable in the imaging evaluation of patients with suspected RCC.

II. BLADDER CANCER

Bladder cancer is the most frequent malignant tumor of the urinary tract and more common in patients aged 50 to 80. Typical presentation is hematuria. Depth of tumor penetration into the bladder wall forms the basis for disease staging and is the most important prognostic factor. Transitional cell carcinoma is the most common histopathology but squamous cell and adenocarcinoma may also occur (Fig. 2). Diagnostic procedures may include cystoscopy with biopsy, excretory urography or retrograde pyelogram, pelvis ultrasound and CT

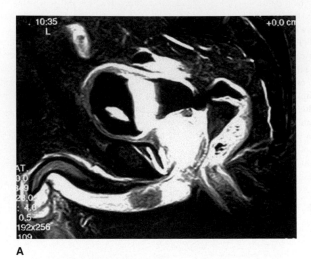

A

B

Figure 2: A 54-year-old male with invasive squamous cell carcinoma of the urethra. A. MRI shows 3 × 2-cm penile mass originating from the bulbous portion of the urethra encroaching upon the corpora cavernosum and spongiosum, located 1 cm anterior to the external sphincter. B. PET shows a corresponding oval-shaped area of elevated tracer uptake in the urethra at midline.

of the chest, abdomen, and pelvis. Superficial lesions may be treated with endoscopic resection, fulguration, or photodynamic therapy. Cystectomy with urinary diversion is indicated when the tumor is invasive. Radiotherapy may be employed as adjuvant therapy, in combination with other therapies, or as a palliative measure. There is no established systemic chemotherapeutic regimen for the treatment metastatic bladder carcinoma. The five-year survival is about 90% for superficial disease and about 60% for invasive disease. Systemic disease has a dismal prognosis.

FDG PET has been found to be modestly accurate in the diagnosis of bladder cancer and in the detection of pelvic lymph node and distant metastases. The intense excreted FDG activity in the urinary bladder is main hindrance in the evaluation of the organ and the adjacent pelvic structures, including the lymph nodes. Use of furosemide (lasix) and/or bladder lavage may help in reducing the urine activity but the exact utility of such intervention is not established. The primary bladder carcinoma and the lymph node metastases may exhibit an SUV in the range 1.7 to 6.2. For lymph node staging, a sensitivity of 67% and a specificity of 86% have been reported. Other PET radiotracers including C-11 methionine and C-11 choline may also be potentially useful in the imaging evaluation of bladder carcinoma.

BIBLIOGRAPHY

Kidney Cancer

1. Bachor R, Kotzerke J, Gottfried HW, et al. Positron emission tomography in diagnosis of renal cell carcinoma. Urologe 1996; 35:146–50.

2. Chang CH, Shiau YC, Shen YY, et al. Differentiating solitary pulmonary metastases in patients with renal cell carcinomas by 18F-fluoro-2-deoxyglucose positron emission tomography—a preliminary report. Urol Int 2003; 71:306–9.

3. Frank IN, Graham Jr S, Nabors WL 1991. Urologic and Male Genital Cancers. In: Holleb AI, Fink DJ, Murphy GP (eds). Clinical Oncology. American Cancer Society, pp. 272–74.

4. Goldberg MA, Mayo-Smith WW, Papanicolaou N, et al. FDG PET characterization of renal masses: preliminary experience. Clin Radiol 1997; 52:510–5.

5. Hain SF, Maisey MN. Positron emission tomography for urological tumors. BJU Int 2003; 92:159–64.

6. Jadvar H, Kherbache HM, Pinski JK, Conti PS. Diagnostic role of [F-18]-FDG positron emission tomography in restaging renal cell carcinoma. Clin Nephrol 2003; 60:395–400.

7. Majhail NS, Urbain JL, Albani JM, et al. F-18 fluorodeoxyglucose positron emission tomography in the evaluation of distant metastases from renal cell carcinoma. J Clin Oncol 2003; 21:3995–4000.

8. Mankoff DA, Thompson JA, Gold P, et al. Identification of interleukin-2-induced complete response in metastatic renal cell carcinoma by FDG PET despite radiographic evidence suggesting persistent tumor. AJR Am J Roentgenol 1997; 169:1049–50.

9. Matthews D, Oz OK. Positron emission tomography in prostate and renal cell carcinoma. Curr Opin Urol 2002; 12:381–5.

10. Miyakita H, Tokunaga M, Onda H, et al. Significance of 18F-fluorodeoxyglucose positron emission tomography (FDG-PET) for detection of renal cell carcinoma and immunohistochemical glucose transporter 1 (GLUT-1) expression in the cancer. Int J Urol 2002; 9:15–8.

11. Montravers F, Grahek D, Kerrou K, et al. Evaluation of FDG uptake by renal malignancies (primary tumor or metastases) using a coincidence detection gamma camera. J Nucl Med 2002; 41:78–84.

12

12. Nagase Y, Takata K, Moriyama N, et al. Immunohistochemical localization of glucose transporters in human renal cell carcinoma. J Urol 1995; 153(3 Pt 1):798–801

13. Poggi MM, Patronas N, Buttman JA, et al. Intramedullary spinal cord metastasis from renal cell carcinoma: detection by positron emission tomography. Clin Nucl Med 2001; 26:837–9.

14. Ramdave S, Thomas GW, Berlangieri SU, et al. Clinical role of F-18 fluorodeoxyglucose positron emission tomography for detection and management of renal cell carcinoma. J Urol 2001; 166:825–30.

15. Safaei A, Figlin R, Hoh CK, et al. The usefulness of F-18 deoxyglucose whole-body positron emission tomography (PET) for re-staging of renal cell cancer. Clin Nephrol 2002; 57:56–62.

16. Seto E, Segall GM, Terris MK. Positron emission tomography detection of osseous metastases of renal cell carcinoma not identified on bone scan. Urology 2000; 55:286.

17. Shreve P, Chiao PC, Humes HD, et al. Carbon-11-acetate PET imaging in renal disease. J Nucl Med 1995; 36:1595–601.

18. Wahl RL, Harney J, Hutchins G, Grossman HB. Imaging of renal cancer using positron emission tomography with 2-deoxy-2-(18F)-fluoro-D-glucose: pilot animal and human studies. J Urol 1991; 146(6):1470–4.

19. Wu HC, Yen RF, Shen YY, et al. Comparing whole body 18F-2-deoxyglucose positron emission tomography and technetium-99m methylene diphosphate bone scan to detect bone metastases in patients with renal cell carcinomas—a preliminary report. J Cancer Res Clin Oncol 2002; 128:503–6.

20. Zhuang H, Duarte PS, Pourdehand M, et al. Standardized uptake value as an unreliable index of renal disease on fluorodeoxyglucose PET Imaging. Clin Nucl Med 2000; 25:358–60.

Bladder Cancer

1. Ahlstrom H, Malmstrom PU, Letocha H, et al. Positron emission tomography in the diagnosis and staging of urinary bladder cancer. Acta Radiol 1996; 37:180–5.

2. Bachor R, Kotzerke J, Reske SN, Hautmann R. Lymph node staging of bladder neck carcinoma with positron emission tomography. Urologe A 1999; 38:46–50.

3. de Jong IJ, Pruim J, Elsinga PH, et al. Visualization of bladder cancer using (11)C-choline PET: first clinical experience. Eur J Nucl Med Mol Imaging 2002; 29:1283–8.

4. Harney JV, Wahl RL, Liebert M, et al. Uptake of 2-deoxy, 2-(18F) fluoro-D-glucose in bladder cancer: animal localization and initial patient positron emission tomography. J Urol 1991; 145:279–83.

5. Heicappell R, Muller-Mattheis V, Reinhardt M, et al. Staging of pelvic lymph nodes in neoplasms of the bladder and prostate by positron emission tomography with 2-[(18)F]-2-deoxy-D-glucose. Eur Urol 1999; 36:582–7.

6. Kosuda S, Kison PV, Greenough R, et al. Preliminary assessment of fluorine-18 fluorodeoxyglucose positron emission tomography in patients with bladder cancer. Eur J Nucl Med 1997; 24:615–20.

7. Letocha H, Ahlstrom H, Malmstrom PU, et al. Positron emission tomography with L-methyl-11C-methionine in the monitoring of therapy response in muscle-invasive transitional cell carcinoma of the urinary bladder. Br J Urol 1994; 74:767–74.

Oncology—Bone and Soft Tissue Tumors

I. BONE TUMORS

The malignant tumors of the bone include osteosarcoma, Ewing's sarcoma, lymphoma, chondrosarcoma, and parosteal osteosarcoma. Central osteosarcoma is the most common primary bone malignancy in childhood and at all ages if multiple myeloma is excluded. The lesion is usually metaphyseal and most frequently involves the distal femur and proximal tibia. The natural history of osteosarcoma involves a rapid enlargement of the primary tumor with propensity for metastatic disease in the lungs, other bones, and lymph nodes. Long-term survival has improved with the introduction of multidrug adjuvant and neoadjuvant chemotherapy.

The principal traditional imaging findings demonstrate a productive lesion with bone disruption and production, soft tissue component, and marked tumor accumulation of bone-seeking radiotracers. Skeletal scintigraphy occasionally demonstrates extraosseous (e.g., lung) metastases due to osteoid production by the metastatic deposits. MRI is used to define the local extent of osteosarcoma in bone and soft tissue. However, signal abnormalities caused by peritumoral edema can result in an overestimation of tumor extension. Due to nonspecific appearance of viable tumor on MRI, variable results have been reported for assessing chemotherapeutic response in planning for limb salvage surgery. Scintigraphy with Tl-201 and Tc-99m MIBI have been shown to be useful for assessing therapeutic response in osteosarcoma.

The exact role of FDG PET in bone tumors is unclear (Fig. 1). However, current experience suggests that in patients with bone sarcomas, FDG PET may play an important role in guiding biopsy, detecting local recurrence in amputation

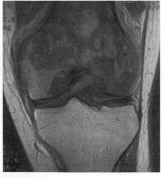
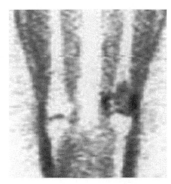

A   **B**

Figure 1: A male patient with isolated distal left femoral osseous lymphoma. **A.** MRI demonstrates a heterogeneous abnormality involving the distal left femoral bone marrow. **B.** PET sows relatively intense hypermetabolism corresponding to the MRI lesion.

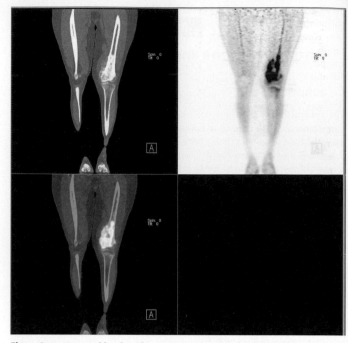

Figure 2: An 18-year-old male with osteogenic carcinoma of the left distal femur treated with chemotherapy. PET-CT shows a large bulky extensive primary tumor with post-treatment central necrosis and some extension within the diaphysis superiorly and along the medial condylar cortical surface.

stumps, evaluating patients with suspected metastatic disease, monitoring response to therapy, and assessing for prognosis (Fig. 2).

There appears to be a statistically significant difference in SUV between benign and malignant lesions. However, lesions such as giant cell tumors and fibrous dysplasias may not display statistically significant difference in SUV compared with osteosarcomas. Therefore, FDG PET may be limited in distinguishing accurately malignant from benign bone tumors due to the high accumulation of FDG in some benign bone lesions. FDG-PET SUV analysis may, however, be useful in histologic grading and guiding biopsy toward the most metabolically active regions of large masses.

FDG PET may have some limitation in detecting local recurrence in the amputation stump. Focal hypermetabolism may be associated with pressure areas and skin breakdown without evidence of disease recurrence. For detecting lung metastases, FDG PET may not be as sensitive as CT (50% vs. 75%), although due to the high specificity of FDG PET (98% vs. 100%), a positive FDG PET result can be used to confirm abnormalities seen on CT as metastatic disease. Similarly FDG PET may miss some osseous metastases of osteosarcoma in comparison to skeletal scintigraphy.

FDG PET has been reported to be useful in evaluating treatment response in patients with osteosarcoma. A ratio of post-therapy SUV to pre-treatment

SUV less than about 40% predicts a favorable histologic response to chemotherapy (defined as ≥90% necrosis). The prognostic utility of FDG PET in osteosarcoma has also been investigated. Overall and event-free survivals are significantly better in patients with tumors that display low FDG uptake in comparison to those patients with tumors that demonstrate high FDG accumulation.

II. SOFT TISSUE TUMORS

Soft tissue sarcomas compose a diverse group of solid malignancies with varied morphologic and anatomic characteristics. The most common sites of initial presentation are the extremities, followed in decreasing order of frequency by retroperitoneum, abdominal, trunk, genitourinary tract, viscera, and head and

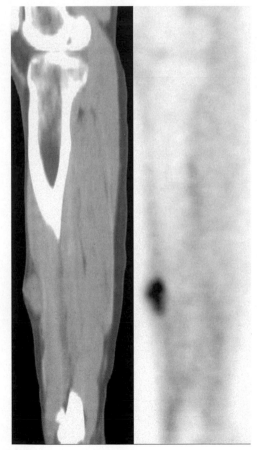

13

Figure 3: A 24-year-old woman with a monophasic synovial sarcoma anterolateral to mid-right tibia. PET-CT shows a hypermetabolic soft tissue mass.

neck. Retroperitoneal and visceral sarcomas are more likely to metastasize than the extremity tumors. High-grade lesions and tumors larger than 5 cm are also more likely to metastasize. The predominant tumor subtypes include liposarcoma, leiomyosarcoma, malignant fibrous histiocytoma (MFH), and fibrosarcoma. Management of soft tissue sarcomas usually involves aggressive tumor resection for local control. For extremity sarcomas, limb sparing surgery is currently the goal of therapy.

Functional imaging with FDG PET has been shown to be useful in directing biopsy, differentiating benign from malignant soft tissue masses, predicting tumor grade, staging, restaging, and prognosis (Figs. 3–7). Sarcomas in general tend to be highly FDG-avid, although significant heterogeneity in glucose metabolism may be evident. FDG PET has been used to direct biopsy to the most metabolically active area of the lesion in order to improve the diagnostic yield. FDG PET has also been used in characterizing soft tissue masses with

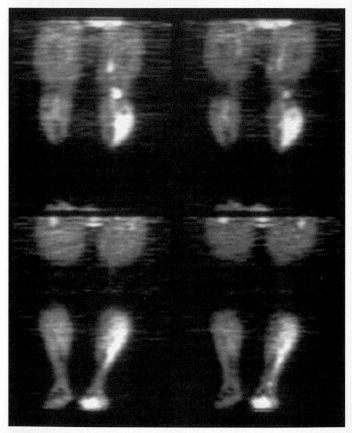

Figure 4: A 25-year-old man with left lower extremity rhabdomyosarcoma. PET shows hypermetabolic disease crossing the left knee joint.

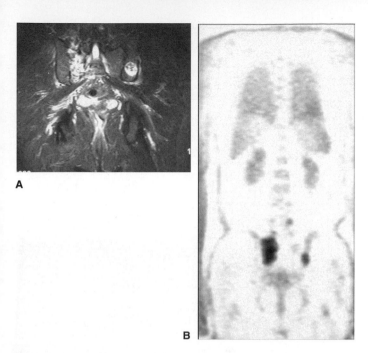

A

B

Figure 5: A 60-year-old man with metastatic angiosarcoma of the pelvis. **A.** Coronal inversion recovery sequence MRI of the sacrum demonstrates tumor foci in right sacral ala and the left posterior ilium. **B.** PET shows hyermetabolism in these same lesions and also demonstrated a left lower paralumbar metastatic retroperitoneal lymph node.

reported sensitivity of 95% and specificity of 75% in diagnosing sarcoma. FDG PET may also identify unexpected sites of metastases.

A systematic review and meta-analysis of 29 clinical studies on the diagnostic utility of FDG-PET in soft tissue and bone sarcomas reported a pooled sensitivity of 91%, specificity of 85%, and accuracy of 88% in detecting sarcomas. The differences between the mean SUV in malignant and benign tumors and that between low- and high-grade sarcomas were statistically significant. Another meta-analysis reviewed the diagnostic performance of FDG PET in grading of soft-tissue sarcomas in 15 clinical studies encompassing 441 soft-tissue lesions (227 malignant, 214 benign). For diagnosis of malignant versus benign lesions, typical pairs of sensitivity and specificity estimates from the summary receiver operating characteristic curves were 92% and 73% for qualitative visualization, 87% and 79% for SUV of 2.0, 70% and 87% for SUV of 3.0. Diagnostic performance was similar for both primary and recurrent lesions. Although FDG PET may be helpful in tumor grading, low-grade tumors and benign lesions may not be adequately discriminated.

An important diagnostic utility of FDG PET has been in the prediction and evaluation of therapy response in soft tissue sarcoma). In one example, FDG PET has been shown to be a sensitive method for evaluating an early

13

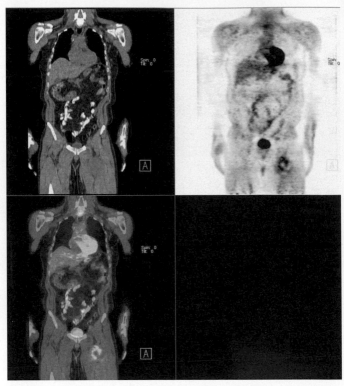

Figure 6: A 50-year-old male with newly diagnosed sarcoma of the left thigh. PET-CT shows relatively heterogeneous hypermetabolism in the anterior left proximal thigh soft tissue mass compatible with a mixture of viable tumor and necrosis.

response to imatinib mesylate (Gleevec/Glivec) treatment in gastrointestinal stromal tumors (GISTs), which are soft tissue sarcomas of the gastrointestinal tract originating from mesenchymal cells. Successful treatment results in a decline in tumor glucose metabolism in comparison to the high level of glucose metabolism in the tumor prior to therapy. Other studies have demonstrated the diagnostic utility of FDG PET in distinguishing viable tumor from changes caused by therapy in areas associated with equivocal MRI findings. However, occasionally prominent FDG accumulation may be observed in benign therapy-related fibrous tissue presumably due to local inflammation and healing. Despite this potential limitation, the ability to differentiate postoperative changes from local recurrence may impact the clinical management of patients with sarcoma. Additionally, pre-therapy FDG PET may be helpful in predicting overall and disease-free survivals. A multivariate analysis has shown that SUV(max) is a statistically significant independent predictor of patient survival such that tumors with larger SUV(max) have a significantly poorer prognosis.

In conclusion, the published literature suggests that FDG PET may have an important role in the imaging evaluation of patients with bone and soft tissue

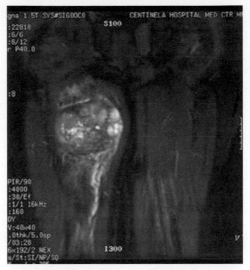

A

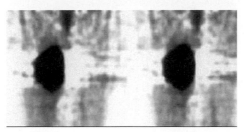

B

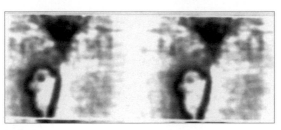

C

13

Figure 7: A 39-year-old female with malignant fibrous histiocytoma of the right thigh diagnosed by incisional biopsy. **A.** MRI shows a heterogeneous soft tissue mass in the right medial thigh. **B.** Pre-treatment PET shows an intensely hypermetabolic tumor. **C.** PET scan after cryoablation shows nodular residual disease in the upper anterolateral aspect of the lesion in combination with extensive subtotal necrosis surrounded by a rim of hypermetabolism which may represent reactive inflammation and residual tumor. The surgical specimen demonstrated 90% tumor necrosis with several areas of residual cancer.

sarcoma. Prospective studies with large patient groups are essential further to evaluate the cost-effectiveness and the short-term and long-term benefits of FDG-PET in these patients.

BIBLIOGRAPHY

Bone and Soft Tissue Tumors

1. Adler LP, Blair HF, Williams RP, et al. Grading liposarcomas with PET using [18F]FDG. J Comput Assist Tomogr 1990; 14:960–2.
2. Antoch G, Kanja J, Bauer S, et al. Comparison of PET, CT, and Dual-Modality PET/CT Imaging for Monitoring of Imatinib (STI571) Therapy in Patients with Gastrointestinal Stromal Tumors. J Nucl Med 2004; 45:357–365.
3. Aoki J, Endo K, Watanabe H, et al. FDG-PET for evaluating musculoskeletal tumors: a review. J Orthop Sci 2003; 8:435–41.
4. Aoki J, Inoue T, Tomiyoshi K, et al. Nuclear imaging of bone tumors: FDG-PET. Semin Musculoskelet Radiol 2001; 5:183–7.
5. Aoki J, Watanabe H, Shinozaki T, et al. FDG PET of primary benign and malignant bone tumors: standardized uptake value in 52 lesions. Radiology 2001; 219:774–7.
6. Aoki J, Watanabe H, Shinozaki T, et al. FDG-PET in differential diagnosis and grading of chondrosarcomas. J Comput Assist Tomogr 1999; 23:603–8.
7. Bastiaannet E, Groen H, Jager PL, et al. The value of FDG-PET in the detection, grading and response to therapy of soft tissue and bone sarcomas; a systematic review and meta-analysis. Cancer Treat Rev 2004; 30:83–101.
8. Bredella MA, Caputo GR, Steinbach LS. Value of FDG positron emission tomography in conjunction with MR imaging for evaluating therapy response in patients with musculoskeletal sarcomas. AJR Am J Roentgenol 2002; 179:1145–50.
9. Brenner W, Bohuslavizki KH, Eary JF. PET imaging of osteosarcoma. J Nucl Med 2003; 44:930–42.
10. Eary JF, Mankoff DA. Tumor metabolic rates in sarcoma using FDG PET. J Nucl Med 1998; 39:250–4.
11. Eary JF, O'Sullivan F, Powitan Y, et al. Sarcoma tumor FDG uptake measured by PET and patient outcome: a retrospective analysis. Eur J Nucl Med Mol Imaging 2002; 29:1149–54.
12. el-Zeftawy H, Heiba SI, Jana S, et al. Role of repeated F-18 fluorodeoxyglucose imaging in management of patients with bone and soft tissue sarcoma. Cancer Biother Radiopharm 2001; 16:37–46.
13. Feldman F, van Heertum R, Manos C. 18FDG PET scanning of benign and malignant musculoskeletal lesions. Skeletal Radiol 2003; 32:201–8.
14. Folpe AL, Lyles RH, Sprouse JT, et al. (F-18) fluorodeoxyglucose positron emission tomography as a predictor of pathologic grade and other prognostic variables in bone and soft tissue sarcoma. Clin Cancer Res 2000; 6:1279–87.
15. Franzius C, Bielack S, Flege S, et al. Prognostic significance of (18)F-FDG and (99m)Tc-methylene diphosphonate uptake in primary osteosarcoma. J Nucl Med 2002; 43:1012–7.
16. Franzius C, Daldrup-Link HE, Sciuk J, et al. FDG-PET for detection of pulmonary metastases from malignant primary bone tumors: comparison with spiral CT. Ann Oncol 2001; 12:479–86.
17. Franzius C, Schulte M, Hillmann A, et al. Clinical value of positron emission tomography (PET) in the diagnosis of bone and soft tissue tumors. 3rd Interdisciplinary Consensus Conference "PET in Oncology": results of the Bone and Soft Tissue Study Group. Chirurg 2001; 72:1071–7.
18. Franzius C, Sciuk J, Brinkschmidt C, et al. Evaluation of chemotherapy response in primary bone tumors with F-18 FDG positron emission tomography compared with histologically assessed tumor necrosis. Clin Nucl Med 2000; 25:874–81.

19. Garcia R, Kim EE, Wong FC, et al. Comparison of fluorine-18-FDG PET and technetium-99m-MIBI SPECT in evaluation of musculoskeletal sarcomas. J Nucl Med 1996; 37:1476–9.

20. Hain SF, O'Doherty MJ, Bingham J, et al. Can FDG PET be used to successfully direct preoperative biopsy of soft tissue tumors? Nucl Med Commun 2003; 24:1139–43.

21. Hain SF, O'Doherty MJ, Lucas JD, Smith MA. Fluorodeoxyglucose PET in the evaluation of amputations for soft tissue sarcoma. Nucl Med Commun 1999; 20:845–8.

22. Hawkins DS, Rajendran JG, Conrad EU 3rd, et al. Evaluation of chemotherapy response in pediatric bone sarcomas by [F-18]-fluorodeoxy-D-glucose positron emission tomography. Cancer 2002; 94(12):3277–84.

23. Ioannidis JP, Lau J. 18F-FDG PET for the diagnosis and grading of soft-tissue sarcoma: a meta-analysis. J Nucl Med 2003; 44:717–24.

24. Israel-Mardirosian N, Adler LP. Positron emission tomography of soft tissue sarcomas. Curr Opin Oncol 2003; 15:327–30.

25. Jones DN, McCowage GB, Sostman HD, et al. Monitoring of neoadjuvant therapy response of soft-tissue and musculoskeletal sarcoma using fluorine-18-FDG PET. J Nucl Med 1996; 37:1438–44.

26. Kern KA, Brunetti A, Norton JA, et al. Metabolic imaging of human extremity musculoskeletal tumors by PET. J Nucl Med 1988; 29:181–6.

27. Kole AC, Nieweg OE, van Ginkel RJ, et al. Detection of local recurrence of soft-tissue sarcoma with positron emission tomography using [18F]fluorodeoxyglucose. Ann Surg Oncol 1997; 4:57–63.

28. Lodge MA, Lucas JD, Marsden PK, et al. A PET study of 18FDG uptake in soft tissue masses. Eur J Nucl Med 1999; 26:22–30.

29. Lucas JD, O'Doherty MJ, Cronin BF, et al. Prospective evaluation of soft tissue masses and sarcomas using fluorodeoxyglucose positron emission tomography. Br J Surg 1999; 86:550–6.

30. Lucas JD, O'Doherty MJ, Wong JC, et al. Evaluation of fluorodeoxyglucose positron emission tomography in the management of soft-tissue sarcomas. J Bone Joint Surg Br 1998; 80:441–7.

31. Mankin HJ, Willett CG, Harmon DC. Malignant Tumors of Bone, in Holleb AI, Fink DJ, Murphy GP (eds): Clinical Oncology. Atlanta, American Cancer Society, 1991.

32. Miraldi F, Adler LP, Faulhaber P. PET imaging in soft tissue sarcomas. Cancer Treat Res 1997; 91:51–64.

33. Nair N, Ali A, Green AA, et al. Response of Osteosarcoma to Chemotherapy. Evaluation with F-18 FDG-PET Scans. Clin Positron Imaging 2000; 3:79–83.

34. Nieweg OE, Pruim J, van Ginkel RJ, et al. Fluorine-18-fluorodeoxyglucose PET imaging of soft-tissue sarcoma. J Nucl Med 1996; 37:257–61.

35. Posner MC, Brennan MF. Soft tissue Sarcomas, in Holleb AI, Fink DJ, Murphy GP (eds): Clinical Oncology. Atlanta, American Cancer Society, 1991.

36. Schulte M, Brecht-Krauss D, Heymer B, et al. Fluorodeoxyglucose positron emission tomography of soft tissue tumors: is a non-invasive determination of biological activity possible? Eur J Nucl Med 1999; 26:599–605.

37. Schulte M, Brecht-Krauss D, Werner M, et al. Evaluation of neoadjuvant therapy response of osteogenic sarcoma using FDG PET. J Nucl Med 1999; 40:1637–43.

38. Schwarzbach M, Willeke F, Dimitrakopoulou-Strauss A, et al. Functional imaging and detection of local recurrence in soft tissue sarcomas by positron emission tomography. Anticancer Res 1999; 19:1343–9.

39. Schwarzbach MH, Dimitrakopoulou-Strauss A, Mechtersheimer G, et al. Assessment of soft tissue lesions suspicious for liposarcoma by F18-deoxyglucose (FDG) positron emission tomography (PET). Anticancer Res 2001; 21:3609–14.

40. Schwarzbach MH, Dimitrakopoulou-Strauss A, Willeke F, et al. Clinical value of [18-F]] fluorodeoxyglucose positron emission tomography imaging in soft tissue sarcomas. Ann Surg 2000; 231:380–6.

13

41. Tse N, Hoh C, Hawkins R, et al. Positron emission tomography diagnosis of pulmonary metastases in osteogenic sarcoma. Am J Clin Oncol 1994; 17:22–5.
42. Van den Abbeele AD, Badawi RD. Use of positron emission tomography in oncology and its potential role to assess response to imatinib mesylate therapy in gastrointestinal stromal tumors (GISTs). Eur J Cancer 2002; 38 Suppl 5:S60–5.
43. van Ginkel RJ, Hoekstra HJ, Pruim J, et al. FDG-PET to evaluate response to hyperthermic isolated limb perfusion for locally advanced soft-tissue sarcoma. J Nucl Med 1996; 37:984–90.
44. Vernon CB, Eary JF, Rubin BP, et al. FDG PET imaging guided re-evaluation of histopathologic response in a patient with high-grade sarcoma. Skeletal Radiol 2003; 32:139–42.
45. Watanabe H, Shinozaki T, Yanagawa T, et al. Glucose metabolic analysis of musculoskeletal tumors using 18fluorine-FDG PET as an aid to preoperative planning. J Bone Joint Surg Br 2000; 82:760–7.

Oncology—Lymphoma

Lymphoma is divided into Hodgkin's disease and non-Hodgkin's lymphoma. **Hodgkin's disease** has had a relatively stable incidence. The estimated incidence for 2003 is 7,600 patients in the United States, with estimated deaths of 1,300. **Non-Hodgkin's lymphoma** (NHL) has been increasing in incidence. Part of the increase is due to HIV associated non-Hodgkin's lymphoma, but non-HIV-associated non-Hodgkin's lymphoma has also been increasing. The estimated incidence for 2003 is 53,400 patients with 23,400 deaths. FDG-PET is important in diagnosis, staging, monitoring therapy, and follow-up for both Hodgkin's disease and for non-Hodgkin's lymphoma.

The incidence of Hodgkin's disease has a peak in the third decade of life and then a second peak in about the sixth or seventh decade. The magnitude of the second peak has been decreasing due to classification of some of these older patients as non-Hodgkin's lymphoma using more modern immunohistological techniques. The incidence of non-Hodgkin's lymphoma increases with age, although enough patients present with non-Hodgkin's lymphoma at an early age that it is an important cause of cancer in young adults. The various subtypes of both Hodgkin's and non-Hodgkin's lymphoma have specific age and sex distributions.

Hodgkin's disease tends to follows an orderly progression along adjacent lymph node groups. Thus, it can be successfully treated with local radiotherapy when we know sites of bulk disease and adjacent sites, which may have microscopic disease. Non-Hodgkin's lymphoma can occasionally be treated with local radiotherapy, but its progression is less orderly and it usually presents at an advanced stage (see Figure 13). Generally, systemic therapy is needed in non-Hodgkin's lymphoma.

The treatment of Hodgkin's disease was an early success for both radiotherapy and chemotherapy. More recently, Hodgkin's disease has been a great success for bone marrow and stem cell transplantation. Initial therapy is often successful, and when it is not, successful salvage therapies are often curative. With either initial therapy or salvage therapy, about 75% of patients with Hodgkin's disease are cured. Results are less good with non-Hodgkin's lymphoma, with cures rates closer to 35%; but both radiotherapy and chemotherapy are quite efficacious when compared with treatment results for most solid tumors.

CLASSIFICATION

The classification of lymphoma has undergone several modifications. The World Health Organization (WHO) modification of the Revised European-American Lymphoma (REAL) classification is the classification that has become the most widely used. Lymphoma, particularly non-Hodgkin's lymphoma, is a complicated group of diseases. The following will describe the more common types of lymphoma.

Hodgkin's Disease. The cancer cell that defines Hodgkin's disease is the **Reed-Sternberg cell**, which appears to be of B-cell origin (bone marrow-derived). It is classically a large multinucleated cell with abundant cytoplasm, but there is a mononuclear variant of the Reed-Sternberg cell. Each of the nuclei has a prominent nucleolus. Hodgkin's disease is unusual in that the tumor cells compose a minority of the cells in a mass. In some cases, there are only very rare Reed-Sternberg cells. The background cells, which make up the majority of the cells, have different characters in the different Hodgkin's disease histologies. In order of frequency, the four classic categories of Hodgkin's disease are nodular sclerosis Hodgkin's disease, mixed cellularity Hodgkin's disease, lymphocyte-depleted Hodgkin's disease, and lymphocyte-rich Hodgkin's disease. Mixed cellularity Hodgkin's disease is most common in patients over 40 years of age. Between 16 and 40 years old, nodular sclerosis Hodgkin's disease is most common. Under 16 years old, lymphocyte-predominant Hodgkin's disease is most common.

Nodular sclerosis Hodgkin's disease is seen in 60–70% of patients with Hodgkin's disease. It has bands of collagen, which divide the cells into nodules. A variant of the Reed-Sternberg cell called a lacunar cell is seen in moderate numbers in a background of lymphocytes. Unlike most types of Hodgkin's disease, where males predominate, the male to female ratio is 1:1. This type of Hodgkin's disease affects adolescents and young adults; it is unusual in patients over 50 years old. **Mixed cellularity Hodgkin's disease**, which affects about one-quarter of patients, is usually found in older patients. Frequently Reed-Sternberg cells are seen in a background of inflammatory cells. There may be generalized lymphadenopathy, and B-symptoms—fevers, night sweats, and weight loss—are common. **Lymphocyte-rich Hodgkin's disease** has infrequent Reed-Sternberg cells with a background of mature lymphocytes. There are few Reed-Sternberg cells, with a background that is predominantly polyclonal B-cells. **Lymphocyte-depleted Hodgkin's disease** is rarely seen. Reed-Sternberg cells are more frequent than normal lymphocytes. Lymphocyte-depleted Hodgkin's disease is often advanced at presentation. It has been associated with HIV.

Nodular lymphocyte-predominant Hodgkin's disease (NLPHD) is somewhat similar histologically to classic lymphocyte-predominant Hodgkin's disease; however, immunophenotypically the cells are CD20 and CD45 positive, whereas classical Hodgkin's disease is CD15 and CD 30 positive. Nodular lymphocyte-predominant Hodgkin's disease accounts for 5–10% of patients, with a 4:1 male predominance. It has a long natural history. It is more common in patients under 15 or over 40 years old.

Non-Hodgkin's Lymphoma. The classification of non-Hodgkin's lymphomas is complex, but the details are often important for determining optimal therapy. Some lymphomas are derived from the **B-cells**, bone marrow-derived lymphocytes, and some are derived from the **T-cells**, thymus-derived lymphocytes. Most non-Hodgkin's lymphoma in adults is of B-cell origin, whereas in children most is of T-cell origin.

Many non-Hodgkin's lymphomas are indolent. Some patients with indolent lymphoma may be followed for relatively long periods without any therapy. Once it is decided to treat a patient, there are many efficacious chemotherapeutic regimes for the indolent lymphomas. Chemotherapy often results in remissions greater than one year, but sequential courses of chemotherapy often have lower response rates and shorter response durations. Radiotherapy can be used for localized disease sites. Immunotherapy can be performed with Rituximab, an antibody against CD20. Since February of 2002, radio-immunotherapy has been approved for treatment of indolent lymphomas and for transformed lymphomas. However, even with all of these efficacious therapies, the indolent lymphomas are generally incurable. One hopeful fact is that there is a subset of patients treated with radioimmunotherapy who are still under observation with durable remissions over several years.

Follicular lymphoma is the most common type of indolent lymphoma, comprising about 22% of non-Hodgkin's lymphoma. Morphologically, follicular lymphoma recapitulates the normal germinal centers of the secondary lymph follicles. The median age for follicular lymphoma is about 60 years. The disease course is quite variable. About 60% of the time, follicular lymphoma transforms to diffuse large B-cell lymphoma, an aggressive lymphoma. The indolent lymphomas also include **small lymphocytic lymphoma** (the solid component of chronic lymphocytic leukemia), **lymphoplasmacytic lymphoma** (immunocytoma) and the marginal zone lymphomas, including **mucosal-associated lymphoid tissue** (MALT) lymphoma.

The aggressive lymphomas have more rapid progression, but about 40% are curable. The most common of these lymphomas is **diffuse large B-cell lymphoma** (DLBCL), which comprises about 30% of non-Hodgkin's lymphoma. It is most common in young adults. Other aggressive lymphomas include **mantle cell lymphoma** and **peripheral T-cell lymphoma**. Some of the most rapidly growing tumors are the highly aggressive lymphomas, such as **Burkitt's lymphoma** and Burkitt's-like lymphoma and precursor T- or B-cell lymphoblastic leukemia/lymphoma.

FDG Avidity. The lymphomas are generally FDG-avid. Hodgkin's disease is highly FDG-avid. The non-Hodgkin's lymphomas have some tendency to have FDG uptake that is similar to their aggressiveness (see Figure 12). The aggressive non-Hodgkin's lymphomas are more FDG-avid than the indolent non-Hodgkin's lymphomas. But, follicular lymphoma, the most common type of indolent lymphoma, is usually easily detected on FDG-PET. The small lymphocytic lymphomas; marginal zone lymphomas, including MALT lymphoma; and peripheral T-cell lymphomas may not be FDG-avid. Figure 1 shows a patient with nodular sclerosis Hodgkin's disease in the neck and mediastinum, which is very FDG-avid. Figure 2 shows a patient with grade 1, follicular non-Hodgkin's lymphoma, which is also very FDG-avid. Figure 3 shows a patient who presented with a single pulmonary nodule that turned out to be an extranodal marginal zone B-cell lymphoma of the MALT type. The nodule is not FDG-avid.

Elstrom et al. compared the sensitivity of FDG-PET in 172 patients with various types of lymphoma. The sensitivity was 100% for large B-cell lymphoma (51/51) and for mantle cell lymphoma (7/7). The sensitivity was 98% for Hodgkin's disease (46/47) and follicular lymphoma (41/42). But the sensitivity was only 67% for marginal zone lymphoma (8/12) and 40% for peripheral T-cell lymphoma (2/5). Other lymphoma categories included only one or two patients. FDG-PET was not accurate for diagnosis of bone marrow involvement in any subtype of lymphoma; however, it did identify unknown sites of bone marrow involvement in Hodgkin's disease (4/32) and large B-cell

14

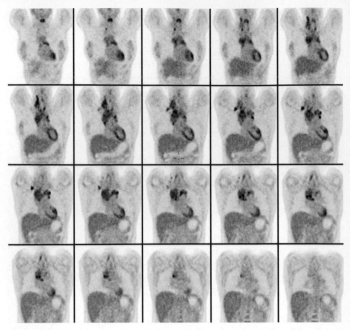

Figure 1: Hodgkin's Disease. Coronal FDG-PET slices of a patient with nodular sclerosis Hodgkin's disease in the neck and mediastinum.

lymphoma (4/32) when iliac crest biopsy was negative. Hoffmann et al. found FDG-PET was negative in 10/10 patients with mucosal-associated lymphoid tissue lymphoma. Jerusalem et al. found FDG-PET detected less than 58% of abnormal lymph node areas in small lymphocytic lymphoma.

DIAGNOSIS

Given its high sensitivity, FDG-PET can be used for detecting most types of lymphoma. However, the specificity of FDG-PET is less good. Any granulomatous disease can be very FDG-avid. For example, sarcoidosis and Castleman's disease show intense FDG uptake. Often the pattern of uptake is typical for a particular diagnosis, and that diagnosis can be favored in a differential. Reactive nodes often show moderate FDG-avidity, and they may have intense uptake. It is common to see moderate uptake in axillary or inguinal nodes related to peripheral infections.

However, even if the FDG-PET scan is positive in a pattern that is highly suggestive of lymphoma, diagnosis of lymphoma requires histological confirmation. The major utility of FDG-PET in diagnosis is often in directing a biopsy. A patient may present with a suspicious mass that is relatively inaccessible for biopsy. FDG-PET may identify other involved regions, which can be biopsied at much lower morbidity. FDG-PET imaging used for diagnosis simultaneously provides staging information.

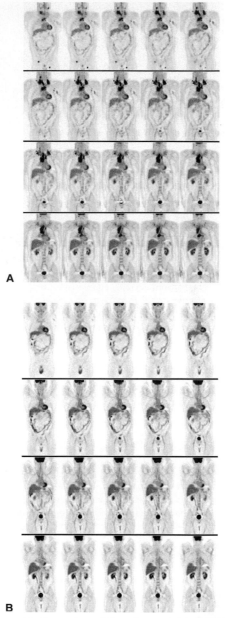

Figure 2: Response to Therapy. Coronal slices of a patient with grade1, follicular non-Hodgkin's lymphoma are shown in A. Note the good uptake of FDG in this type of indolent lymphoma. Response after three of six cycles of chemotherapy is shown in B. Note the good response to therapy at mid-course.

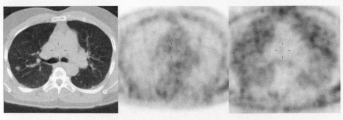

Figure 3: Lymphoma Presenting as a Single Pulmonary Nodule. The CT on the left shows a single pulmonary nodule. The attenuation corrected image in the center and the non-corrected image on the right show that the nodule is not FDG-avid. It turned out that the nodule was an extranodal marginal zone B-cell lymphoma of the mucosa associated lymphoid tissue (MALT) type. Marginal zone B-cell lymphomas may not be FDG-avid.

STAGING

The staging system used for lymphoma is shown in Table 1. Staging was orig-inally introduced for Hodgkin's disease. It identifies patients who can be suc-cessfully treated with radiotherapy and defines the extent of the radiation ports. Hodgkin's disease often involves lymph nodes in the neck or mediastinum. Patients with no disease below the diaphragm on a staging laparotomy have a considerably better prognosis than those with more extensive disease. Therapy for Hodgkin's disease, including salvage therapy for patients who fail first-line treatment, has become so effective that the recent emphasis has been on limit-ing the toxicity of first-line therapy. These regimes often involve systemic ther-apy with well-tolerated chemotherapy, so that detection of microscopic disease by staging laparotomy is less important than in the past. Thus, staging laparo-tomy is less commonly employed, and radiological staging has become even more important.

Non-Hodgkin's lymphoma is less well localized, but the same staging system is used for it (see Figure 11). Staging has some prognostic and thera-peutic implications for non-Hodgkin's lymphoma, but staging is less central in non-Hodgkin's lymphoma than it is in Hodgkin's disease.

Compared to Gallium Scintigraphy. The consensus is that gallium scintigraphy does not add substantially to anatomic imaging with CT during the initial staging of lymphoma. It has been shown to be very useful for moni-toring therapy and during follow-up of both Hodgkin's disease and aggressive non-Hodgkin's lymphoma. Its role in indolent non-Hodgkin's lymphoma is more complex, and it can be used in combination with thallium scintigraphy. Although gallium scintigraphy is not useful for staging, nuclear medicine physi-cians tend to recommend a baseline gallium scan in order to assess gallium-avidity for interpretation of post-therapy studies.

Gallium's role in the evaluation of lymphoma has been supplanted by FDG-PET imaging. Bar-Shalom et al. found a statistically significant difference in sensitivity, specificity, and accuracy between Anger camera-based FDG-PET and gallium scintigraphy on both a patient and site basis. Gallium scintigraphy accurately defined the disease state in 63% of 84 patients and 33% of 219 sites,

Table 1: Lymphoma Staging

Stage	
I	Involvement of a single lymph node region or lymphoid structure (spleen, thymus, Waldeyer's ring)
II	Involvement of two or more lymph node regions or lymphoid structures on the same side of the diaphragm; the number of sites is indicated by a subscript, e.g., II_2
III	Involvement of lymph node regions or lymphoid structures on both sides of the diaphragm III_1: Upper abdomen, without involvement of para-aortic, iliac, and mesenteric nodes III_2: With involvement of para-aortic, iliac, or mesenteric nodes
IV	Involvement of one or more extranodal sites other than an "E" site

Modifiers	
A	No symptoms.
B	Fever (> 38ºC), drenching night sweats, unexplained loss > 10% of body weight within the preceding 6 months
X	Bulky disease (> 1/3 the width of the mediastinum, or a nodal mass with maximal dimension greater than 10 cm)
E	Involvement of a single extranodal site that is contiguous or proximal to the known nodal site
CS	Clinical stage
PS	Pathological stage

Node Regions
Waldeyer's ring
Cervical, supraclavicular, occipital, and preauricular
Epitrochlear and brachial
Axillary and pectoral
Infraclavicular
Mediastinal
Hilar
Para-aortic
Splenic
Mesenteric
Iliac
Inguinal and femoral
Popliteal

14

whereas Anger camera-based FDG-PET accurately defined the disease state in 83% of patients and 87% of sites. Kostakoglu et al. found that the target-to-background ratios were significantly higher for camera based FDG-PET than for gallium. FDG-PET showed disease at all 158 sites in 51 patients, while gallium scintigraphy showed 113 sites of disease in 41 patients. Thus, even using Anger camera-based PET scanning, FDG is more accurate than gallium scintigraphy.

Wirth et al. compared gallium scintigraphy, FDG-PET, and conventional staging, including CT scanning in 50 patients. The case positivity for conventional assessment was 90%; for gallium scanning, 88%; and for PET scanning, 100%. The positivity for conventional assessment plus gallium scintigraphy was 98%, and for conventional assessment plus FDG-PET it was 100%. The per site positivity rate for PET, 82%, was significantly better than for conventional assessment, 68%, or for gallium, 69%. In 19 patients, FDG-PET identified 25 sites of disease missed by gallium, while gallium identified only 10 sites of disease missed by PET.

In monitoring therapy (see below) Zijlstra et al. found that there was less inter-observer variation in FDG-PET interpretation than gallium scintigraphy. Furthermore, 64% of patients who had negative FDG-PET studies after two cycles of chemotherapy were free from progression of disease after 25 ± 5 months compared to 50% of patients with a negative gallium scan. Only 25% of patients with positive FDG-PET scans remained free of disease, while 42% of patients with positive gallium scintigraphy remained free of disease. Thus, FDG-PET also appears to a better agent for monitoring patients during therapy.

In addition to gallium, positron-emitting radiopharmaceuticals other than FDG have shown uptake in lymphoma. Hustinx et al. studied ten patients with lymphoma using F-18 labeled fluoro-L-tyrosine, a marker of protein synthesis. Sutinen et al. studied nodal staging in 19 patients with lymphoma using C-11 labeled methionine, another marker of protein synthesis. Neither of these tracers showed superiority to FDG. Thus, FDG is the most valuable radiopharmaceutical for lymphoma.

Compared to Computed Tomography (CT).   Summarizing a number of studies, Schiepers et al. estimate that FDG-PET is about 15% more sensitive than CT for staging disease. This may be particularly true for identification of extranodal sites of disease such as the spleen. Now that staging laparotomy is no longer being used in the staging of Hodgkin's disease, more accurate assessment of the spleen will be important in initial staging. (FDG-PET does not reliably detect extranodal bone marrow involvement; see below). Thus, unlike gallium, initial FDG imaging is valuable not only for assessing FDG-avidity of the tumor, but also for the initial staging of lymphoma.

Although FDG-PET appears more sensitive than CT, the radiological community has rapidly become aware of the synergistic relation of FDG-PET and CT. Integrated interpretation of FDG-PET with CT data provides better diagnosis of lymphoma than use of either alone.

PROGNOSIS

In Hodgkin's disease, staging is used not only to determine therapy, but it also is important for determining prognosis. FDG-PET has a role in the prognosis of Hodgkin's disease by better defining the stage of disease. Limited-stage non-Hodgkin's lymphoma can be cured by local radiation therapy. However, except for this case, staging has less impact on prognosis. In non-Hodgkin's lymphoma prognosis is generally provided by the international prognostic index (IPI). The international prognostic index is based on age, tumor stage, serum lactate dehydrogenase (LDH), performance status, and number of extranodal sites of disease. The prognostic information provided by the international prognostic index is modest. Four risk groups can be identified using these factors with five-year survivals of 73%, 51%, 43%, and 26%.

In several cancers, the intensity of uptake as measured by the SUV provides prognostic information. In lymphoma, therapy is often quite successful, especially in the more aggressive forms of lymphoma. Therefore, prognosis can be more accurately defined by incorporating the response of the lymphoma to therapy. As described in the following section, FDG-PET has a major role in determining the response to therapy, and in turn this response provides valuable prognostic information.

MONITORING THERAPY

A major indication for FDG-PET is monitoring therapy for lymphoma. It is clear that FDG-PET imaging either at the end of a course of therapy or at some point during therapy provides valuable prognostic information. The precise details of when FDG-PET should be obtained and how the information should be used are still being worked out. But algorithms are already being developed which incorporate FDG-PET in decisions about modification of therapy regimes.

Figure 4 shows a sequence of FDG-PET/CT scans in a patient undergoing therapy for diffuse large B-cell non-Hodgkin's lymphoma. The FDG information was used at several points to help to make a therapeutic decision. Unfortunately, this patient responded only partially to initial chemotherapy, and FDG-PET provided information that allowed prompt progression to an autologous stem-cell transplantation.

Post-Therapy. Guay et al. studied 48 patients with Hodgkin's disease after the completion of therapy. FDG-PET prediction of relapse over a median follow up of 605 days had a sensitivity of 79% and a specificity of 97% compared to CT with a sensitivity of 83% and a specificity of 40%. Lavely et al. studied 40 patients, 20 patients with Hodgkin's disease and 20 patients with non-Hodkin's lymphoma after completion of therapy. FDG-PET prediction of relapse had a sensitivity of 100% and a specificity of 84%. Reske reviewed 15 other studies reporting results on differentiation of viable lymphoma from scar tissue in 723 patients. The sensitivity for detection of active disease was 71–100% with a specificity of 69–100%. The sensitivity of CT was high, 84–100%, but the specificity was poor, 4–31%.

A major problem with anatomic evaluation of therapy for lymphoma is that after successful therapy there is often a residual mass. For example, prominent residual masses are commonly seen in young adults with nodular sclerosis Hodgkin's disease. This is the reason that the specificity of anatomic imaging is poor post-therapy. The only way to differentiate residual mass from residual disease at the end of therapy using anatomic imaging is to follow the size of the mass over time. Thus, tumor-specific imaging with FDG-PET provides a much more specific diagnosis.

It appears that there is a fraction of patients, who have durable remissions but have persistently positive FDG-PET studies post therapy. The presence of disease at a new site should especially raise the possibility of a benign cause for the uptake. In patients with persistently positive studies, it is wise to follow up the finding closely or confirm the presence of disease prior to altering therapy.

14

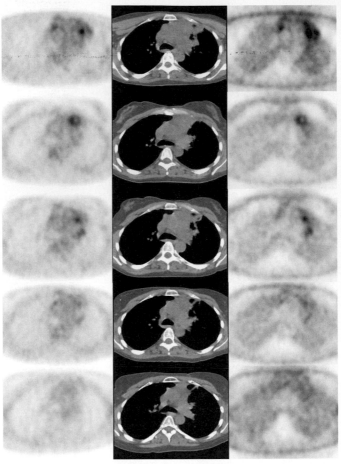

Figure 4: Therapy Monitoring. This sequence of FDG-PET scans shows a progressive response to several therapies. On the left is the attenuation-corrected FDG-PET, in the center is the corresponding CT, and on the right is the non-attenuation-corrected FDG-PET. The first line shows a mid-course FDG-PET/CT study after four cycles of R-CHOP. Because of the residual bulk disease it was decided to intensify therapy with two cycles of RIME. The second line shows a mixed response, so an additional two cycles of DHAP were given. The third line shows progression of disease, thus it was decided to progress to an autologous stem-cell transplant. The fourth line shows only low-level residual FDG activity. The fifth line shows no residual uptake after consolidative radiation therapy.

Figure 5 shows a patient with faint residual disease near the end of therapy. Follow-up confirms progression of residual disease.

Mid-Course. Because of finite resolution, tumor-specific imaging with gallium or with FDG can only detect bulk disease. It is not able to detect residual

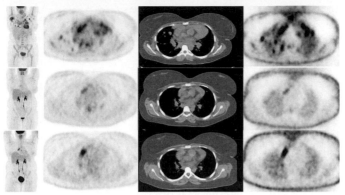

Figure 5: Residual Disease. The top line shows a baseline FDG-PET/CT in a patient with stage IV (pulmonary involvement), nodular sclerosis Hodgkin's disease. The second line shows a study near the end of the Stanford V regime. Although there has been marked improvement, there appears to be faint residual disease. The last line shows a study three months later confirming residual disease. On the left are a anterior MIP images; in the center-left are attenuation-corrected FDG-PET images; in the center-right are CT slices; and on the right are non-corrected FDG-PET images.

microscopic disease. The concept of mid-course imaging was developed with gallium scintigraphy. In order to affect a cure by the end of therapy, the bulk disease needs to be under control early in the course of therapy. Early evaluation of the effect of therapy has the potential for indicating the likelihood that not only the bulk disease, but also the microscopic disease, will be successfully treated by the end of therapy.

Figure 2 shows a good response to therapy at after three of six cycles of chemotherapy. Figure 6 shows a patient with a high-grade, diffuse large B-cell non-Hodgkin's lymphoma at baseline and again after four of six cycles of therapy with R-CHOP. Initially there is very extensive disease. At mid-course all of the abnormal sites of FDG uptake have disappeared, except for an area in the rectum that had worsened in the interval. Clinically, the patient was found to have a benign finding, a very inflamed hemorrhoid in this region.

Spaepen et al. studied 70 patients with aggressive non-Hodgkin's lymphoma at the middle of their chemotherapy. None of the 33 patients who had positive studies achieved a durable remission. Thirty-one of the 37 patients who had negative studies remain in remission after a mean follow-up of 1,107 days. In multivariate analysis, FDG-PET was a stronger predictor of progression-free survival than the international prognostic index.

Kostakoglu et al. studied 13 patients with Hodgkin's disease and 17 patients with non-Hodgkin's lymphoma after one cycle and at the end of chemotherapy. Both time points correlated with follow-up over a mean of 19 months. There was a better correlation (r^2 = 0.45 versus 0.17) with the study after one cycle than with the study at the end of therapy.

Torizuka et al. studied 20 patients, 3 with Hodgkin's disease and 17 with aggressive non-Hodgkin's lymphoma after one or two cycles of chemotherapy. Visual assessment showing persistent FDG uptake was sensitive, but not specific

14

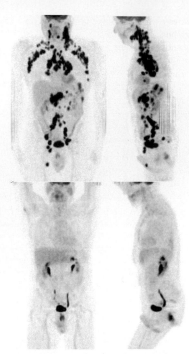

Figure 6: Inflamed Hemorrhoid. Anterior and lateral MIP images form FDG-PET scans before and after four of six cycles of R-CHOP therapy for a high-grade, diffuse B-cell non-Hodgkin's lymphoma. At baseline, there is very widespread intensely FDG-avid disease. At follow-up the only abnormal area was in the rectum, corresponding to intensely inflamed hemorrhoids.

for 24-month clinical outcome. A 60% reduction in SUV form baseline to the early post-therapy study provides the best separation of responders from non-responders.

Pre-Transplant.   Schot et al. studied 68 patients with persistent or recurrent lymphoma (both Hodgkin's disease and non-Hodgkin's lymphoma) in an attempt to predict the response to autologous stem-cell transplantation. An FDG-PET scan was obtained before and after three courses of induction chemotherapy. Of 46 patients who responded to chemotherapy, 39 went on to transplant. The two-year progression-free survival was 62% for the 15 of 39 patients with negative FDG-PET scans, whereas it was 32% for the 31 patients with a positive FDG-PET.

Spaepen et al. studied 60 patients after salvage therapy before high-dose chemotherapy with stem-cell transplantation. Of 30 patients with negative studies, 25 remain in complete remission a mean follow-up of 1,510 days. Two patients died of therapy complications, and the three patients who relapse had a median progression-free survival of 1,083 days. Twenty-six of 30 patients with a positive scan progressed with a median progression free survival of 402 days. Four patients with a positive scan remain in complete remission.

Filmont et al. studied 20 patients (6 with Hodgkin's disease and 14 with non-Hodgkin's lymphoma) after salvage cytoreductive chemotherapy but before high-dose chemotherapy and autologous stem-cell transplantation. Seven of eight patients with negative studies had a disease-free follow-up over a median of 13.3 months. Eleven of 12 patients with positive studies relapsed. These authors also studied 23 patients (6 with Hodgkin's disease and 14 with non-Hodgkin's lymphoma) after autologous stem-cell transplantation. Eight of nine patients with negative studies had a disease-free follow-up over a median of 16.5 months. Thirteen of 14 patients with positive studies had progression of disease.

These studies all suggest that the response to salvage cytoreductive chemotherapy is highly predictive of the response after stem-cell transplantation. So far, this information has been used for prognosis; however, it raises the question whether it should be used to help direct therapy.

FOLLOW-UP

There are efficacious therapies for patients with recurrent lymphoma. It is believed that early therapy for recurrent disease is more effective than delayed therapy, especially for Hodgkin's disease. Therefore, early detection of disease with frequent follow-up is believed to have an important affect on outcome.

Jerusalem et al. studied 36 patients with Hodgkin's disease every four- to six months for two to three years after the end of chemotherapy. Positive FDG-PET findings were confirmed on a short, four- to six-week, follow-up. There was one patient with persistent disease. Four patients relapsed, two at one month and one each at five and nine months. Two patients had B-symptoms at relapse; the other three were asymptomatic. FDG-PET identified all five patients with residual or relapsed disease. Clinical examination, laboratory findings, or CT were never first to identify relapse. The confirmatory four- to six week follow-up study was important since six patients had transient findings on FDG-PET which otherwise would have been mistaken for relapse.

Freudenberg et al. found that anatomic plus metabolic imaging with PET/CT was more effective than either procedure alone in restaging 27 patients with lymphoma (9 with Hodgkin's disease and 18 with non-Hodgkin's lymphoma). The sensitivities for CT alone, FDG-PET alone, side-by-side FDG-PET and CT, and integrated FDG-PET/CT were 78%, 86%, 93%, and 93% with specificities of 54%, 100%, 100%, and 100%, respectively. On a per region basis the sensitivities were 61%, 78%, 91%, and 96% with specificities of 89%, 98%, 99%, and 99%, respectively. Figure 7 shows a small lymph node near the bladder in the pelvis on PET/CT. The CT shows that the focal FDG activity is located in a non-pathologically enlarged lymph node.

The indolent non-Hodgkin's lymphomas may be watched without therapy or treated with a relatively non-toxic regime. The indolent non-Hodgkin's lymphoma often transforms to a more aggressive form requiring more intensive therapy. A change in the avidity of FDG uptake of a lesion may be the first clue of transformation.

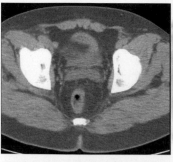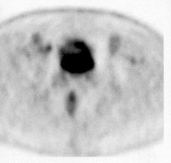

Figure 7: Perivesicular Lymph Node. The CT scan shows that the small perivesicular region of increased uptake is localized to a non-pathologically enlarged lymph node. Interpretation of the FDG-PET study would be difficult without the anatomic information provided by the CT.

IMPACT OF FDG-PET

Several studies have shown a considerable impact of FDG-PET on both staging and on management of disease. Shah et al. found that FDG-PET added extra information to clinical evaluation and CT scan in 10 of 29 (41%) patients with lymphoma. Furthermore, there was a change in clinical management in 10 (34%).

Schoder et al. assessed the impact of FDG-PET on staging and management of lymphoma using a questionnaire. Fifty-two of 108 questionnaires (48%) were returned. FDG-PET resulted in a change in clinical stage in 44% of patients—21% were up-staged and 23% were down-staged. There was a change in intermodality management in 42%, a change in intramodality management in 10%, and a combination of changes in 10%. Other management changes occurred in 6% of patients. There was no change in management in only 32% of patients.

Dizendorf et al. studied a number of tumors, including lymphoma, which were to be treated with radiation therapy. In 55 of 202 patients (27%), FDG-PET changed the management. In 18 cases (9%), radiation therapy was canceled due to detection of either previously unknown disease (16) or the absence of active disease (2). In 21 cases (10%) there was a change in the intent of therapy (curative or palliative). Radiation dose was changed in 25(12%) and radiated volume was changed in 12 (6%).

Naumann et al. compared therapy decisions for 88 patients with Hodgkin's disease based on staging with and without FDG-PET imaging. Similar treatment decisions would have been made in 70/88 (80%) patients. Management would have changed with intensification of therapy in 9/88 (10%) and minimization of therapy in 7/88 (8%). In nine out of 44 patients (20%) with early-stage disease, therapy would have been intensified.

LIMITATIONS OF FDG-PET

Benign Uptake of FDG. There are several benign causes for FDG uptake. Benign uptake is usually a problem for specificity; however, if there is widespread benign uptake as is sometimes seen with muscle or brown fat uptake,

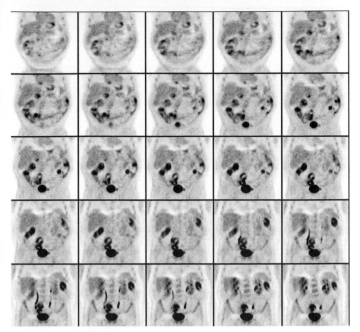

Figure 8: Bowel Lymphoma. The FDG-PET coronal images of the abdomen show widespread, intense (greater than liver), regional uptake in the bowel due to lymphomatous involvement of the bowel.

then real disease may get lost in the benign findings. Close anatomical correlation, with, for example, PET/CT, can help in many of these circumstances. Uptake in normal muscle or in fat can be discounted, and uptake corresponding to a lymph node will receive greater importance.

There is avid normal uptake of FDG in the gray matter of the brain. FDG-PET is relatively insensitive to brain involvement with lymphoma. Uptake in the bowel is variable. Diffuse intense bowel uptake is not unusual. Bowel involvement with lymphoma can be difficult to identify, although the index of suspicious should be higher when there is intense focal or regional uptake, especially in someone with bowel symptoms (Figure 8).

Chemotherapy for lymphoma often results in immunocompromising the patient and an increase in infections. These infections can be seen on FDG-PET, and it is important to distinguish them from new sites of disease (see Figure 6).

Bone Marrow.   Bone marrow uptake is variable in patients without disease in the marrow. Rebound from therapy, particularly when the marrow has been stimulated by growth factors, can result in marked bone marrow uptake. In some cases, focal bone marrow involvement can be accurately identified on FDG-PET, and it may be valuable for upstaging the patient (Figure 9). However, identification of bone marrow involvement is not reliable on FDG-PET. In the indolent non-Hodgkin's lymphomas, the bone marrow involvement can be relatively diffuse with a small volume of disease at any one site, making it

14

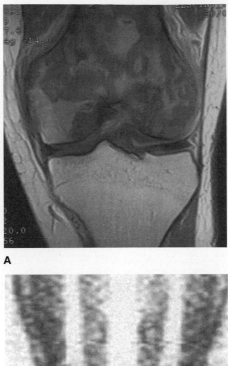

A

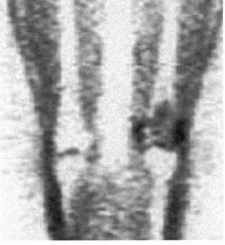

B

Figure 9: Bone Lymphoma. A male patient with isolated distal left femoral osseous lymphoma. **A.** MRI demonstrates a heterogeneous abnormality involving the distal left femoral bone marrow. **B.** PET shows relatively intense hypermetabolism corresponding to the MRI lesion.

technically difficult to identify the marrow involvement. Thus, FDG-PET is not a reliable tool for identifying bone marrow involvement.

Thymic Rebound. After chemotherapy, there may be a rebound in the thymus. A histologically normal thymus may increase in size and become FDG-avid. Since the anterior mediastinum is also an important location of recurrent lymphoma, thymic rebound can easily be confused with relapse. Thymic uptake is common in younger patients. Nakahara et al. found moderate thymic uptake in 34% of 94 patients with a mean age of 25.4 (19–29) years. Thymic rebound is seen in young adults. Brink et al. found thymic uptake in 11 of 15 (73%) children (11.9 ± 3.7 years) prior to chemotherapy; in 9 of 12 (75%) children (10.3 ± 5 years) after chemotherapy; in none of 37 (0%) of adults (43.9 ± 16.7 years) before chemotherapy; and in 5 of 104 adults (40.9 ± 14.6 years) after chemotherapy. The oldest patient with thymic uptake was 25 years old. The average SUV for visible thymic uptake was four.

There are some clues that help in interpretation. In thymic rebound, the thymus usually retains its normal shape, whereas with lymphomatous involvement, it often will show a mass-like shape. The time course of thymic rebound is usually within months of the end of therapy. On subsequent FDG-PET imaging, the thymic uptake decreases in intensity. Moderate FDG uptake in a normally shaped thymus gland in a child or in a young adult after chemotherapy is

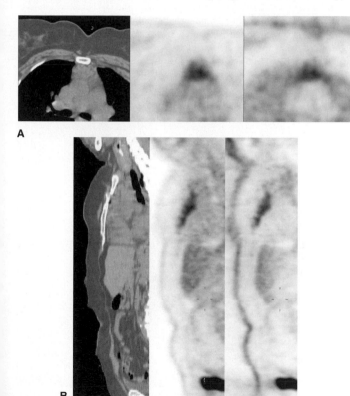

A

B

Figure 10: FDG-avid Thymus. An FDG-PET/CT scan of a 54-year old-woman with myasthenic syndrome in the axial (**A**) and sagittal (**B**) projections. The CT shows an enlarged somewhat nodular thymus that retains the general thymic shape. Attenuation-corrected and non-corrected FDG images show moderate FDG-avidity.

14

easily identified as physiologic uptake. Intense FDG uptake in a rounded mass in an older adult is easily identified as disease. In less clear-cut cases, follow-up studies are needed to establish the correct diagnosis.

Figure 10 shows moderate FDG-avidity in a patient who presented with an enlarged thymus. The thymus is somewhat nodular on the CT scan, but although enlarged, it generally retains a normal shape. This patient was 54 years old; therefore, both the enlargement and the FDG avidity were abnormal. Histology showed extensive follicular B-cell hyperplasia and focal cyst formation, findings that are typically seen in patients with myasthenia gravis. This patient had clinical and laboratory findings that allowed her to be classified as myasthenic syndrome, but not as myasthenia gravis.

SUMMARY

FDG-PET is a major tool in diagnosis, staging, follow-up, restaging, and monitoring therapy in both Hodgkin's disease and non-Hodgkin's lymphoma. Except for some of the indolent non-Hodgkin's lymphomas (small lymphocytic lymphoma; marginal zone lymphoma, including MALT lymphoma; and peripheral T-cell lymphoma) lymphoma has a very high rate of FDG-avidity. The simultaneous interpretation of FDG-PET and anatomic imaging should improve both the ability to identify disease and to identify regions of benign

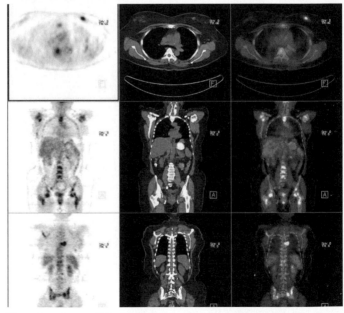

Figure 11: A 56-year-old female with non-Hodgkin's lymphoma diagnosed by CT-guided biopsy of a T5-T6 paraspinal soft tissue mass. PET-CT shows numerous hypermetabolic lesions, including the medial aspect of the left breast, a right internal mammary node, soft tissue mass with extension to the adjacent thoracic spine at the level between T5 and T6, and multiple osseous structures.

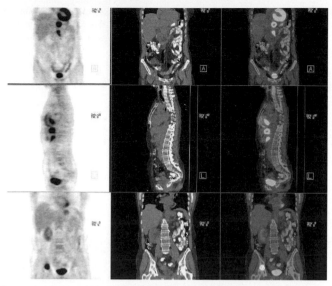

Figure 12: A 59-year-old female with lymphoma with subsequent chemotherapy and radiation. PET-CT shows hypermetabolic lesions in the right hilum, left hepatic lobe, celiac axis, and right supra-acetabular area consistent with tumor recurrence.

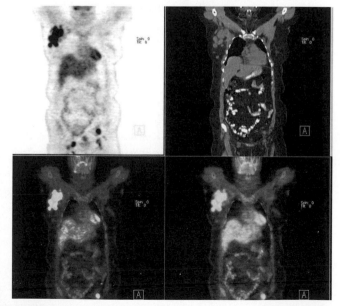

Figure 13: A 50-year-old female with non-Hodgkin's lymphoma diagnosed by biopsy of a right axillary node. PET-CT shows hypermetabolic disease involving the right axilla, left iliac, and bilateral inguinal nodal basins.

uptake. It is likely that there will be continuing development of therapeutic regimes which incorporate FDG-PET imaging in therapeutic algorithms. These algorithms may reduce toxicity in some patients and allow for early intensification of therapy in others.

BIBLIOGRAPHY

1. A predictive model for aggressive non-Hodgkin's lymphoma. The International Non-Hodgkin's Lymphoma Prognostic Factors Project. *N Engl J Med* 1993; 329(14):987–94.
2. Alavi A, Gupta N, Alberini JL, et al. Positron emission tomography imaging in non-malignant thoracic disorders. *Semin Nucl Med* 2002; 32(4):293–321.
3. Bar-Shalom R, Yefremov N, Haim N, et al. Camera-based FDG PET and 67Ga SPECT in evaluation of lymphoma: comparative study. *Radiology* 2003; 227(2):353–60.
4. Dizendorf EV, Baumert BG, von Schulthess GK, et al. Impact of whole-body 18F-FDG PET on staging and managing patients for radiation therapy. *J Nucl Med* 2003; 44(1):24–9.
5. Elstrom R, Guan L, Baker G, et al. Utility of FDG-PET scanning in lymphoma by WHO classification. *Blood* 2003; 101(10):3875–6.
6. Filmont JE, Czernin J, Yap C, et al. Value of F-18 fluorodeoxyglucose positron emission tomography for predicting the clinical outcome of patients with aggressive lymphoma prior to and after autologous stem-cell transplantation. *Chest* 2003; 124(2):608–13.
7. Freudenberg LS, Antoch G, Schutt P, et al. FDG-PET/CT in re-staging of patients with lymphoma. *Eur J Nucl Med Mol Imaging* 2004; 31:325–9.
8. Friedberg JW, Chengazi V. PET scans in the staging of lymphoma: current status. *Oncologist* 2003; 8(5):438–47.
9. Guay C, Lepine M, Verreault J, Benard F. Prognostic value of PET using 18F-FDG in Hodgkin's disease for posttreatment evaluation. *J Nucl Med* 2003; 44(8):1225–31.
10. Hoffmann M, Kletter K, Diemling M, et al. Positron emission tomography with fluorine-18-2-fluoro-2-deoxy-D-glucose (F18-FDG) does not visualize extranodal B-cell lymphoma of the mucosa-associated lymphoid tissue (MALT)-type. *Ann Oncol* 1999; 10(10):1185–9.
11. Hong SP, Hahn JS, Lee JD, et al. 18F-fluorodeoxyglucose-positron emission tomography in the staging of malignant lymphoma compared with CT and 67Ga scan. *Yonsei Med J* 2003; 44(5):779–86.
12. Hustinx R, Lemaire C, Jerusalem G, et al. Whole-body tumor imaging using PET and 2-18F-fluoro-L-tyrosine: preliminary evaluation and comparison with 18F-FDG. *J Nucl Med* 2003; 44(4):533–9.
13. Jemal A, Murray T, Samuels A, et al. Cancer statistics, 2003. *CA Cancer J Clin* 2003; 53(1):5–26.
14. Jerusalem G, Beguin Y, Fassotte MF, et al. Early detection of relapse by whole-body positron emission tomography in the follow-up of patients with Hodgkin's disease. *Ann Oncol* 2003; 14(1):123–30.
15. Jerusalem G, Beguin Y, Najjar F, et al. Positron emission tomography (PET) with 18F-fluorodeoxyglucose (18F-FDG) for the staging of low-grade non-Hodgkin's lymphoma (NHL). *Ann Oncol* 2001; 12(6):825–30.
16. Kostakoglu L, Coleman M, Leonard JP, et al. PET predicts prognosis after 1 cycle of chemotherapy in aggressive lymphoma and Hodgkin's disease. *J Nucl Med* 2002; 43(8):1018–27.
17. Kostakoglu L, Leonard JP, Kuji I, et al. Comparison of fluorine-18 fluorodeoxyglucose positron emission tomography and Ga-67 scintigraphy in evaluation of lymphoma. *Cancer* 2002; 94(4):879–88.
18. Lavely WC, Delbeke D, Greer JP, et al. FDG PET in the follow-up management of patients with newly diagnosed Hodgkin and non-Hodgkin lymphoma after first-line chemotherapy. *Int J Radiat Oncol Biol Phys* 2003; 57(2):307–15.

19. Lister TA, Crowther D, Sutcliffe SB, et al. Report of a committee convened to discuss the evaluation and staging of patients with Hodgkin's disease: Cotswolds meeting. *J Clin Oncol* 1989; 7(11):1630–6.

20. Moog F, Bangerter M, Diederichs CG, et al. Extranodal malignant lymphoma: detection with FDG PET versus CT. *Radiology* 1998; 206(2):475–81.

21. Nakahara T, Fujii H, Ide M, et al. FDG uptake in the morphologically normal thymus: comparison of FDG positron emission tomography and CT. *Br J Radiol* 2001; 74(885):821–4.

22. Naumann R, Beuthien-Baumann B, Reiss A, et al. Substantial impact of FDG PET imaging on the therapy decision in patients with early-stage Hodgkin's lymphoma. *Br J Cancer* 2004; 90(3):620–5.

23. O'Doherty MJ, Macdonald EA, Barrington SF, et al. Positron emission tomography in the management of lymphomas. *Clin Oncol (R Coll Radiol)* 2002; 14(5):415–26.

24. Reddy MP, Graham MM. FDG positron emission tomographic imaging of thoracic Castleman's disease. *Clin Nucl Med* 2003; 28(4):325–6.

25. Reske SN. PET and restaging of malignant lymphoma including residual masses and relapse. *Eur J Nucl Med Mol Imaging* 2003; 30 Suppl 1:S89–96.

26. Rini JN, Leonidas JC, Tomas MB, Palestro CJ. 18F-FDG PET versus CT for evaluating the spleen during initial staging of lymphoma. *J Nucl Med* 2003; 44(7):1072–4.

27. Schiepers C, Filmont JE, Czernin J. PET for staging of Hodgkin's disease and non-Hodgkin's lymphoma. *Eur J Nucl Med Mol Imaging* 2003; 30 Suppl 1:S82–8.

28. Schoder H, Larson SM, Yeung HW. PET/CT in oncology: integration into clinical management of lymphoma, melanoma, and gastrointestinal malignancies. *J Nucl Med* 2004; 45 Suppl 1:72S–81S.

29. Schoder H, Meta J, Yap C, et al. Effect of whole-body (18)F-FDG PET imaging on clinical staging and management of patients with malignant lymphoma. *J Nucl Med* 2001; 42(8):1139–43.

30. Schot B, van Imhoff G, Pruim J, et al. Predictive value of early 18F-fluoro-deoxyglucose positron emission tomography in chemosensitive relapsed lymphoma. *Br J Haematol* 2003; 123(2):282–7.

31. Spaepen K, Stroobants S, Dupont P, et al. Prognostic value of pretransplantation positron emission tomography using fluorine 18-fluorodeoxyglucose in patients with aggressive lymphoma treated with high-dose chemotherapy and stem cell transplantation. *Blood* 2003; 102(1):53–9.

32. Spaepen K, Stroobants S, Dupont P, et al. Early restaging positron emission tomography with (18)F-fluorodeoxyglucose predicts outcome in patients with aggressive non-Hodgkin's lymphoma. *Ann Oncol* 2002; 13(9):1356–63.

33. Sutinen E, Jyrkkio S, Varpula M, et al. Nodal staging of lymphoma with whole-body PET: comparison of. *J Nucl Med* 2000; 41(12):1980–8.

34. Tatsumi M, Kitayama H, Sugahara H, et al. Whole-body hybrid PET with 18F-FDG in the staging of non-Hodgkin's lymphoma. *J Nucl Med* 2001; 42(4):601–8.

35. Torizuka T, Nakamura F, Kanno T, et al. Early therapy monitoring with FDG-PET in aggressive non-Hodgkin's lymphoma and Hodgkin's lymphoma. *Eur J Nucl Med Mol Imaging* 2004; 31(1):22–8.

36. Wirth A, Seymour JF, Hicks RJ, et al. Fluorine-18 fluorodeoxyglucose positron emission tomography, gallium-67 scintigraphy, and conventional staging for Hodgkin's disease and non-Hodgkin's lymphoma. *Am J Med* 2002; 112(4):262–8.

37. Wittram C, Fischman AJ, Mark E, et al. Thymic enlargement and FDG uptake in three patients: CT and FDG positron emission tomography correlated with pathology. *AJR Am J Roentgenol* 2003; 180(2):519–22.

38. Zijlstra JM, Hoekstra OS, Raijmakers PG, et al. 18FDG positron emission tomography versus 67Ga scintigraphy as prognostic test during chemotherapy for non-Hodgkin's lymphoma. *Br J Haematol* 2003; 123(3):454–62.

14

Oncology—Melanoma

Melanoma develops from the malignant transformation of the melanocyte, which is a cell of neural crest origin and produces the pigment melanin. Melanoma is a potentially curable disease if discovered at an early stage. The disease is more frequent among whites that nonwhites and the incidence rises with increasing age. Diagnosis is established by biopsy, either excisional or by a core-punch technique. Important histopathologic factors include the lesion thickness (Breslow's microstaging) and level of invasion (Clark's microstaging). Staging is according to the tumor microstaging as adopted by the American Joint Committee on Cancer (AJCC). Melanoma can metastasize to almost any organ site. However, metastatic spread to the regional lymph nodes, lung, liver, bone, and brain is more common. Wide surgical excision is standard treatment for early-stage disease. Surgical excision of the regional nodes, as directed by mapping the sentinel lymph node, and accessible isolated distant metastases are also indicated in selected patients. Radiation therapy is considered for bone, brain, skin, and soft tissue metastases. There is a lack of effective chemotherapy, but immunotherapy with a variety of immunological and biological agents has been promising for metastatic disease. The five-year survival rates are 92.5%, 49%, and 17.9% for early disease (stages I and II), stage III, and stage IV disease, respectively.

The optimal management of melanoma depends on the accurate determination of the extent of disease. Whole-body FDG PET is cost-effective in the imaging evaluation of patients at high risk for metastatic disease (Breslow thickness greater than 1.5 cm). FDG PET impacts the clinical management of patients with melanoma by detecting unknown metastases prior to planned surgical intervention. PET can also be useful in evaluating treatment response. In fact, FDG PET is evolving as a standard diagnostic imaging tool in patients with melanoma and is an approved indication by the Centers for Medicare and Medicaid Services.

FDG PET provides more accurate assessment of the extent of disease in comparison to conventional imaging techniques, leading to significant alterations in treatment planning (Fig. 1). From the referring physician's perspective, FDG PET has a major impact on the management of patients with melanoma by either down-staging or up-staging the disease leading to changes in treatment strategy in up to 53% of patients. However, false-positive results may occur with unrelated benign and malignant lesions, infection, and inflammation. PET may also miss small-volume disease in the lungs and the brain due to spatial resolution limitations. PET may be falsely negative in detecting micrometastatic lymph nodal disease. Sensitivities of 22% and 100% have been reported for PET and sentinel node biopsy, respectively, for detecting lymph node metastatic involvement in ≥1-mm Breslow thickness melanoma. One study determined the tumor volume threshold for successful PET imaging of melanoma nodal metastases. The observed 90% sensitivity threshold for detection of nodal metastases was ≥78 mm^3. The sensitivity of PET was only 14% for detection of tumor volumes <78 mm^3. In another study, PET detected 100% of metastases ≥10 mm, 83% of metastases 6–10 mm, and only 23% of

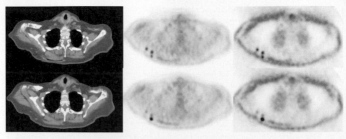

Figure 1: Melanoma Satellite Lesions. Sequential CT/FDG-PET slices in a 58-year-old woman with a 16-mm ulcerated melanoma with microsatellite lesions on pathology. Adjacent to the sit e of wide surgical excision, three FDG-avid subcutaneous nodules are identified. On the left are the CT slices; in the center are the corresponding attenuation-corrected FDG-PET slices; on the right are the corresponding uncorrected FDG-PET slices.

metastases ≥5 mm. Therefore, FDG PET can reliably detect lymph node tumor deposits greater than approximately 80 mm^3 in volume, which is most likely to occur in patients with AJCC stage III and IV disease, and cannot substitute for sentinel lymph node mapping and tissue sampling.

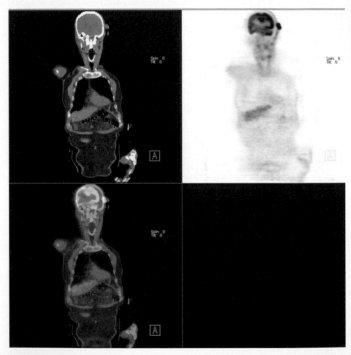

Figure 2: A 77-year-old man with a history of resection of left scalp melanoma who now presents with exophytic local recurrence and metastatic left cervical lymph nodes. There is some misregitration of the brain activity in the fused PET-CT image.

FDG PET offers a diagnostic advantage over CT for the detection of metastatic disease (Figs. 2–7). PET is particularly more sensitive than CT in detecting metastatic deposits in the soft tissues and the small bowel. In a retrospective study of 104 patients with primary or recurrent melanoma who had a median follow-up of 24 months, the sensitivity and specificity were 84% (95% CI: 78–89%) and 97% (95% CI: 95–99%), respectively, for PET, and 58% (95% CI: 49–66%) and 70% (95% CI: 51–84%), respectively, for CT. The sensitivity of CT increased to 69% (95% CI: 59–77%), still inferior to PET, when sites not routinely evaluated by CT were excluded from comparative analysis.

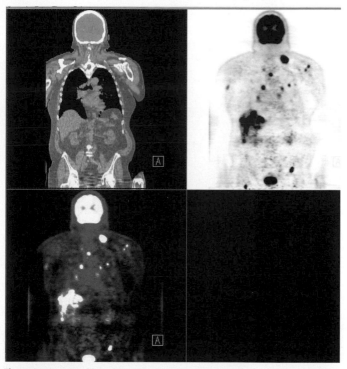

Figure 3: A 74-year-old man with a history of an excised melanoma of the upper back. He now presents with advanced metastatic disease involving the left supraclavicular nodes, both hila, lungs, numerous bones, and subtotal replacement of the liver.

15

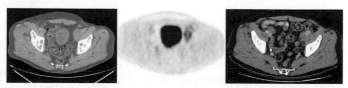

Figure 4: Necrotic Lymph Node Metastasis. On the left is a non-contrast CT and in the center is an FDG-PET from a PET/CT scan. On the right is a contrast CT from six weeks earlier. The necrotic left inguinal lymph node shows peripheral FDG uptake.

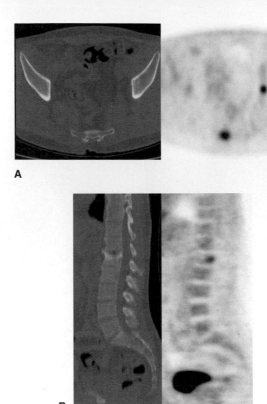

Figure 5: Melanoma Bone Metastases. **A.** focal FDG uptake is seen in the sacrum corresponding to a lytic lesion on CT. (Intense activity is also seen in a normal left ureter.) **B.** Focal FDG uptake is seen in the L1 vertebral body in association with a sclerotic lesion on CT.

In a study that reviewed the published literature between 1980 and 2000, an overall sensitivity of 74–100% and specificity of 67–100% were reported. PET was considered particularly valuable when surgical intervention was being considered and for clarification of the abnormal radiological findings at follow-up. In another, more rigorous systematic review and meta-analysis of the diagnostic accuracy of FDG PET in cutaneous melanoma that included 11 studies, the pooled sensitivity and specificity of PET were reported to be 79% (95% CI: 66–99%) and 86% (95% CI: 78–95%). Subgroup analysis revealed that PET was more accurate for systemic staging than for regional staging.

In summary, FDG PET provides a single imaging tool for surveying the whole body in patients with melanoma and is superior to CT for the detection of metastatic disease. Although PET cannot detect micrometastases, this is a common limitation with any imaging modality. In patients at high risk for metastases (Breslow thickness more than 1.5 mm), PET may be performed first

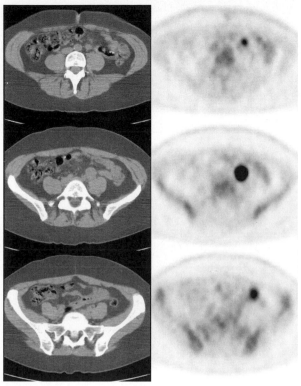

Figure 6: Mesenteric Melanoma Metastases. FDG-PET/CT abdominal slices showing three mesenteric melanoma metastases.

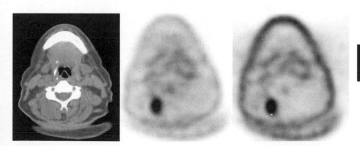

15

Figure 7: Melanoma Metastasis in Muscle. FDG-PET/CT in a patient with a prior history of recurrent melanoma shows intense focal uptake in the posterior neck corresponding to an asymmetric muscle mass. On the left is the CT; in the center is the attenuation-corrected PET; on the right is the non-attenuation-corrected PET.

to evaluate for distant metastatic disease. In patients with negative PET studies, sentinel lymph node mapping and tissue sampling may be performed to assess for micrometastatic nodal disease. In patients with PET demonstration of extensive disease, therapeutic decisions may be made in a cost-effective manner without additional diagnostic work-up.

BIBLIOGRAPHY

1. Acland KM, Healy C, Calonje E, et al. Comparison of positron emission tomography scanning and sentinel lymph node biopsy in the detection of micrometastases of primary cutaneous malignant melanoma. J Clin Oncol 2001; 19:2674–78.
2. Acland KM, O'Doherty MJ, Russell-Jones R. The value of positron emission tomography scanning in the detection of subclinical metastatic melanoma. J Am Acad Dermatol 2000; 42:606–11.
3. Argenyi EE, Dogan AS, Urdaneta LF, et al. Detection of unsuspected metastases in a melanoma patient with positron emission tomography. Clin Nucl Med 1995; 20:744.
4. Baum RP, Rinne D, Zollner TM, et al. F-18 FDG PET for staging of high risk melanoma and restaging of recurrences: results of a prospective study and influence on therapeutic management. J Nucl Med 1996; 37(5):137P.
5. Belhocine T, Pierard G, De Labrassinne M, et al. Staging of regional nodes in AJCC stage I and II melanoma: 18FDG PET imaging versus sentinel node detection. Oncologist 2002; 7:271–8.
6. Blessing C, Feine U, Geiger L, et al. Positron emission tomography and ultrasonography. A comparative retrospective study assessing the diagnostic validity in lymph node metastases of malignant melanoma. Arch Derm 1995; 131(12):1394–8.
7. Boni R, Boni RA, Steinert H, et al. Staging of metastatic melanoma by whole-body positron emission tomography using 2-fluorine-18-fluoro-2-deoxy-D-glucose. Br J Derm 1995; 132:556-62.
8. Boni R, Huch-Boni RA, Steinert H, et al. Early detection of melanoma metastasis using fluorodeoxyglucose F 18 positron emission tomography. Arch Dermatol 1996; 132:875–6.
9. Carlini M, Lonardo MT, Boschetto A, et al. Adrenal glands metastases from malignant melanoma. Laparoscopic bilateral adrenalectomy. J Exp Clin Cancer Res 2003; 22:141–5.
10. Chang AE, Karnell LH, Menck HR. The National Cancer Data Base report on cutaneous and noncutaneous melanoma. A summary of 84,836 cases from the past decade. Cancer 1998; 83:1664–78.
11. Cobben DC, Jager PL, Elsinga PH, et al. 3'-18F-fluoro-3'-deoxy-L-thymidine: a new tracer for staging metastatic melanoma? J Nucl Med 2003; 44:1927–32.
12. Crippa F, Leutner M, Belli F, et al. Which kinds of lymph node metastases can FDG PET detect? A clinical study in melanoma. J Nucl Med 2000; 41:1491–4.
13. Daiman DL, Fulham MJ, Thompson E, Thompson JF. Positron emission tomography in the detection and management of metastatic melanoma. Melanoma Research 1996; 6:325–329.
14. Dalrymple-Hay MJ, Rome PD, Kennedy C, et al. Pulmonary metastatic melanoma—the survival benefit associated with positron emission tomography scanning. Eur J Cardiothorac Surg 2002; 21:611–4.
15. Dietlein M, Krug B, Groth W, et al. Positron emission tomography using 18F-fluorodeoxyglucose in advanced stages of malignant melanoma: a comparison of ultrasonographic and radiological methods of diagnosis. Nucl Med Commun 1999; 20:255–61.
16. Eigtved A, Andersson AP, Dahlstrom K, et al. Use of fluorine-18 fluorodeoxyglucose positron emission tomography in the detection of silent metastases from malignant melanoma. Eur J Nucl Med 2000; 27:70–5.

17. Gritters LS, Francis IR, Zasadny KR, Wahl RL. Initial assessment of positron emission tomography using 2-fluorine-18-fluoro-2-deoxy-D-glucose in the imaging of malignant melanoma. J Nucl Med 1993; 34:1420–7.

18. Gulec SA, Faries MB, Lee CC, et al. The role of fluorine-18 deoxyglucose positron emission tomography in the management of patients with metastatic melanoma: impact on surgical decision making. Clin Nucl Med 2003; 28:961–5.

19. Havenga K, Cobben DC, Oyen WJ, et al. Fluorodeoxyglucose-positron emission tomography and sentinel lymph node biopsy in staging primary cutaneous melanoma. Eur J Surg Oncol 2003; 29:662-4.

20. Holder WD Jr, White RL Jr, Zuger JH, et al. Effectiveness of positron emission tomography for the detection of melanoma metastases. Ann Surg 1998; 227:764–9.

21. Hustinx R, Benard F, Alavi A. Whole-body FDG-PET imaging in the management of patients with cancer. Semin Nucl Med 2002; 32:35–46.

22. Jadvar H, Johnson DL, Segall GM. The effect of fluorine-18 fluorodeoxyglucose positron emission tomography on the management of cutaneous malignant melanoma. Clin Nucl Med 2000; 25:48–51.

23. Kabalka GW, Nichols TL, Smith GT, et al. The use of positron emission tomography to develop boron neutron capture therapy treatment plans for metastatic malignant melanoma. J Neurooncol 2003; 62:187–95.

24. Klein M, Freedman N, Lotem M, et al. Contribution of whole body F-18-FDG-PET and lymphoscintigraphy to the assessment of regional and distant metastases in cutaneous malignant melanoma. A pilot study. Nuklearmedizin 2000; 39:56–61.

25. Krug B, Dietlein M, Groth W, et al. Fluor-18-fluorodeoxyglucose positron emission tomography (FDG-PET) in malignant melanoma. Diagnostic comparison with conventional imaging methods. Acta Radiol 2000; 41:446–52.

26. Lindholm P, Leskinen S, Nagren K, et al. Carbon-11-methionine PET imaging of malignant melanoma. J Nucl Med 1995; 36:1806–10.

27. Longo MI, Lazaro P, Bueno C, et al. Fluorodeoxyglucose-positron emission tomography imaging versus sentinel node biopsy in the primary staging of melanoma patients. Dermatol Surg 2003; 29:245–8.

28. Lucignani G, Paganelli G, Modorati G, et al. MRI, antibody-guided scintigraphy, and glucose metabolism in uveal melanoma. J Comput Assist Tomogr 1992; 16:77–83.

29. Macfarlane DJ, Sondak V, Johnson T, Wahl RL. Prospective evaluation of 2-[18F]-2-deoxy-D-glucose positron emission tomography in staging of regional lymph nodes in patients with cutaneous malignant melanoma. J Clin Oncol 1998; 16:1770–6.

30. Mijnhout GS, Comans EF, Raijmakers P, et al. Reproducibility and clinical value of 18F-fluorodeoxyglucose positron emission tomography in recurrent melanoma. Nucl Med Commun 2002; 23:475–81.

31. Mijnhout GS, Hoekstra OS, van Tulder MW, et al. Systematic review of the diagnostic accuracy of (18)F-fluorodeoxyglucose positron emission tomography in melanoma patients. Cancer 2001; 91:1530–42.

32. Mishima Y, Imahori Y, Honda C, et al. In vivo diagnosis of human malignant melanoma with positron emission tomography using specific melanoma-seeking 18F-DOPA analogue. J Neurooncol 1997; 33:163–9.

33. Nguyen AT, Akhurst T, Larson SM, et al. PET scanning with (18)F 2-Fluoro-2-Deoxy-D-Glucose (FDG) in patients with melanoma. Benefits and limitations. Clin Positron Imaging 1999; 2:93–98.

34. Paquet P, Henry F, Belhocine T, et al. An appraisal of 18-fluorodeoxyglucose positron emission tomography for melanoma staging. Dermatology 2000; 200:167 9.

35. Paquet P, Hustinx R, Rigo P, Pierard GE. Malignant melanoma staging using whole-body positron emission tomography. Melanoma Res 1998; 8:59–62.

36. Prichard RS, Hill AD, Skehan SJ, O'Higgins NJ. Positron emission tomography for staging and management of malignant melanoma. Br J Surg 2002; 89:389–96.

15

37. Rinne D, Baum RP, Hor G, Kaufmann R. Primary staging and follow-up of high risk melanoma patients with whole-body 18F-fluorodeoxyglucose positron emission tomography: results of a prospective study of 100 patients. Cancer 1998; 82:1664–71.
38. Schoder H, Larson SM, Yeung HW. PET/CT in oncology: integration into clinical management of lymphoma, melanoma, and gastrointestinal malignancies. J Nucl Med 2004; 45 Suppl 1:72S–81S.
39. Schwimmer J, Essner R, Patel A, et al. A review of the literature for whole-body FDG PET in the management of patients with melanoma. Q J Nucl Med 2000; 44:153–67.
40. Singletary SE, Balch CM. Malignant Melanoma. In: Holleb AI, Fink DJ, Murphy GP (eds): Clinical Oncology. Atlanta, American Cancer Society, 1991.
41. Stas M, Stroobants S, Dupont P, et al. 18-FDG PET scan in the staging of recurrent melanoma: additional value and therapeutic impact. Melanoma Res 2002; 12:479–90.
42. Steinert HC, Huch Boni RA, Buck A, Boni R, et al. Malignant melanoma: staging with whole-body positron emission tomography and 2-[F-18]-fluoro-2-deoxy-D-glucose. Radiology 1995; 195:705–9.
43. Swetter SM, Carroll LA, Johnson DL, Segall GM. Positron emission tomography is superior to computed tomography for metastatic detection in melanoma patients. Ann Surg Oncol 2002; 9:646–53.
44. Tatlidil R, Mandelkern M. FDG-PET in the detection of gastrointestinal metastases in melanoma. Melanoma Res 2001; 11:297–301.
45. Tyler DS, Onaitis M, Kherani A, et al. Positron emission tomography scanning in malignant melanoma. Cancer 2000; 89:1019–25.
46. Valk PE, Pounds TR, Tesar RD, et al. Cost-effectiveness of PET imaging in clinical oncology. Nucl Med Biol 1996; 23:737–743.
47. Wagner JD, Schauwecker D, Davidson D, et al. Prospective study of fluorodeoxyglu-cose-positron emission tomography imaging of lymph node basins in melanoma patients undergoing sentinel node biopsy. J Clin Oncol 1999; 17:1508–15.
48. Wagner JD, Schauwecker D, Hutchins G, Coleman III JJ. Initial assessment of positron emission tomography for detection of nonpalpable regional lymphatic metastases in melanoma. J Surg Oncol 1997; 64: 181–189.
49. Wagner JD, Schauwecker DS, Davidson D, et al. FDG-PET sensitivity for melanoma lymph node metastases is dependent on tumor volume. J Surg Oncol 2001; 77:237–42.
50. Wong C, Silverman DH, Seltzer M, et al. The impact of 2-deoxy-2[18F] fluoro-D-glu-cose whole body positron emission tomography for managing patients with melanoma: the referring physician's perspective. Mol Imaging Biol 2002; 4:185–90.

Infection and Inflammation

Infectious and non-infectious inflammatory conditions may demonstrate high FDG uptake. Elevated FDG accumulation in inflammatory tissues is related to increased glucose metabolism by the stimulated inflammatory cells, macrophage proliferation, and healing.

Although FDG accumulation in inflammatory or infectious tissue may reduce specificity in patients with cancer, in the group of patients with suspected infection and no known history of cancer, FDG PET may be quite useful for imaging localization of infectious disease. In difficult clinical cases (e.g., a postoperative patient after resection of a tumor), the differentiation of FDG uptake in cancer versus an infectious or inflammatory lesion may become possible using various more sophisticated methods such as kinetic analysis and dual or more time-point PET scans. FDG PET avoids many of the disadvantages associated with radiolabeled leukocyte scans, including complexities of the cell-labeling procedure, handling and cross-contamination of blood samples, high radiation dose, low counts, and time to imaging diagnosis.

BASIC SCIENCE STUDIES

Several studies have investigated the uptake, distribution, and cellular localization of FDG in infection and inflammation. One study performed animal model studies of soft tissue abscesses after intramuscular inoculation of *Staphylococcus aureus* suspension into the calves of rats. Autoradiography was performed on days 2, 5, and 9 after intraperitoneal administration of FDG. Detailed histopathologic and autoradiographic images showed that the highest FDG uptake is within the areas of inflammatory cell infiltrate, which were largely neutrophils in the acute phase and in macrophages in the chronic phase soft tissue infection. Another study reported similar results in an animal *E. coli* infection and turpentine-induced inflammation model. These investigators also showed in other studies that intra-tumoral macrophages (which may increase after anti-neoplastic treatment because of tumor cell destruction) could also result in high FDG uptake. A recent study, reported FDG specifically accumulated in concanavalin A-lymphocyte activation and the resultant acute inflammation. FDG localization in inflammatory and infectious lesions appears to be due to increased expression of the glucose transporters (mainly GLUT-1 and Glut-3). The expression of these transports also decreases by about 70% with glucose loading. Radiolabeling of human leukocytes with FDG has also been explored to increase the specificity of FDG PET for imaging of infection.

CLINICAL STUDIES

Many investigators have reported the utility of FDG PET in the imaging evaluation of patients with infectious and inflammatory diseases. Zhuang and Alavi present an excellent review of the literature on this topic in addition to their clinical experience at the University of Pennsylvania.

Clinical case examples have been reported for many infectious and inflammatory conditions, including but not limited to pneumonia; pulmonary cryptococcoma, tuberculoma, and clostridium perfringens and pseudomonas infections; aortitis; infected vascular graft; allergen-invoked airway inflammation in atopic asthma; detection of disseminated mycobacterium avium complex (DMAC) and active lymphoid tissues as well as differentiation of central nervous system lymphoma from toxoplasmosis infection in patients with acquired immunodeficiency syndrome (AIDS); assessment of viability of echinococcus multilocularis (Buck 2002), detection of abdominal abscess; infectious mononucleosis; infected hepatic and renal cysts in autosomal dominant polycystic kidney disease; differentiation of degenerative and infectious endplate disease in lumbar spine; Crohn's disease activity; breast infection and inflammation; pancreatitis; enterocolitis; arthritis; osteomyelitis; chronic tonsillitis; and sarcoidosis (Figs. 1–4).

FDG PET has also been used in the imaging evaluation of patients with fever of unknown origin (FUO). A recent study reported a positive predictive value of 87% and a negative predictive value of 95% in detecting sites of infection or inflammation. PET offers many advantages over gallium scintigraphy in this clinical setting, which include better image spatial resolution and hence quality as well as decreased time-to-imaging results.

One major area of recent interest has been in the evaluation of patients with suspected osteomyelitis and infected limb prosthesis implants. One report studied 39 patients with suspected soft tissue and bone infections. Pooled sensitivity and specificities of 98% and 75% were found, respectively, for FDG PET in the imaging evaluation of these conditions. FDG PET has high negative predictive value in osteomyelitis, such that a negative scan effectively excludes osteomyelitis. High sensitivity (100%) and specificity (88%) have also been reported for the diagnosis of chronic musculoskeletal infections in both the axial and appendicular skeleton.

In another report, PET was highly sensitive but not specific for detection of suspected infection in 31 joint replacements (12 hips, 19 knees). The positive predictive value and negative predictive values were 55% and 100%, respective-

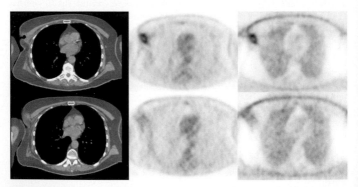

Figure 1: Surgical Healing. The CT/PET-FDG on top line shows a surgical bed with an open wound cavity after surgical remove of right axillary nodes. There is intense FDG uptake. The CT/PET-FDG on the bottom line shows the same region two months later after considerable healing has taken place.

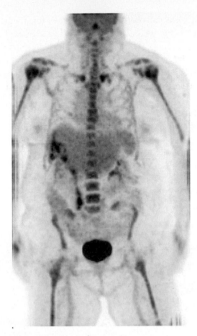

A

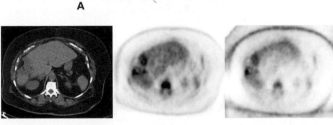

B

Figure 2: Post-Operative Abscess. **A.** An anterior reprojection of an FDG scan shows marked bone marrow uptake and focal uptake in the right upper quadrant with a linear region of uptake extending down and medially. **B.** Axial CT and PET slices show that the right upper quadrant uptake was associated with a defect post-hepatic resection with surrounding low density in the liver. The linear region of FDG uptake corresponded to the tract of a previous drainage catheter, which had recently begun to drain purulent material spontaneously. The bone marrow uptake is due to stimulation from the abscess. The absence of central pelvic bone marrow is due to prior radiation therapy for rectal carcinoma.

16

ly. In another study, PET was compared to the combined WBC/BM imaging method. Although PET was 100% sensitive (94% for WBC/BM), the specificity was low at only 11% (100% for WBC/BM). The specificity of PET could be improved with different interpretation criteria for infection, but the improvement in specificity was at the expense of some loss in sensitivity.

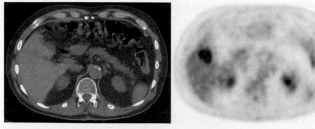

Figure 3: Cholecystitis. FDG-PET/CT in a patient with lung cancer shows intense uptake in the region of the gall bladder fossa. Gall bladder pathology showed acute and chronic cholecystitis with severe fibrosis.

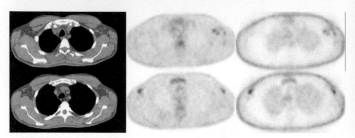

Figure 4: Lymph Nodes in HIV. FDG-PET/CT in a patient with lung cancer shows mild increased uptake in axillary nodes bilaterally with a maximum SUV of 3.0. The patient was HIV positive with a CD4 count of 680. Mild increased FDG uptake can be seen in patients with benign HIV lymphadenopathy.

In contrast to these reports, the Penn group compared FDG PET to the standard combined radiolabeled WBC, bone marrow scintigraphy, and bone scan (WBC/BM/BS) for detection of orthopedic infections in 25 patients. Diagnostic validation was by surgical findings, culture, and clinical follow-up. The negative predictive value was 93% for PET and 87% for the standard method. The positive predictive value was 100% for PET and 90% for the combined standard method. Therefore, PET was shown to be an effective and simple alternative to the cumbersome combined WBC/BM/BS imaging for the evaluation of suspected osteomyelitis. Another comparative study of BS, Tc-99m HMPAO leukocyte scintigraphy, and FDG PET for the detection of infected hip prosthesis demonstrated that PET has same sensitivity (88%) as the combined BS and leukocyte scintigraphy, although the specificity was slightly lower (78% for combined studies vs. 67% for PET alone). In another study in patients suspected of having metallic implant-associated infections with the microbiologic evaluation of the surgical specimens as the standard of reference, FDG PET demonstrated a sensitivity of 100%, and a specificity of 93%.

The seemingly different accuracy of PET in this clinical setting may stem from the differences in patient selection and in image interpretation criteria for the presence or absence of infection. The location of the prosthesis may also be a factor, since higher sensitivity and specificity have been reported for infected hip replacement (90% and 90%) in comparison to infected knee replacement (90% and 72%). Additionally, since FDG may accumulate around the arthroplasty in response to non-infectious inflammatory reactions, discrimination from infection may be challenging. Therefore, in order to minimize the false-positive results for infection with PET in the evaluation of painful hip prosthesis, the FDG uptake around the head and neck portion of the prosthesis, which may last for many years after arthroplasty, should be interpreted with caution. In fact, the location of the increased FDG uptake is more important than the intensity of the uptake in differential diagnosis with hypermetabolism around the head (acetabulum) or neck of the prosthesis associated with loosening and tracer localization around the shaft at the interface between bone and prosthesis likely to represent infection.

In summary, FDG PET avoids many of the disadvantages of current techniques used in the imaging evaluation of patients with infectious and inflammatory diseases and provides a high degree of diagnostic accuracy in these clinical settings. Future investigations will define the exact role of FDG PET in the imaging evaluation of infection and inflammation.

BIBLIOGRAPHY

1. Alavi A, Zhuang H. Finding infection—help from PET. Lancet 2001; 358:1386.
2. Bakheet SM, Powe J, Kandil A, et al. F-18 FDG uptake in breast infection and inflammation. Clin Nucl Med 2000; 25(2):100–3.
3. Bakheet SM, Saleem M, Powe J, et al. F-18 fluorodeoxyglucose chest uptake in lung inflammation and infection. Clin Nucl Med 2000; 25(4):273–8.
4. Bandoh S, Fujita J, Ueda Y, et al. Uptake of fluorine-18-fluorodeoxyglucose in pulmonary Mycobacterium avium complex infection. Intern Med 2003; 42:726–9.
5. Bleeker-Rovers CP, Sevaux RG, Van Hamersvelt HW, et al. Diagnosis of renal and hepatic cyst infections by 18-F-fluorodeoxyglucose positron emission tomography in autosomal dominant polycystic kidney disease. Am J Kidney Dis 2003; 41:E18–21.
6. Bleeker-Rovers CP, De Kleijn EM, Corstens FH, et al. Clinical value of FDG PET in patients with fever of unknown origin and patients suspected of focal infection or inflammation. Eur J Nucl Med Mol Imaging 2003. [electronic publication ahead of print]
7. Brudin LH, Valind S-O, Phodes CG, et al. Fluorine-18 deoxyglucose uptake in sarcoidosis measured with positron emission tomography. Eur J Nucl Med 1994; 21(4): 297–305.
8. Buck AK, Reuter S, Schirrmeister H, et al. FDG-PET for assessment of viability of echinococcus multilocularis. J Nucl Med 2002; 43(5 Suppl):128P.
9. Chacko TK, Moussavian B, Zhuang HM, et al. Critical role of FDG-PET imaging in the management of patients with suspected infection in diverse settings. J Nucl Med 2002; 43(5 Suppl):126P.
10. Chacko TK, Zhuang H, Nakhoda KZ, et al. Applications of fluorodeoxyglucose positron emission tomography in the diagnosis of infection. Nucl Med Commun 2003; 24:615–24.
11. Chacko TK, Zhuang H, Stevenson K, et al. The importance of the location fluorodeoxyglucose uptake in periprosthetic infection in painful hip prostheses. Nucl Med Commun 2002; 23:851–5.
12. Chacko TK, Zhuang HM, Alavi A. FDG-PET is an effective alternative to WBC imaging in diagnosing and excluding orthopedic infections. J Nucl Med 2002; 43(5 Suppl): 126P.
13. De Winter F, van de Wiele C, Vogelaers D, et al. Fluorine-18 fluorodeoxyglucose positron emission tomography: a highly accurate imaging modality for the diagnosis of chronic musculoskeletal infections. J Bone Joint Surg Am 2001; 83-A(5):651–60.

16

14. De Winter F, Vogelaers D, Gemmel F, et al. Promising role of 18-F-fluoro-D-deoxyglucose positron emission tomography in clinical infectious diseases. Eur J Clin Microbiol Infect Dis 2002; 21:247–57.

15. El-Zeftawy H, LaBombardi V, Dakhel M, et al. Evaluation of 18F-FDG PET Imaging in diagnosis of disseminated mycobacterium avium complex (DMAC) in AIDS patients. J Nucl Med 2002; 43(5 Suppl):127P.

16. Forstrom LA, Mullan BP, Hung JC, et al. 18F-FDG labeling of human leukocytes. Nucl Med Commun 2000; 21(7):691–4.

17. Goo JM, Im JG, Do KH, et al. Pulmonary tuberculoma evaluated by means of FDG PET: findings in 10 cases. Radiology 2000; 21(6):117–21.

18. Hsu CH, Lee CM, Wang FC, et al. F-18 fluorodeoxyglucose positron emission tomography in pulmonary cryptococcoma. Clin Nucl Med 2003; 28:791–3.

19. Hustinx R, Smith RJ, Benard F, et al. Dual time point fluorine-18 fluorodeoxyglucose positron emission tomography: a potential method to differentiate malignancy from inflammation and normal tissue in the head and neck. Eur J Nucl Med 1999; 26(10): 1345–1348.

20. Ichiya Y, Kuwabara Y, Sasaki M, et al. FDG-PET in infectious lesions: the detection and assessment of lesion activity. Ann Nucl Med 1996; 10(2):185–91.

21. Ishimori T, Saga T, Mamede M, et al. Increased 18F-FDG uptake in a model of inflammation: Concanavalin A-mediated lymphocyte activation. J Nucl Med 2002; 43(5):658–63.

22. Jadvar H, Bading JR, Yu X, et al. Kinetic analysis of inflammation and cancer with dynamic 18F-FDG PET. J Nucl Med 2002; 43(5 Suppl): 271P.

23. Kaim AH, Weber B, Kurrer MO, et al. Autoradiographic quantification of 18F-FDG uptake in experimental soft-tissue abscesses in rats. Radiology 2002; 223:446–51.

24. Kalicke T, Schmitz A, Risse JH, et al. Fluorine-18 fluorodeoxyglucose PET in infectious bone diseases: results of histologically confirmed cases. Eur J Nucl Med 2000; 27:524–38.

25. Kapucu LO, Meltzer CC, Townsend DW, et al. Fluorine-18-fluorodeoxyglucose uptake in pneumonia. J Nucl Med 1998; 39:1267–69.

26. Kawabe J, Okamura T, Shakudo M, et al. Two cases of chronic tonsillitis studied by FDG-PET. Ann Nucl Med 13(4):277–9.

27. Keidar Z, Engel A, Nitecki S, et al. PET/CT using 2-deoxy-2-[18F]fluoro-D-glucose for the evaluation of suspected infected vascular grafts. Mol Imaging Biol 2003; 5:23–5.

28. Kisielinski K, Cremerius U, Reinartz P, et al. Fluorodeoxyglucose positron emission tomography detection of inflammatory reactions due to polyethylene wear in total hip arthroplasty. J Arthroplasty 2003; 18:528–32.

29. Kresnik E, Gallowitsch HJ, Mikosch P, et al. (18)F-FDG positron emission tomography in the early diagnosis of enterocolitis: preliminary results. Eur J Nucl Med Mol Imaging 2002; 29:1389–92.

30. Krupnick AS, Lombardi V, Engels FH, et al. 18-fluorodeoxyglucose positron emission tomography as a novel imaging tool for the diagnosis of aortoenteric fistula and aortic graft infection—a case report. Vasc Endovascular Surg 2003; 37:363–6.

31. Kubota R, Kubota K, Yamada S, et al. Microautoradiographic study for the differentiation of intratumoral macrophages, granulation tissues and cancer cells by the dynamics of fluorine-18-fluorodeoxyglucose uptake. J Nucl Med 1994; 35:104–112.

32. Kubota R, Yamada S, Kubota K, et al. Intra-tumoral distribution of fluorine-18-fluorodeoxyglucose in vivo: high accumulation in macrophages and granulation tissues studied by microautoradiography. J Nucl Med 1992; 33:1972–80.

33. Larson SM. Cancer or inflammation? A holy grail for nuclear medicine. J Nucl Med 1994; 35(10): 1653–1655.

34. Liu RS, Shei HR, Feng CF, et al. Combined 18F-FDG and 11C-Acetate PET imaging in diagnosis of pulmonary tuberculosis. J Nucl Med 2002; 43(5 Suppl):127P.

35. Lorenzen J, Buchert R, Bohuslavizki KH. Value of FDG PET in patients with fever of unknown origin. Nucl Med Commun 2001; 22:779–83.

36. Love C, Marwin SE, Tomas MB, Palestro CJ. Improving the specificity of 18F-FDG imaging of painful joint prostheses. J Nucl Med 2002; 43(5 Suppl):126P.

37. Love C, Pugliese PV, Afriyie MO, et al. Utility of F-18 FDG imaging for diagnosing the infected joint replacement. Clin Positron Imaging 2000; 3(4):159.

38. Manthey N, Reinhard P, Moog F, et al. The use of [18F]fluorodeoxyglucose positron emission tomography to differentiate between synovitis, loosening and infection of hip and knee prostheses. Nucl Med Commun 2002; 23:645–53.

39. Meller J, Strutz F, Siefker U, et al. early diagnosis and follow-up of aortitis with [(18)F]FDG PET and MRI. Eur J Nucl Med Mol Imaging 2003; 30:730–6.

40. Mochizuki T, Tsukamoto E, Kuge Y, et al. FDG uptake and glucose transporter subtype expression in experimental tumor and inflammation models. J Nucl Med 2001; 42:10551–5.

41. Neurath MF, Vehling D, Schunk K, et al. Noninvasive assessment of Crohn's disease activity: a comparison of 18F-fluorodeoxyglucose positron emission tomography, hydromagnetic resonance imaging, and granulocyte scintigraphy with labeled antibodies. Am J gastroenterol 2002; 97:1978–85.

42. Palmer WE, Rosenthal DI, Schoenberg OI, et al. Quantification of inflammation in the wrist with gadolinium-enhanced MR imaging and PET with 2-[F-18]-fluoro-2-deoxy-D-deoxyglucose. Radiology 1995; 196:647–55.

43. park CH, Lee MH, Oh CG. F-18 FDG positron emission tomographic imaging in bilateral iliopsoas abscesses (Park 2002).

44. Scharko AM, Perlman SB, Pyzalski RW, et al. Whole-body positron emission tomography in patients with HIV-1 infection. Lancet 2003; 362:959–61.

45. Schiesser M, Stumpe KD, Trentz O, et al. Detection of metallic implant-associated infections with FDG PET in patients with trauma: correlation with microbiologic results. Radiology 2003; 226:391–8.

46. Schuster DP, Kozlowski J, Hogue L. Imaging lung inflammation in a murine model of pseudomonas infection: a positron emission tomography study. Exp Lung Res 2003; 29:45–57.

47. Shreve PD. Focal fluorine-18 fluorodeoxyglucose accumulation in inflammatory pancreatic disease. Eur J Nucl Med 1998; 25(3):259–64.

48. Sorbara LR, Maldarelli F, Chamoun G, et al. Human immudeficiency virus type 1 infection of H9 cells induces increased glucose transporter expression. J Virol 1996; 70:7275–9.

49. Stumpe KD, Dazzi H, Schaffner A, von Schulthess GK. Infection imaging using whole-body FDG-PET. Eur J Nucl Med 2000; 27(7):822–32.

50. Stumpe KD, Zanetti M, Weishaupt D, et al. FDG positron emission tomography for differentiation of degenerative and infectious endplate abnormalities in the lumbar spine detected on MR imaging. AJR Am J Roentgenol 2002; 179:1151–7.

51. Sugawara Y, Braun DK, Kison PV, et al. Rapid detection of human infections with fluorine-18 fluorodeoxyglucose and positron emission tomography: preliminary results. Eur J Nucl Med 1998; 25(9):1238–43.

52. Tahara T, Ichiya Y, Kuwabara Y, et al. High [18F]-fluorodeoxyglucose uptake in abdominal abscesses: PET study. J Comput Assist Tomogr 1989; 13(5):829–31.

53. Taylor IK, Hill AA, Hayes M, et al. Imaging allergen-invoked airway inflammation in atopic asthma with [18-F]-fluorodeoxyglucose and positron emission tomography. Lancet 347:937–40.

54. Temmerman OP, Heyligers IC, Hoekstra OS, et al. detection of osteomyelitis using FDG and positron emission tomography. J Arthroplasty 2001; 16(2):243–46.

55. Tomas MB, Tronco GG, Karayalcin G, Palestro CJ. FDG uptake in infectious mononucleosis. Clin Positron Imaging 2000; 3(4):176.

56. Vanquickenborne B, Maes A, Nuyts J, et al. The value of (18)FDG-PET for the detection of infected hip prosthesis. Eur J Nucl Med Mol Imaging 2003; 30:705–15.

57. Yamada S, Kubota K, Ido T, Tamahashi N. High accumulation of fluorine-18-fluorodeoxyglucose in terpentine-induced inflammatory tissue. J Nucl Med 1995; 36:1301–06.

16

58. Yamada S, Kubota K, Kubota R, et al. Accumulation of Fluorine-18 fluorodeoxyglucose in inflammation tissue. J Nucl Med 1993; 34:103P.

59. Yang CM, Hsu CH, Lee CM, et al. Intense uptake of [F-18]-fluoro-2-deoxy-D-glucose in active pulmonary tuberculosis. Ann Nucl Med 2003; 17:407–10.

60. Zhao S, Kuge Y, Tsukamoto E, et al. Fluorodeoxyglucose uptake and glucose transporter expression in experimental inflammatory lesions and malignant tumors: effects of insulin and glucose loading. Nucl Med Commun 2002; 23:545–50.

61. Zhuang H, Alavi A. 18-fluorodeoxyglucose positron emission tomography imaging in the detection and monitoring of infection and inflammation. Semin Nucl Med 2002; 32(1):47–59.

62. Zhuang H, Chacko TK, Hickeson M, et al. Persistent non-specific FDG uptake on PET imaging following hip arthroplasty. Eur J Nucl Med Mol Imaging 2002; 29:1328–33.

63. Zhuang H, Duarte PS, Pourdehand M, et al. Exclusion of chronic osteomyelitis with F-18 fluorodeoxyglucose positron emission tomographic imaging. Clin Nucl Med 2000; 25(4):281–4.

64. Zhuang HM Lee JH, Lambright E, et al. Experimental evidence in support of dual time point FDG-PET imaging for differentiating malignancy from inflammation. J Nucl Med 2000; 41(5 Suppl):114P.

65. Zhunag H, Duarte PS, Pourdehnad M, et al. The promising role of 18F-FDG PET in detecting infected lower limb prosthesis implants. J Nucl Med 2001; 42:44–48.

66. Zhunag H, Duarte PS, Rebenstock A, et al. Pulmonary clostridium perfringens infection detected by FDG positron emission tomography. Clin Nucl Med 2003; 28:517–8.

17

Pediatrics

PET is recognized as a powerful imaging technique for a variety of disease conditions, mainly cancer, in adults. PET is also emerging as an important tool in evaluating children with a number of disease states. This chapter briefly reviews the current status of PET with FDG in pediatric diseases.

Patient Preparation

Patients should fast for at least four hours prior to imaging. The administered FDG dose is 0.144 mCi/kg (minimum 1 mCi, maximum 15 mCi). Imaging is initiated 40–60 min after radiotracer injection. Sheets wrapped around the body, sandbags, and/or special holding devices are often sufficient for immobilization. Sedation is indicated when it is anticipated that the methods described above will prove inadequate. Specific sedation protocols vary from institution to institution.

Radiation Dosimetry.   Radiation dose from intravenous injection of FDG has been studied in adults. One study has investigated the radiation dose to infants from FDG. The bladder wall, which is the target organ, is estimated to receive 1.03 ± 2.10 mGy/MBq (3.81 ± 7.77 rad/mCi). Good hydration and rapid drainage of radioactive urine helps to reduce this absorbed dose, which is higher by a factor of about 4 than the absorbed bladder wall dose per unit of administered activity in adults. In comparison to adults, infants also receive a higher absorbed dose to the brain per unit of administered activity. The estimated absorbed dose per unit of administered activity to the infant brain (0.24 ± 0.05 mGy/MBq or 0.93 rad/mCi ± 0.18 rad/mCi) is higher by a factor of nearly 10 than that estimated to be received by the adult brain. This reflects a slightly higher percent uptake of FDG in the infant brain (8.8%) as compared to the adult brain (6.9%) and a differing distribution of FDG in the infant brain. Due to the low administered doses of FDG in infants, however, an infant's total absorbed radiation dose is lower than or similar to that of an adult undergoing FDG PET and is also lower than or similar to that of children being studied with other widely used radionuclides.

PET in Pediatric Cardiology.   Currently, PET plays a relatively minor role in pediatric cardiology. PET with N-13 ammonia has been employed to measure myocardial perfusion in infants after anatomic repair of congenital heart defects, after Norwood palliation for hypoplastic left heart syndrome, and arterial switch operation. A major application of PET in adult cardiology is the assessment of myocardial viability with FDG as the tracer for glucose metabolism. A recent study evaluated the regional glucose metabolism and contractile function by gated FDG PET in infants and children after arterial switch operation and suspected myocardial infarction. Gated FDG PET was found to contribute pertinent information to guide additional revascularization procedure. In another study in children with Kawasaki disease, PET with N-13 ammonia and FDG showed abnormalities during various stages of the disease and was specifically valuable in assessing immunoglobulin therapy response. PET has also been employed to assess mitochondrial dysfunction in children with hypertrophic and dilated cardiomyopathy which demonstrated diminished oxidative metabolism and enhanced glycolysis.

PET in Pediatric Neurology. An understanding of the normal brain development and evolution of cerebral glucose utilization is important when FDG PET is considered as a diagnostic functional imaging study in pediatrics. Glucose metabolism is initially high in the sensorimotor cortex, thalamus, brainstem, and cerebellar vermis. During the first three months of life, glucose metabolism gradually increases in the basal ganglia and in the parietal, temporal, calcarine, and cerebellar cortices. Maturation of the frontal cortex and the dorsolateral cortex occur during the second six months of life. Cerebral FDG distribution in children after the age of one year resembles that of adults.

Epilepsy is a relatively common neurologic condition during childhood. Accurate preoperative localization of the epileptogenic region is an essential but difficult task. Computed tomography (CT) and magnetic resonance imaging (MRI) are used to detect anatomic lesions that may cause the seizures. However, structural lesions occur in a relatively small percentage of patients with epilepsy and when such lesions are detected, they may not necessarily represent the epileptogenic region. Ictal or interictal single-photon emission tomography (SPECT) evaluation of regional cerebral blood flow (rCBF) with tracers such as Tc-99m hexamethylpropylene (Tc-99m HMPAO) and Tc-99m ethyl cysteinate dimer (Tc-99m ECD) can localize the epileptogenic region regardless of the presence or absence of structural abnormalities. The characteristic appearance of an epileptogenic region is relative zonal hyperperfusion on ictal SPECT and relative zonal hypoperfusion on interictal SPECT. The sensitivity of ictal rCBF tracer SPECT may approach 90%, while that of interictal SPECT is in the range of 50%. The utility of ictal SPECT is somewhat reduced by difficulty in coordinating tracer administration with seizures.

FDG PET has proven useful in preoperative localization of the epileptogenic region. FDG PET is generally performed following an interictal injection. Although metabolic alterations might be localized better ictally than interictally, the relatively short half-life of F-18 limits the window of opportunity during which it can be administered ictally. Even when FDG can be administered at seizure onset, the approximately 30-min brain-uptake time of FDG means that the study may depict periictal as well as ictal FDG distribution. For interictal PET, FDG should be administered in a setting, such as a quiet room and dim lights. During the 30 min following FDG administration, it is best to have the child remain awake with minimal parental interaction during this period. Pharamacologic sedation, if needed for imaging, is best withheld during this 30-min interval to avoid unwanted effects of sedation on cerebral metabolism during the uptake interval. EEG monitoring during the uptake period is essential to detect seizure activity that might affect FDG distribution. The sensitivity of interictal FDG PET approaches that of ictal rCBF SPECT in localizing the epileptogenic region, which is indicated by regional hypometabolism. Importantly, the hypometabolism may predominantly affect cortex bordering the epileptogenic focus. The best results have been obtained in epilepsy of temporal lobe origin, for which metabolic abnormalities may be evident in as many as 90% of surgical candidates. Extratemporal epileptogenic regions are more difficult to identify but some success has been achieved in children with intractable frontal lobe epilepsy. FDG PET has particularly helpful in the evaluation of infantile spasms, which is a subtype of seizure disorder. Incorporation of FDG PET into the evaluation of children with infantile spasms has resulted in identification of a significant number of children who benefit from cortical resection. FDG PET has revealed marked focal cortical glucose hypometabolism associated with malformative or dysplastic lesions that are not evident on anatomic imaging. Patients with bitemporal hypometabolism on FDG PET have poor prognosis and are typically not candidates for resection. It should also be noted that PET tracers, other than FDG, that assess altered abundance or function of receptors, enzymes, and neurotransmitters in epileptogenic regions have also been applied to localizing the epileptogenic region.

PET has also been employed to study the pathophysiology of many other childhood brain disorders such as Rasmussen's syndrome, hypoxic-ischemic encephalopathy, traumatic brain injury, autism, attention deficit hyperactivity disorder, schizophrenia, sickle cell encephalopathy, and anorexia and bulimia nervosa. However, the exact role of PET in these clinical settings remains unclear.

PET in Pediatric Oncology. Although childhood cancer can be considered relatively rare, cancer is second only to trauma as a cause of death in children. There is marked variation in the incidence rates of specific cancers at different ages in children. It is important consider potential causes of misinterpretation of FDG PET that relate to physiologic FDG distribution in children. High FDG uptake is typically seen in thymus and in skeletal growth centers (Figs. 1, 2). Elevated bone marrow FDG uptake has been observed in patients as many as four weeks following completion of treatment with granulocyte colony-stimulating factor (GCSF).

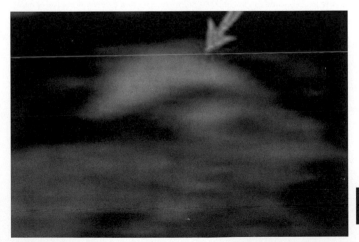

17

Figure 1: Coronal PET shows physiologic hypermetabolism in the normal thymus (arrow) of a child.

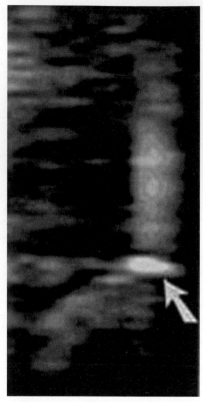

Figure 2: Coronal PET shows physiologic hypermetabolism in the growth plate of distal ulna and radius (arrow) in a child.

Central Nervous System Tumors

FDG PET has been applied to tumor grading and prognostic stratification. Higher-grade aggressive tumors typically have higher FDG uptake than do lower grade tumors. The development of hypermetabolism as evidenced by increased FDG uptake in a low-grade tumor that appeared hypometabolic at diagnosis indicates degeneration to a higher grade. Shorter survival times have been reported for patients whose tumors show the highest degree of FDG uptake. Decreased FDG uptake relative to normal brain is observed in areas of necrosis. Increased FDG uptake indicates residual or recurrent tumor. Combined PET-guided stereotactic brain biopsy may also improve the diagnostic yield of the biopsy while reducing the sampling in high-risk functional brain areas.

Lymphoma.   In numerous studies of patient populations including predominantly adults, FDG has been shown to accumulate in non-Hodgkin's and Hodgkin's lymphomas. FDG uptake is generally higher in high-grade than in

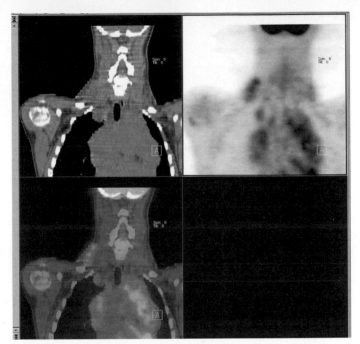

Figure 3: A 14-year-old female with newly diagnosed Hodgkin's lymphoma status post-biopsy of the right cervical lymph node. There is moderate hypermetabolism involving the nodal basins of the right posterior cervical triangle and anterior and superior mediastinum.

low-grade lymphomas. For staging, FDG PET has been shown to be useful in showing sites of nodal and extranodal disease that are not detected by conventional staging methods, including CT and gallium-67 imaging (Fig. 3). Identification of areas of intense FDG uptake within the bone marrow can be particularly useful in directing the site of biopsy or even eliminating the need for biopsy at staging (Fig. 4). Following therapy, FDG PET can be useful for assessing residual soft tissue masses shown by CT. Absence of FDG uptake in a residual mass is predictive of remission. FDG PET is particularly useful in monitoring the rare pediatric patient whose lymphoma does not show avidity for gallium-67. In summary, PET is expected to play an important role in staging, evaluating tumor response, planning radiation treatment fields, restaging, and surveillance monitoring after completion of therapy in pediatric lymphoma.

Neuroblastoma. In one study, neuroblastomas and/or their metastases avidly concentrated FDG prior to chemotherapy or radiation therapy in 16 of 17 patients studied with FDG PET and MIBG imaging. Uptake after therapy was variable but tended to be lower. In most instances, FDG and MIBG results were concordant, but overall, MIBG imaging was considered superior to FDG PET particularly in delineation of residual disease. Initiation of imaging 60 min

17

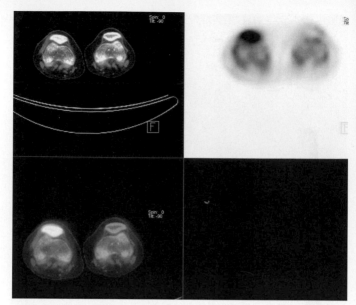

Figure 4: A 14-year-old girl with ALL diagnosed at age four treated with chemotherapy and bone marrow transplantation. She presents with right knee pain. PET-CT shows intense hypermetabolism of the right patella with marrow sclerosis and soft tissue extension along the anterolateral retinaculum to the lateral aspect of the knee. Right patellar biopsy revealed lymphoid leukemia.

after FDG administration was a definite advantage of FDG PET over MIBG imaging, which is performed one or more days following administration. An important consideration regarding the potential application of FDG PET in neuroblastoma is FDG accumulation by normal bone marrow constituents, which limits FDG PET in assessing skeletal disease. The primary role of FDG PET in neuroblastoma is likely to be evaluation of known or suspected neuroblastomas that do not demonstrate MIBG uptake.

Wilms Tumor. Wilms tumor is the most common renal malignancy of childhood. Uptake of FDG by Wilms tumor has been described but a role for FDG PET in Wilms tumor has not been established. Normal excretion of FDG through the kidney is a potential limiting factor. Careful correlation with anatomic cross-sectional imaging should allow distinction of tumor uptake from normal renal excretion in difficult cases.

Bone Tumors. Osteosarcoma and Ewing's sarcoma are the two primary bone malignancies of childhood. The exact role of FDG PET in osteosarcoma and Ewing's sarcoma is not established. It has been suggested, however, that FDG PET will come to play an important role in assessing therapeutic response

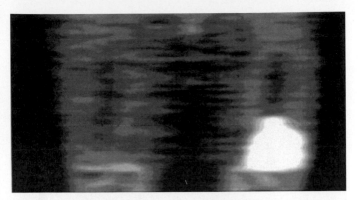

A

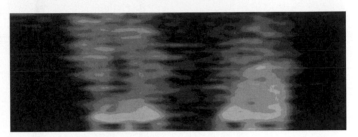

B

Figure 5: Left distal femoral osteosarcoma in a young patient. **A.** Pre-treatment coronal PET shows a large hypermetabolic lesion in the distal left femur. **B.** Coronal PET after radiation treatment shows marked decline in the metabolic activity. Surgical specimen demonstrated 95% tumor necrosis.

prior to surgery. A second potential role is in assessing patients with suspected or known pulmonary metastases (Figs. 5–7).

Soft Tissue Tumors.   Rhabdomyosarcomas show variable degrees of FDG accumulation. Cases showing the clinical utility of FDG PET have been described but a definite role for FDG PET in rhabdomyosarcoma has not been established.

Summary

PET has been shown to be useful in the imaging evaluation of many pediatric diseases. However, the expansion of PET and PET-CT imaging systems to children's hospitals will facilitate the multi-institutional trials that are necessary to define the precise roles of this powerful imaging technology in pediatrics. Also there may be potential challenges in the incorporation of the new PET-CT in imaging children and adolescents which will be another important areas of future investigations.

17

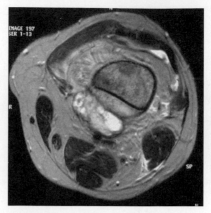

A

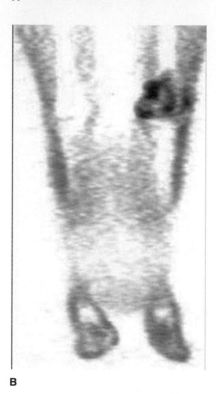

B

Figure 6: A 16-year-old M with left distal femoral osteosarcoma. **A.** Axial T1-weighted MRI of the distal left femur demonstrate large tumor extending out into the posterior soft tissues to the neurovascular bundle. **B.** PET demonstrates heterogeneous hypermetabolic tumor with intensely hypermetabolic posteromedial soft tissue component. There was no evidence for distant metastatic disease.

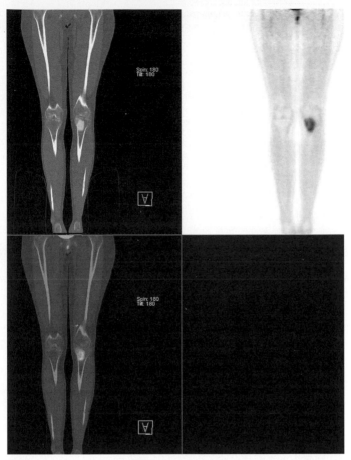

Figure 7: An 18-year-old female with osteogenic sarcoma of the left proximal tibia.

BIBLIOGRAPHY

1. Borgwardt L, Carstensen H, Schmiegelow K, Hojgaard L. Increased FDG uptake in childhood CNS tumors is associated with tumor malignancy. Clin Positron Imaging 2000; 3(4):175.
2. Borgwardt L, Larsen HJ, Pedersen K, Hojgaard L. Practical use and implementation of PET in children in a hospital PET Center. Eur J Nucl Med Mol Imaging 2003; 30(10):1389–97.
3. Chugani HT, Conti JR. Etiologic classification of infantile spasms in 140 cases: role of positron emission tomography. J Child Neurol 1996; 11:44–48.
4. Chugani HT, Phelps ME, Mazziotta JC. Positron emission tomography study of human brain functional development. Ann Neurol 1987; 22:487–497.
5. Chugani HT, Phelps ME. Maturational changes in cerebral function in infants determined by 18FDG positron emission tomography. Science 1986; 231:840–843.

6. Chugani HT, Da Silva E, Chugani DC. Infantile spasms: III. Prognostic implications of bitemporal hypometabolism on positron emission tomography. Ann Neurol 1996; 39:643–649.

7. Chugani HT. Positron emission tomography scanning: applications in newborns. Clin Perinatol 20(2): 395–409; 1993.

8. Cummings TJ, Chugani DC, Chugani HT. Positron emission tomography in pediatric epilepsy. Neurosurg Clin North Am 1995; 6:465–472.

9. da Silva EA, Chugani DC, Muzik O, et al. Identification of frontal lobe epileptic foci in children using positron emission tomography. Epilepsia 1997; 38:1198–1208.

10. Delvenne V, Goldman S, Simon Y, et al. Brain hypometabolism of glucose in bulimia nervosa. Int J Eat Disord 1997; 21(4):313–20.

11. Delvenne V, Lotstra F, Goldman S, et al. Brain hypometabolism of glucose in anorexia nervosa: a PET scan study. Biol Psychiatry 1995; 37(3):161–9.

12. Donnelly JP, Raffel DM, Shulkin BL, et al. Resting coronary flow and coronary flow reserve in human infants after repair or palliation of congenital heart defects as measured by positron emission tomography. J Thorac Cardiovasc Surg 1998; 115(1):103–10.

13. Engel J Jr, Kuhl DE, Phelps ME. Patterns of human local cerebral glucose metabolism during epileptogenic seizures. Science 1982; 218:64–66.

14. Ernst M, Zametkin AJ, Matochik JA, et al. High midbrain [18F]DOPA accumulation in children with attention deficit hyperactivity disorder. Am J Psychiatry 1999; 156(8):1209–15.

15. Franzius C, Schober O. Assessment of therapy response by FDG PET in pediatric patients. Q J Nucl Med 2003; 47(1):41–5.

16. Hawkins DS, Rajendran JG, Conrad EU III, et al. Evaluation of chemotherapy response in pediatric bone sarcomas by [F-18]-fluorodeoxy-D-glucose positron emission tomography. Cancer 2002; 97(12):3277–84.

17. Hudson MM, Krasin MJ, Kaste SC. PET imaging in pediatric Hodgkin's lymphoma. Pediatr Radiol; 2004; 34(3):190–8.

18. Hwang B, Liu RS, Chu LS, et al. Positron emission tomography for the assessment of myocardial viability in Kawasaki disease using different therapies. Nucl Med Commun 2000; 21(7):631–6.

19. Jacobson LK, Hamburger SD, Van Horn JD, et al. Cerebral glucose metabolism in childhood onset schizophrenia. Psychiatry Res 1997; 75(3):131–44.

20. Jadvar H, Connolly LP, Shulkin BL, Treves ST, Fischman AJ. Positron emission tomography in pediatrics. In: Nuclear Medicine Annual. LM Freeman (ed.), Lippincott Williams & Wilkins, Philadelphia, PA, pp. 53–83; 2000. (ISBN 0-7817-2573-9)

21. Jadvar H, Connolly LP, Shulkin BL. Pediatrics. In: Principles and Practice of Positron Emission Tomography. Wahl RL (ed.), Lippincott Williams & Wilkins, Philadelphia, PA, pp. 395–410; 2002. (ISBN 0-7817-2904-1)

22. Jadvar H, Connolly LP, Shulkin BL. PET imaging in pediatric disorders. In: Positron Emission Tomography: Basic Science and Clinical Practice. Valk PE, Bailey DL, Townsend DW, Maisey MN (eds), Springer-Verlag, London, UK, pp. 755–774; 2003. (ISBN 1-85233-485-1)

23. Juhasz C, Chugani DC, Muzik O, et al. Is epileptogenic cortex truly hypometabolic on interictal positron emission tomography? Ann Neurol 2000; 48(1):88–96.

24. Kaste SC. Issues specific to implementing PET-CT for pediatric oncology: what we have learned along the way. Pediatr Radiol; 2004; 34(3):205–13.

25. Krasin MJ, Hudson MM, Kaste SC. Positron emission tomography in pediatric radiation oncology: integration in the treatment-planning process. Pediatr Radiol 2004; 34(3):214–21.

26. Lee JS, Juhasz C, Kaddurah AK, Chugani HT. Patterns of cerebral glucose metabolism in early and late stages of Rasmussen's syndrome. J Child Neurol 2001; 16(11):798–805.

27. Meltzer CC, Adelson PD, Brenner RP, et al. Planned ictal FDG PET imaging for localization of extratemporal epileptic foci. Epilepsia 2000; 41(2):193–200.

28. Mohan KK, Chugani DC, Chugani HT. Positron emission tomography in pediatric neurology. Semin Pediatr Neurol 1999; 6(2):111–9.

29. O'Hara SM, Donnelly LF, Coleman RE. Pediatric body applications of FDG PET. AJR 172: 1019–1024; 1999.

30. Patel PM, Alibazoglu H, Ali A, Fordham E and LaMonica G. Normal thymic uptake of FDG on PET imaging. Clin Nucl Med 1996; 21:772–775.

31. Pirotte B, Goldman S, Salzberg S, et al. Combined positron emission tomography and magnetic resonance imaging for the planning of stereotactic brain biopsies in children: experience in 9 cases. Pediatr Neurosurg 2003; 38(3):146–55.

32. Quinlivan RM, Robinson RO, Maisey MN. Positron emission tomography in pediatric cardiology. Arch Dis Child 1998; 79(6):520–2.

33. Reed W, Jagust W, Al-Mateen M, Vichinsky E. Role of positron emission tomography in determining the extent of CNS ischemia in patients with sickle cell disease. Am J Hematol 1999; 60(4):268–72.

34. Richardson MP, Koepp MJ, Brooks DJ, et al. 11C-flumanezil PET in neocortical epilepsy. Neurology 1998; 51:485–492.

35. Rickers C, Sasse K, Buchert R, et al. Myocardial viability assessed by positron emission tomography in infants and children after the arterial switch operation and suspected infarction. J Am Coll Cardiol 2000; 36(5):1676–83.

36. Roberts EG, Shulkin BL. Technical issues in performing PET studies in pediatric patients. J Nucl Med Technol 2004; 32(1):5–9.

37. Ruotsalainen U, Suhonen-Povli H, Eronen E, et al. Estimated radiation dose to the newborn in FDG-PET studies. J Nucl Med 1996; 37(2):387–93.

38. Schelbert HR, Schawiger M, Phelps ME. Positron emission tomography and its applications in the young. J Am Coll Cardiol 1985; 5(1 Suppl):140S–149S.

39. Shulkin BL, Chang E, Strouse PJ, Bloom DA, Hutchinson RJ. PET FDG studies of Wilms tumors. J Pediatr Hematol Oncol 1997; 19(4):334–8.

40. Shulkin BL, Mitchell DS, Ungar DR, Parkash D, Dole MG, Castle VP, Hernandez RJ, Koeppe RA, Hutchinson RJ. Neoplasms in a pediatric population: 2-[F-18]-fluoro-2-deoxy-D-glucose PET studies. Radiology 1995; 194(2):495–500.

41. Shulkin BL. PET applications in pediatrics. Q J Nucl Med 1997; 41(4):281–91.

42. Shulkin BL. PET imaging in pediatric oncology. Pediatr Radiol 2004; 34(3):199–204.

43. Snead OC III, Chen LS, Mitchell WG, et al. Usefulness of [18F]fluorodeoxyglucose positron emission tomography in pediatric epilepsy surgery. Pediatr Neurol 1996; 14:98–107.

44. Treves ST, Connolly LP. Single photon emission computed tomography in pediatric epilepsy. Neurosurg Clin North Am 1995; 6:473–480.

45. Volpe JJ, Herscovitch P, Perlman JM, et al. Positron emission tomography in the asphyxiated term newborn: parasagittal impairment of cerebral blood flow. Ann Neurol 1985; 17(3):287–96.

46. Weinblatt ME, Zanzi I, Belakhlef A, et al. False-positive FDG-PET imaging of the thymus of a child with Hodgkin's disease. J Nucl Med 1997; 38(6):888–90.

47. Worley G, Hoffman JM, Paine SS, et al. 18-fluorodeoxyglucose positron emission tomography in children and adolescents with traumatic brain injury. Dev Med Child Neurol 1995; 37(3):213–20.

48. Yanai K, Iinuma K, Matsuzawa T, et al. Cerebral glucose utilization in pediatric neurological disorders determined by positron emission tomography. Eur J Nucl Med 1987; 13(6):292–6.

49. Yates RW, Marsden PK, Badawi RD, et al. Evaluation of myocardial perfusion using positron emission tomography in infants following a neonatal arterial switch operation. Pediatr Cardiol 2000; 21(2):111–8.

50. Zilbovicius M, Boddaert N, Belin P, et al. Temporal lobe dysfunction in childhood autism: A PET study. Am J Psychiatry 2000; 157(12):1988–93.

17

Variants and Pitfalls

Several technical and clinical factors may result in false-negative and false-positive findings on FDG PET and PET-CT (Table 1). *False-negative* causes may be related to small lesion size (less than 1 cm), type of neoplasm (e.g., hepatocellular carcinoma, lymphoma of the mucosa-associated lymphoid tissue or MALT, bronchioloalveolar carcinoma, carcinoid and other neuroendocrine tumors), tumor histologic grade (e.g., low-grade gliomas and low-grade lymphomas), and lesion location. *False-positive* examples include high tracer localization in the working muscles and the urinary tract, skin contamination with the tracer or urine, infectious (e.g., abscess, granulomatous disease) and non-infectious inflammatory conditions (e.g., sarcoid), and particular physiologic states (e.g., lactating breast, sweat glands in hyperhidrosis, bone marrow after treatment with hematopoietic factors, thymus and bone growth plates in children). Recognition of these pitfalls is important for the accurate evaluation and interpretation of clinical FDG PET and PET-CT images.

Normal FDG Biodistribution

Brain (gray matter) normally displays high FDG uptake. The heart can have variable uptake, depending on its metabolic state at the time of the study. The urinary system may show high activity due to excretion of FDG in urine. High tracer uptake in the stomach and bowel is seen occasionally. In children, thymus and growth plates display relatively high uptake. The rest of the body normally has low FDG uptake.

Causes of False-Negative Results. Lesion Physical Factors: The in-plane spatial resolution of dedicated PET scanners is 4–6 mm FWHM. Small lesions

Table 1: Summary of Factors that May Result in False-Negative and False-Positive Findings

False-Negative Causes	False-Positive Causes
Small lesion size	Gastrointestinal and urinary activity
Lesion location	Myocardial activity
Tumor type	Breast, thymus, physis activity
Tumor histologic grade	Autoimmune thyroiditis/parathyroid adenoma
Respiratory motion	Inflammation (infectious and non-infectious)
	Trauma, surgery, fracture
	treatment-related marrow hyperplasia
	Skin contamination (urine) or infiltration (lymph nodes)
	Reconstruction artifacts
	Radiodense and metallic materials (PET-CT)
	Respiratory motion
	Skeletal muscle and brown fat

(less than 1 cm) may not be detected due to volume averaging with the adjacent background activity. Even very small lesions, however, may be detected if they are very hypermetabolic with high regional target-to-background ratios (TBR).

Lesion location is also an important factor. If the lesion is located in a region with normally low background activity (e.g., lung), the TBR may be sufficient for a very small lesion to be seen. However, if the lesion is located in regions of adjacent high activity (e.g., renal collecting system, urinary bladder), detection may be problematic due to diminished TBR.

Lesion Histologic Factors: Other important factors in false-negative findings relate to the type and grade of neoplasm. Some tumors may not be hypermetabolic and may be missed on FDG PET imaging. Examples include hepatocellular carcinoma, renal cell carcinoma, bronchioloalveolar carcinoma, carcinoid, and other neuroendocrine tumors. Tumor histologic grade is also an important factor. Low-grade tumors (e.g., gliomas and lymphomas) may have low to moderate FDG uptake in comparison to high-grade histologies, which show high FDG uptake.

Causes of False-Positive Results.   Physiologic Variants: Urine shows normal high activity due to FDG excretion by the kidneys. This activity may be present in the renal collecting systems, which may be asymmetric, and in the ureters, which may be focal, as well as in the urinary bladder. The bladder urine activity may obscure detection of lesions in the adjacent structures such as the rectum. In such cases, a Foley catheter with continuous saline bladder washing may be useful. Lasix has also been employed to drain and decrease the activity

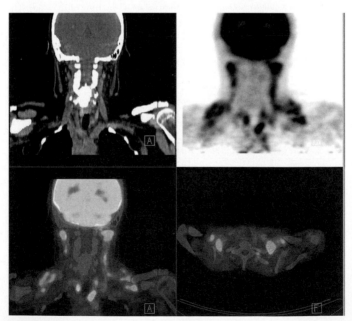

Figure 1: Relatively intense hypermetabolism in bilateral neck and supraclavicular brown fat and muscles.

in the urinary system. In general, the patient should empty his/her bladder before the imaging study.

High activity may also be seen in the working skeletal muscles, which may be asymmetric (Fig. 1). The high uptake is due to the hypermetabolic state of working muscle and may hinder lesion detection (e.g., soft tissue sarcoma, lymphadenopathy, melanoma). In the head and neck, high uptake by the salivary glands, tongue, as well as mastication, pharyngeal, cervical, and shoulder muscles also pose a problem in lesion detection. The patient should be instructed to relax and restrain from physical exercise, talking, swallowing, eating, and chewing after FDG injection for the duration of the imaging study. Some investigators have suggested the use of muscle relaxants (e.g., benzodiazepines) given before FDG administration to limit or eliminate skeletal muscle FDG uptake.

Another problem is the normal FDG uptake by the heart, which can be variable. High cardiac activity may cause problems in evaluating the adjacent mediastinum or the lung.

Moderate breast uptake, which is usually symmetric, can be seen at the time of menstruation as well as in lactating women. High thymic and physis activities may also be seen in the young patients.

Normal bowel activity can make it more difficult to detect lesions in the abdomen and pelvis (Figs. 2–4). Normal activity in the stomach may be high,

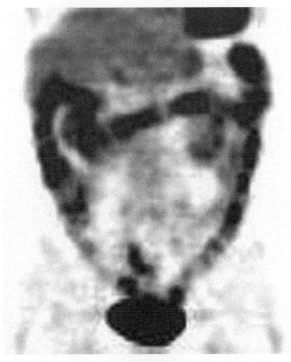

Figure 2: Physiologic colonic activity in a patient with normal colonoscopy.

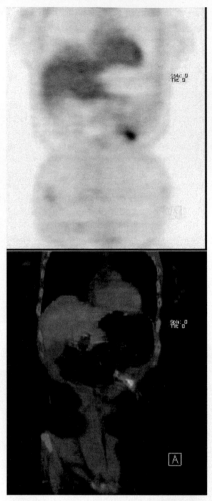

Figure 3: Physiologic focal moderate hypermetabolism at the bowel ostomy site.

mimicking neoplasm. The exact origin of the uptake is unknown but it may be related to uptake by the mucosa or the smooth muscle.

Artifacts: Reconstruction artifacts and noise are usually self-evident. A common artifact is due to skin contamination with urine, especially in patients who are incontinent. Placement of a Foley catheter will lessen the problem. Inadvertent tracer extravasation and subcutaneous infiltration of FDG in the arm may also result in axillary lymph node uptake unrelated to metastasis.

Other Non-Neoplastic Conditions: There are several clinical conditions which may result in high FDG accumulation and mimic malignancy.

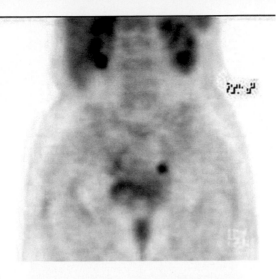

A

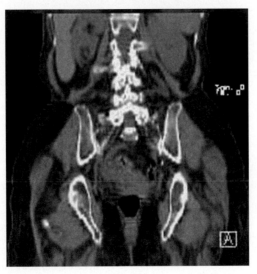

B

Figure 4: Left pelvic focal hypermetabolism on PET (A) corresponding to sigmoid colonic wall on CT (B) and determined to be due to adenomatous polyp on sigmoidoscopy.

Inflammation is a common cause of FDG accumulation unrelated to neoplasm. Active infections such as pneumonia, tuberculosis, histoplasmosis, toxoplasmosis, cryptococcoma, and coccidiomycosis may demonstrate very high FDG uptake, thereby diminishing the specificity of PET in characterizing lesions

18

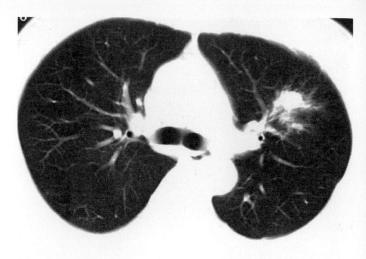

A

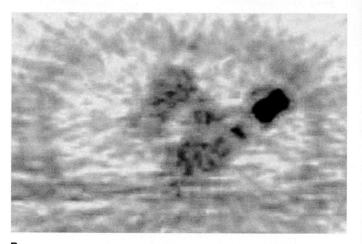

B

Figure 5: CT (a) and PET (b) demonstrate a metabolically active left lung lesion in a male patient from Southeast Asia that was confirmed by biopsy to be a tuberculoma.

(Figs. 5, 6). The patient's clinical history and the regional prevalence of granulomatous disease may aid in correct interpretation. Noninfectious inflammatory conditions such as atherosclerosis, arthritis, eosinophilic granuloma, sarcoid, bleomycin-induced pneumonitis, and pleuritis have also been shown to result in high FDG uptake (Figs. 7, 8).

Other causes of non-neoplastic high FDG uptake include iatrogenic pulmonary microembolism, active Paget's disease (increased bone activity),

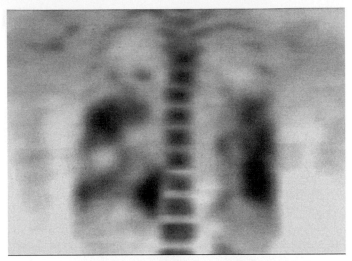

Figure 6: A male patient with neutropenic fever. PET shows bilateral multifocal hypermetabolic lesions determined to represent pneumonia.

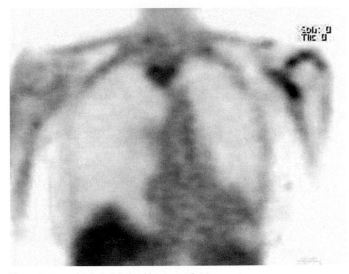

Figure 7: Hypermetabolic left shoulder osteoarthritis.

retroperitoneal fibrosis, neurofibroma, thyroiditis, parathyroid adenoma, chemotherapy-induced inflammation and marrow hyperplasia, fracture, hyperhidrosis, soft tissue dermatome prior to herpes zoster eruption, and non-paralyzed vocal cord (Fig. 9).

18

Figure 8: PET shows bihilar hypermetabolism related to metabolically active sarcoidosis.

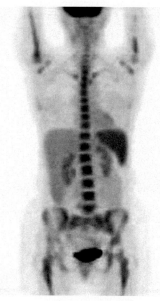

Figure 9: Diffuse bone marrow and splenic hypermetabolism induced by colony-stimulating factors.

PET-CT Artifacts. PET-CT scanners offer several advantages over PET alone by providing fast and low-noise CT-based transmission scan for attenuation correction, allowing for precise anatomic localization of the metabolic information, and possibly leading to synergistic diagnostic information. However, the use of CT for attenuation correction can result in artifacts and alteration of semi-quantitative measurements.

The artifacts which are unique to the PET-CT imaging may be due to metallic objects, respiration, and oral and intravenous contrast agents. Overcorrection of dense metallic objects may result in hot spot artifacts in the attenuation-corrected PET images (Fig. 10). This situation occurs most commonly with the metallic dental implants, cardiac pacemakers, and the metallic hip prosthesis. Examination of the nonattenuation corrected images can be helpful in distinguishing this technical artifact from physiologic/pathologic hypermetabolism. It is also important to note that attenuation correction

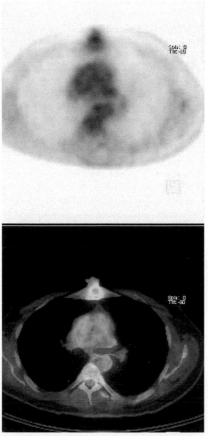

Figure 10: Hot spot artifact in the CT attenuation-corrected PET due to overcorrection of a dense metallic object.

18

of PET emission data using an artifactual CT map can yield false semi-quantitative indices in the regions adjacent to metallic artifacts and probably in the presence of oral contrast.

Similar to the situation with dense metallic objects, radiodense oral and intravenous contrast agents may be expected to cause hot spot artifacts on the CT-based attenuation-corrected PET image. It has been observed that high-density barium causes overestimation of tissue FDG concentration, while low-density barium does not lead to significant artifacts. Similarly, transient hot spot artifacts may be seen on PET as a result of the bolus passage of undiluted intravenous contrast material. Additionally, there may be a modest overestimation bias (less than 15%) on the PET emission images of organs, except the kidneys, which may display higher bias. However, with appropriate imaging protocols, which may include alternative contrast application schemes or variations to the attenuation correction procedure, PET-CT diagnostic capacity may be improved with little or no reduction in PET image quality.

Respiration may also cause misregistration and differential attenuation of structures adjacent to the diaphragm. The artifacts may present as curvilinear cold bands paralleling the dome of the diaphragm at the lung/diaphragm interface. Breath-hold during normal expiration or free-breathing respiratory patterns appears most suitable for PET-CT, while deep inspiration causes severe deterioration in the corrected PET images.

Increased FDG activity has also been noted on PET-CT studies involving the adipose tissue of the supraclavicular area ("USA-Fat") which has been speculated to be due to metabolically active brown adipose tissue. This activity is unrelated to the muscular activity while both the fat and the muscle activities may co-exist. The incidence of this finding increases with the cooler period of the year, which suggests stimulation of brown adipose tissue by increased sympathetic nervous system activity induced by cold temperatures. FDG uptake in neck fat is more commonly seen in female patients and the pediatric population. Increased FDG uptake may also be seen in the adipose tissue of the axillae, mediastinum, perinephric area, and the intercostal spaces in the paravertebral regions. Propranolol or reserpine treatment in rats have resulted in remarkable reduction in brown fat FDG uptake.

BIBLIOGRAPHY

1. Antoch G, Freudenberg LS, Egelhof T, et al. Focal tracer uptake: a potential artifact in contrast-enhanced dual modality PET/CT scans. J Nucl Med 2002; 43:1339–42.
2. Antoch G, Freudenberg LS, Stattaus J, et al. Whole-body positron emission tomography-CT: optimized CT using oral and IV contrast materials. AJR Am J Roentgenol 2002; 179:1555–60.
3. Barrington SF, Maisey MN. Skeletal muscle uptake of fluorine-18-FDG: effect of oral diazepam. J Nucl Med 1996; 37(7):1127–9.
4. Beyer T, Antoch G, Muller S, et al. Acquisition protocol considerations for combined PET/CT imaging. J Nucl Med 2004; 45(Suppl 1):25S–35S.
5. Bujenovic S, Mannting F, Chakrabarti R, et al. Artifactual 2-deoxy-2-[(18)F]fluoro-D-deoxyglucose localization surrounding metallic objects in a PET/CT scanner using CT-based attenuation correction. Mol Imaging Biol 2003; 5:20–2.
6. Chander S, Ergun EL, Chugani HT, et al. High 2-deoxy-2-[18F]fluoro-D-glucose accumulation in a case of retroperitoneal fibrosis following resection of carcinoid tumor. Mol Imaging Biol 2002 4(5):363–8.

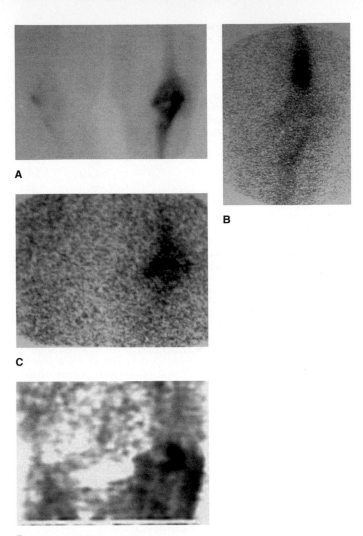

Figure 11: Infected left knee prosthesis. (a) bone, (b) bone marrow, and (c) leukocyte scintigraphic studies are positive for infection, (d) PET scan also demonstrates shows extensive concordant hypermetabolism.

7. Cohade C, Mourtzikos KA, Wahl RL. "USA-Fat": prevalence is related to ambient outdoor temperature-evaluation with 18F-FDG PET/CT. J Nucl Med 2003; 44:1267–70.
8. Cohade C, Osman M, Nakamoto Y, et al. Initial experience with oral contrast in PET/CT: phantom and clinical studies. J Nucl Med 2003; 44:412–6.
9. Cohade C, Osman M, Pannu HK, et al. Uptake in supraclavicular area fat ("USA-Fat"): description on 18F-FDG PET/CT. J Nucl Med 2003; 44:170–6.

10. Cohade C, Wahl RL. Applications of positron emission tomography/computed tomography image fusion in clinical positron emission tomography—Clinical use, interpretation methods, diagnostic improvements. Semin Nucl Med 2003; 33(3):228–37.

11. Cook GJ, Maisey MN, Fogelman I. Normal variants, artifacts and interpretative pitfalls in PET imaging with 18-fluoro-2-deoxyglucose and carbon-11 methionine. Eur J Nucl Med 1999; 26(10):1363–1378.

12. Cook GJ, Fogelman I, Maisey MN. Normal physiological and benign pathological variants of 18-Fluoro-2-Deoxyglucose positron-emission tomography scanning: potential for error in interpretation. Semin Nucl Med 1996; XXVI(4):308–314.

13. De Juan R, Seifert B, Berthold T, et al. Clinical evaluation of a breathing protocol for PET/CT. Eur Radiol 2004; 14(6):1118–23.

14. Dizendorf EV, Treyer V, von Schulthess GK, Hany TF. Application of oral contrast media in coregistered positron emission tomography-CT. AJR Am J Roentgenol 2002; 179(12):477–81.

15. Engel H, Steinert H, Buck A, et al. Whole-body PET: physiological and artifactual fluorodeoxyglucose accumulations. J Nucl Med 1996; 37(3):441–446.

16. Fayad LM, Cohade C, Wahl RL, Fishman EK. Sacral fractures: a potential pitfall of FDG positron emission tomography. AJR Am J Roentgenol 2003; 181(5):1239–43.

17. Goerres GW, Burger C, Kamel E, et al. Respiration-induced attenuation artifact at PET/CT: technical considerations. Radiology 2003; 226:906–10.

18. Goerres GW, Burger C, Schwitter MR, et al. PET/CT of the abdomen: optimizing the patient breathing pattern. Eur Radiol 2003; 13:734–9.

19. Goerres GW, Hany TF, Kamel E, et al. Head and neck imaging with PET and PET/CT: artifacts from dental metallic implants. Eur J Nucl Med Mol Imaging 2002; 29:367–70.

20. Goerres GW, Ziegler SI, Burger C, et al. Artifacts at PET and PET/CT caused by metallic hip prosthetic material. Radiology 2003; 226:577–84.

21. Gordon BA, Flanagan FL, Dehdashti F. Whole-body positron emission tomography: normal variations, pitfalls, and technical considerations. AJR Am J Roentgenol 1997; 169(6):1675–80.

22. Halpern BS, Dahlbom M, Waldherr C, et al. Cardiac pacemakers and central venous lines can induce focal artifacts on CT-corrected PET images. J Nucl Med 2004; 45:290–3.

23. Hanif MZ, Ghesani M, Shah AA, Kasai T. F-18 fluorodeoxyglucose uptake in atherosclerotic plaque in the mediastinum mimicking malignancy: another potential for error. Clin Nucl Med 2004; 29(2):93–5.

24. Hany TF, Heuberger J, von Schulthess GK. Iatrogenic FDG foci in the lungs: a pitfall of PET image interpretation. Eur Radiol 2003; 13(9):2122–7.

25. Hany TF, Gharehpapagh E, Kamel EM, et al. Brown adipose tissue: a factor to consider in symmetrical tracer uptake in the neck and upper chest region. Eur J Nucl Med Mol Imaging 2002; 29:1393–8.

26. Heiba SI, Luo J, Sadek S, et al. Attenuation-correction induced artifact in F-18 FDG PET imaging following total knee replacement. Clin Positron Imaging 2000; 3(6):237–239.

27. Heller MT, Meltzer CC, Fukui MB, et al. Superphysiologic FDG uptake in the non-paralyzed vocal cord. Resolution of a false-positive PET result with combined PET-CT imaging. Clin Positron Imaging 2000; 3(5):207–211.

28. Hsu CH, Lee CM, Wang FC, Lin YH. F-18 fluorodeoxyglucose positron emission tomography in pulmonary cryptococcoma. Clin Nucl Med 2003; 28(9):791–3.

29. Jacobsson H, Celsing F, Ingvar M, et al. Accumulation of FDG in axillary sweat glands in hyperhidrosis: a pitfall in whole-body PET examination. Eur Radiol 1998; 8(3):482–3.

30. Jadvar H, Schambye RB, Segall GM. Effect of atropine and sincalide on the intestinal uptake of F-18 fluorodeoxyglucose. Clin Nucl Med 1999; 24(12):965–7.

31. Joe A, Hoegerle S, Moser E. Cervical lymph node sarcoidosis as a pitfall in F-18 FDG positron emission tomography. Clin Nucl Med 2001; 26(6):542–3.

32. Kamel EM, Burger C, Buck A, et al. Impact of metallic dental implants on CT-based attenuation correction in a combined PET/CT scanner. Eur Radiol 2003; 13:724–8.
33. Kerrou K, Montravers F, Grahek D, et al. [18F]-FDG uptake in soft tissue dermatome prior to herpes zoster eruption: an unusual pitfall. Ann Nucl Med 2001; 15(5):455–8.
34. Kostakoglu L, Hardoff R, Mirtcheva R, Goldsmith SJ. PET-CT fusion imaging in differentiating physiologic from pathologic FDG uptake. Radiographics 2004; 24(5):1411–31.
35. Minotti AJ, Shah L, Keller K. Positron emission tomography/computed tomography fusion imaging in brown adipose tissue. Clin Nucl Med 2004; 29(1):5–11.
36. Nakahara T, Fujii H, Ide M, et al. FDG uptake in the morphologically normal thymus: comparison of FDG positron emission tomography and CT. Br J Radiol 2001; 74(885):821–4.
37. Nakamoto Y, Chin RB, Kraitchman DL, et al. effects of nonionic intravenous contrast agents at PET/CT imaging: phantom and canine studies. Radiology 2003; 227:817–24.
38. Naumann R, Beuthien-Baumann B, et al. Simultaneous occurrence of Hodgkin's lymphoma and eosinophilic granuloma: a potential pitfall in positron emission tomography imaging. Clin Lymphoma 2002; 3(2):121–4.
39. Nehmeh SA, Erdi YE, Kalaigian H, et al. Correction for oral contrast artifacts in CT attenuation-corrected PET images obtained by combined PET/CT. J Nucl Med 2003; 44(12):1940–4.
40. Osman MM, Cohade C, Nakaoto Y, et al. Respiratory motion artifacts on PET emission images obtained using CT attenuation correction on PET-CT. Eur J Nucl Med Mol Imaging 2003; 30:603–6.
41. Patel PM, Alibazoglu H, Ali A, et al. Normal thymic uptake of FDG on PET imaging. Clin Nucl Med 1996; 21:772–775.
42. Pitman AG, Binns DS, Ciavarella F, Hicks RJ. Inadvertent 2-deoxy-2-[18F]fluoro-D-glucose lymphoscintigraphy: a potential pitfall characterized by hybrid PET-CT. Mol Imaging Biol 2002; 4(4):276–8.
43. Sandherr M, von Schilling C, Link T, et al. Pitfalls in imaging Hodgkin's disease with computed tomography and positron emission tomography using fluorine-18-fluorodeoxyglucose. Ann Oncol 2001; 12(5):719–22.
44. Shreve PD, Anzai Y, Wahl RL. Pitfalls in oncologic diagnosis with FDG PET imaging: physiologic and benign variants. Radiographics 1999; 19(1):61–77.
45. Stokkel MP, Bongers V, Hordijk GJ, van Rijk PP. FDG positron emission tomography in head and neck cancer: pitfall or pathology? Clin Nucl Med 1999; 24(12):950–4.
46. Strauss LG. Fluorine-18 deoxyglucose and false-positive results: a major problem in the diagnostics of oncological patients. Eur J Nucl Med 1996; 23(10):1409–15.
47. Tatlidil R, Jadvar H, Bading JR, Conti PS. Incidental colonic fluorodeoxyglucose uptake: correlation with colonoscopic and histopathologic findings. Radiology 2002; 224(3):783–7.
48. Tatsumi M, Cohade C, Nakamoto Y, Wahl RL. Fluorodeoxyglucose uptake in the aortic wall at PET/CT: possible finding for active atherosclerosis. Radiology 2003; 229(3):831–7.
49. Tatsumi M, Engles JM, Ishimori T, et al. Intense (18)F-FDG uptake in brown fat can be reduced pharmacologically. J Nucl Med 2004; 45(7):1189–93.
50. Vesselle HJ, Miraldi FD. FDG PET of the retroperitoneum: normal anatomy, variants, pathologic conditions, and strategies to avoid diagnostic pitfalls. Radiographics 1998; 18(4):805–23.
51. Visvikis D, Costa DC, Croasdale I, et al. CT-based attenuation correction in the calculation of semi-quantitative indices of [18F]FDG uptake in PET. Eur J Nucl Med Mol Imaging 2003; 30(3):344–53.
52. Yeung HW, Grewal RK, Gonen M, et al. Patterns of (18)F-FDG uptake in adipose tissue and muscle: a potential source of false-positives for PET. J Nucl Med 2003; 44(11):1789–96.

18

Index

A

Acceptance angle, and Compton-scattered photon detection, 26
Acetate, carbon-11-labeled
  for studying hepatocellular carcinoma, 156–157
  for studying prostate cancer, 185
Adenocarcinoma
  of the bladder, 192–193
  cervical, 167
  endometrial, uterine, 169
  esophageal, 137
  gastric, 139–142
  of the lung, 117–118
  pancreatic ductal, 153–155
  of the prostate, 183
Adenosine triphosphatase, energy for glucose transportation from, 51
Affine transformation, for image registration, 23
Aging, effects of, on the brain, 87–88
Alpha-fetoprotein (AFP), as a marker for hepatocellular carcinoma, 155–157
Alzheimer's disease (AD), diagnosis of, 91
American College of Radiology Imaging Network (ACRIN), 134
American Joint Committee on Cancer (AJCC), staging for melanoma, 227
Ammonia, nitrogen-13-labeled, 61–62
  for coronary artery evaluation, 69
Anger, Hal, 33
Anger gamma camera
  for fluorodeoxyglucose images, 78–79
  for single photon detection, 6
Anger logic
  defined, 33
  to determine the position of a crystal detector, 7–8
Annihilation photons
  attenuation of, 35
  interaction of
    in the detector, 33
    with tissue, 9–10
Areola, uptake of fluorodeoxyglucose by, 57
Arteriolar blockade, pre-capillary, 63

Artifacts
  diaphragmatic, due to attenuation, 15–16
  due to physiologic motion, 16–17
  positron emission tomography/computed tomography, 263–264
  reconstruction, in positron emission tomography, 258
Attenuation
  independence of depth, in positron emission tomography, 17–18
  of photons by tissue, 9–10
    versus energy of the photons, 21–22
Attenuation coefficient (μ)
  for 511-keV photons, 11
  effect on coronary artery evaluation, 71
  linear, defined, 11–12
  real and apparent, 11
Attenuation correction, 11–24
  artifacts due to, 263–264
  calculated, 18–19
  types of, 18–21
Attenuation equation, 11–12
Axial collimation, 25–29
  degree of, in three-dimensional imaging, 29

B

Barium fluoride (BaF_2), for scintillation crystals, 38
Baryons, protons and neutrons as, 1
B-cells, lymphomas derived from, 206.
  See also Diffuse large B-cell lymphoma (DLBCL)
Becquerel, Henri, 64
Benign prostatic hyperplasia (BPH), fluorodeoxyglucose uptake in, 183
Biodistribution of fluorodeoxyglucose uptake
  altered, 54–60
  normal, 255
Bismuth germinate (BGO), for scintillation crystals, 38
Bladder cancer, 191–193
Blobs, as noise in iterative reconstruction, 32